Dizziness and Vertigo across the Lifespan

Guest Editors

BRADLEY W. KESSER, MD
A. TUCKER GLEASON, PhD

OTOLARYNGOLOGIC CLINICS OF NORTH AMERICA

www.oto.theclinics.com

April 2011 • Volume 44 • Number 2

SAUNDERS an imprint of ELSEVIER, Inc.

W.B. SAUNDERS COMPANY
A Division of Elsevier Inc.

1600 John F. Kennedy Boulevard • Suite 1800 • Philadelphia, Pennsylvania 19103-2899

http://www.theclinics.com

OTOLARYNGOLOGIC CLINICS OF NORTH AMERICA Volume 44, Number 2
April 2011 ISSN 0030-6665, ISBN-13: 978-1-4557-0481-1

Editor: Joanne Husovski
Developmental Editor: Natalie Whitted

Otolaryngologic Clinics of North America (ISSN 0030-6665) is published bimonthly by Elsevier, Inc., 360 Park Avenue South, New York, NY 10010-1710. Months of issue are February, April, June, August, October, and December. Business and Editorial Offices: 1600 John F. Kennedy Blvd., Suite 1800, Philadelphia, PA 19103-2899. Customer Service Office: 6277 Sea Harbor Drive, Orlando, FL 32887-4800. Periodicals postage paid at New York, NY and additional mailing offices. Subscription prices is $310.00 per year (US individuals), $590.00 per year (US institutions), $149.00 per year (US student/resident), $409.00 per year (Canadian individuals), $741.00 per year (Canadian institutions), $459.00 per year (international individuals), $741.00 per year (international institutions), $230.00 per year (international & Canadian student/resident). Foreign air speed delivery is included in all *Clinics'* subscription prices. All prices are subject to change without notice. **POSTMASTER:** Send address changes to *Otolaryngologic Clinics of North America*, Elsevier Health Sciences Division, Subscription Customer Service, 3251 Riverport Lane, Maryland Heights, MO 63043. **Telephone: 1-800-654-2452 (U.S. and Canada); 314-447-8871 (outside U.S. and Canada). Fax: 314-447-8029. E-mail: journalscustomerservice-usa@elsevier.com (for print support); journalsonlinesupport-usa@elsevier.com (for online support).**

Reprints. For copies of 100 or more of articles in this publication, please contact the Commercial Reprints Department, Elsevier Inc., 360 Park Avenue South, New York, NY 10010-1710. Tel.: 212-633-3812; Fax: 212-462-1935; E-mail: reprints@elsevier.com.

Otolaryngologic Clinics of North America is also published in Spanish by McGraw-Hill Interamericana Editores S.A., P.O. Box 5-237, 06500 Mexico D.F., Mexico.

Otolaryngologic Clinics of North America is covered in *MEDLINE/PubMed (Index Medicus), Current Contents/Clinical Medicine, Excerpta Medica, BIOSIS, Science Citation Index,* and *ISI/BIOMED.*

Printed and bound by CPI Group (UK) Ltd, Croydon, CR0 4YY

Transferred to Digital Print 2011

Contributors

GUEST EDITORS

BRADLEY W. KESSER, MD
Associate Professor, Director, Division of Otology/Neurotology, Department of
Otolaryngology—Head and Neck Surgery, University of Virginia Health System,
Charlottesville, Virginia

A. TUCKER GLEASON, PhD
Assistant Professor, Department of Otolaryngology—Head and Neck Surgery,
Division of Audiology and Vestibular & Balance Center, University of Virginia,
Charlottesville, Virginia

AUTHORS

FAITH W. AKIN, PhD
Director, Vestibular/Balance Laboratory, Audiology Service, Veterans Affairs Medical
Center, Mountain Home; Associate Professor, Department of Audiology and Speech
Pathology, Audiology (126), Veterans Affairs Medical Center, East Tennessee State
University, Johnson City, Tennessee

MUHAMMAD ALRWAILY, PT, MS
Doctoral Student, Department of Physical Therapy, University of Pittsburgh, Pittsburgh,
Pennsylvania

KAMRAN BARIN, PhD
Assistant Professor of Otolaryngology—Head and Neck Surgery and Director, Balance
Disorders Clinic, Department of Otolaryngology-Head and Neck Surgery, The Ohio State
University Medical Center, Columbus, Ohio

JOHN P. CAREY, MD
Department of Otolaryngology—Head and Neck Surgery, The Johns Hopkins University
School of Medicine, Baltimore, Maryland

MARCELLO CHERCHI, MD, PhD
Assistant Professor of Neurology, Department of Neurology, Northwestern University
Feinberg School of Medicine; Chicago Dizziness & Hearing, Chicago, Illinois

EDWARD I. CHO, MD
Section of Vestibular and Balance Disorders, The Cleveland Clinic Head and Neck
Institute, Cleveland, Ohio

EDWARD E. DODSON, MD
Associate Professor of Otolaryngology—Head and Neck Surgery and Director, Division
of Otology, Neurotology, and Cranial Base Surgery, Department of Otolaryngology-Head
and Neck Surgery, The Ohio State University Medical Center, Columbus, Ohio

JOSE N. FAYAD, MD
Associate, House Clinic; Associate Professor of Clinical Otolaryngology, University
of Southern California, Los Angeles, California

GERARD J. GIANOLI, MD
The Ear and Balance Institute, Baton Rouge; Clinical Associate Professor, Departments of Otolaryngology and Pediatrics, Tulane University School of Medicine, New Orleans, Louisiana

JOHN C. GODDARD, MD
Clinical Fellow, House Clinic, Los Angeles, California

HOWARD P. GOODKIN, MD, PhD
The Shure Associate Professor of Neurology and Pediatrics, Department of Neurology; Department of Pediatrics, University of Virginia Health Systems, Charlottesville, Virginia

CHRIS GRINDLE, MD
Fellow, Otolaryngology, Alfred I. duPont Hospital for Children, Wilmington, Delaware

JILL M. GRUENWALD, AuD
Audiologist, Division of Audiology, Department of Hearing and Speech Sciences, Vanderbilt Bill Wilkerson Center, Hearing and Speech Sciences, Vanderbilt University Medical Center, Nashville, Tennessee

TIMOTHY C. HAIN, MD
Professor, Departments of Neurology, Otolaryngology - Head and Neck Surgery, and Physical Therapy and Human Movement Sciences, Northwestern University Feinberg School of Medicine; Chicago Dizziness and Hearing, Chicago, Illinois

STEFAN C.A. HEGEMANN, MD
Department of Otorhinolaryngology, Head and Neck Surgery, Zürich University Hospital, Zürich, Switzerland

AKIRA ISHIYAMA, MD
Professor, Division of Head and Neck Surgery, Department of Surgery, UCLA School of Medicine, Los Angeles, California

GAIL ISHIYAMA, MD
Associate Professor of Neurology, Division of Neurotology, UCLA School of Medicine, Reed Neurological Research Center, Los Angeles, California

GARY P. JACOBSON, PhD
Director of Audiology and Professor, Division of Audiology, Department of Hearing and Speech Sciences, Vanderbilt Bill Wilkerson Center, Hearing and Speech Sciences, Vanderbilt University Medical Center, Nashville, Tennessee

DEVIN L. MCCASLIN, PhD
Assistant Professor, Division of Audiology, Department of Hearing and Speech Sciences, Vanderbilt Bill Wilkerson Center, Hearing and Speech Sciences, Vanderbilt University Medical Center, Nashville, Tennessee

CLIFF A. MEGERIAN, MD
FACS, Division of Otology and Neurotology, Department of Otolaryngology–Head and Neck Surgery, University Hospitals Case Medical Center, Case Western Reserve University School of Medicine, Cleveland, Ohio

THIERRY MORLET, PhD
Head, Auditory Physiology and Psychoacoustics Research Laboratory, Alfred I. duPont Hospital for Children, Wilmington, Delaware

OWEN D. MURNANE, PhD
ACOS, Research and Development, Veterans Affairs Medical Center, Mountain Home;
Associate Professor, Department of Audiology and Speech Pathology, Audiology (126),
Veterans Affairs Medical Center, East Tennessee State University, Mountain Home,
Tennessee

ABNER N. NYANDEGE, MS
Geriatric Pharmacotherapy Program, Department of Pharmacotherapy and Outcomes
Science, Virginia Commonwealth University, Richmond, Virginia

ROBERT O'REILLY, MD
Associate Professor of Pediatrics and Otolaryngology, Thomas Jefferson University,
Philadelphia, Pennsylvania; Division Chief, Otolaryngology, Alfred I. duPont Hospital for
Children, Wilmington, Delaware

MAROUN T. SEMAAN, MD
Division of Otology and Neurotology, Department of Otolaryngology–Head and Neck
Surgery, University Hospitals Case Medical Center, Louis Stokes Veteran's Affair Medical
Center, Case Western Reserve University School of Medicine, Cleveland, Ohio

OSAMA A. SHOAIR, BS
Geriatric Pharmacotherapy Program, Department of Pharmacotherapy and Outcomes
Science, Virginia Commonwealth University, Richmond, Virginia

PATRICIA W. SLATTUM, PharmD, PhD
Geriatric Pharmacotherapy Program, Department of Pharmacotherapy and Outcomes
Science, Virginia Commonwealth University, Richmond, Virginia

JAMES S. SOILEAU, MD
The Ear and Balance Institute, Baton Rouge, Louisiana

JENNIE TAYLOR, MD
Resident Physician in Neurology, Department of Neurology, University of Virginia Health
Systems, Charlottesville, Virginia

L. MAUREEN VALENTE, PhD
Director of Audiology Studies, Program in Audiology and Communication Sciences;
Associate Professor, Department of Otolaryngology, Washington University School
of Medicine, St Louis, Missouri

JUDITH A. WHITE, MD, PhD
Head, Section of Vestibular and Balance Disorders, The Cleveland Clinic Head and Neck
Institute; Associate Professor of Surgery, Lerner College of Medicine, Cleveland Clinic,
Cleveland, Ohio

SUSAN L. WHITNEY, PT, PhD
Departments of Physical Therapy and Otolaryngology, University of Pittsburgh,
Pittsburgh, Pennsylvania; Rehabilitation Research Chair, King Saud University,
Riyadh, Saudi Arabia

EMILY F. ZWICKY, AuD, CCC-A
Pediatric Audiologist, Department of Pediatric Audiology, Alfred I. duPont Hospital for
Children, Wilmington, Delaware

Contents

emphasis on migraine headaches, chronic daily headaches, postural orthostatic tachycardia syndrome, and presentations that may require head imaging.

Young adults are more likely to suffer blast injury and traumatic brain injury (TBI) than other age groups. This article reviews the literature on the vestibular consequences of blast exposure and TBI and concussion. In addition, the vestibular test findings obtained from 31 veterans with a history of blast exposure and/or mild TBI are presented. The authors discuss loss of horizontal semicircular canal function and postural instability related to head injury. Preliminary data suggest the novel theory that otolith organs are uniquely vulnerable to head injury and blast exposure.

Section 3: Adult

Evaluation of dizziness in patients who are involved in litigation can deviate significantly from the evaluation of patients who have no ongoing litigation. This article presents the basic principles of the physician's role in the evaluation of litigating patients. Considerations for physical examination, diagnostic testing, and review of medical records are discussed. Topics of malingering and legal "pearls" are presented in the context of providing an objective and unbiased evaluation of the litigating patient.

This article reviews the pathophysiology, diagnosis, and treatment of benign paroxysmal positional vertigo of the posterior and lateral semicircular canals and summarizes the evidence-based outcome data. The authors discuss this common cause of vertigo, its cause and prevalence across the life span, and efficacy of treatment through both physical repositioning maneuvers and surgery.

The epidemiology, diagnostic features, differential diagnosis, and treatment of vestibular neuritis are reviewed. The authors present considerations for physical examination, imaging, and management in both the acute and chronic phases of this disease. The authors also present a dizziness questionnaire in the Appendix of this publication.

This article presents a brief overview of migraine-associated vertigo for the practicing otolaryngologist. Discussion includes the definition of

migraine-associated vertigo and its pathophysiology, clinical features, de-
mographics, findings on physical examination, use of otologic and vestibular testing, differential diagnosis, treatment, and prognosis.

Stefan C.A. Hegemann and John P. Carey

This article presents a detailed case report of a patient who was diagnosed
with superior canal dehiscence at 37 years of age, but who had a suspicious history for that syndrome from at least 10 years of age. The authors
hypothesize several reasons for this late diagnosis, with the goal of helping
pediatricians, otolaryngologists, and neurologists consider this syndrome
in their differential diagnosis of children, adolescents, or adults experiencing dizziness.

Maroun T. Semaan and Cliff A. Megerian

Ménière's disease (MD) is characterized by episodic vertigo, fluctuating
hearing loss and tinnitus, and by the presence of endolymphatic hydrops
on postmortem examination. This disease continues to be a diagnostic
and therapeutic challenge. Patients with MD range from minimally symptomatic, highly functional individuals to severely affected, disabled patients. Current management strategies are designed to control the acute
and recurrent vestibulopathy but offer minimal remedy for the progressive
cochlear dysfunction. Recent research highlights the role of neurotoxicity
in the pathogenesis of the cochleovestibular deterioration. This article discusses a patient with MD, and provides an algorithm for the management
of this disease.

Marcello Cherchi

This content focuses on some of the less common causes of dizziness in
the adult. The diseases have been divided into the 2 broad categories of
those causing chronic symptoms and those causing episodic symptoms.
Presented here are the unusual causes of chronic disequilibrium in the
adult, including bilateral vestibular loss, progressive supranuclear palsy,
spinocerebellar ataxias, and mal de debarquement. Also discussed are
the unusual causes of episodic disequilibrium in the adult, including psychogenic disequilibrium, vestibular paroxysmia, episodic ataxia, vestibular
seizures, and cervicogenic vertigo.

Section 4: Elderly

Gail Ishiyama and Akira Ishiyama

This article discusses the clinical presentation of vertebrobasilar ischemia
and infarcts. Pertinent dizziness intake questions are presented, as well as
key components of the physical examination. The anatomy of the posterior

cerebral circulation is discussed as are syndromes associated with cerebrovascular infarcts in the posterior circulation. A high incidence of recurrence of ischemic attacks or infarcts in vertebrobasilar insufficiency is noted. The authors note that recent developments in imaging and interventions may indicate need for referral or consultation with specialists in some cases.

RELATED INTEREST ARTICLE

In Emergency Medicine Clinics, August 2010, Pages 453–469
Dizzy and Confused: A Step-by-Step Evaluation of the Clinician's Favorite Chief Complaint
Christine Kulstad, MD, and Blaine Hannafin, MD, *Guest Editors*

THE CLINICS ARE NOW AVAILABLE ONLINE!

Access your subscription at:
www.theclinics.com

Preface

Age-Focused Approach to Dizziness

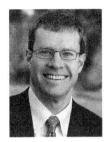 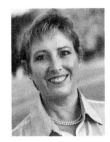

Bradley W. Kesser, MD   A. Tucker Gleason, PhD
Guest Editors

When we otolaryngologists, audiologists, physical therapists, and other allied health professionals evaluate the patient with dizziness, we quickly note the patient's age, but do we consciously use age in building the framework for our differential diagnosis and management?

Dizziness comes in many forms in each age group—some specific to an age group (eg, benign paroxysmal vertigo of childhood), while others span the age spectrum (eg, migraine-associated vertigo). We felt that a publication that organizes the evaluation and management of the dizzy patient by age brings a useful perspective to seeing these often difficult patients. Many texts and references on the care of the dizzy patient are organized by diagnosis—a review on Ménière's disease, a review on benign paroxysmal positional vertigo, etc. We have organized this *Otolaryngology Clinics* issue on the topic of balance and dizziness by *age*—pediatric, adolescent, adult, and elderly.

Diagnosing and treating the patient with dizziness is challenging for a number of reasons—patients do not (often cannot) state clearly the exact symptom complex they are experiencing, the hugely broad differential diagnosis of dizziness, the limited capability we have to test the individual components of the vestibular system, and the seemingly limited treatment options for specific forms of dizziness. Frighteningly, patients presenting with dizziness can harbor serious if not life-threatening conditions such as stroke, brain abscess, or severe chronic ear disease. We must separate the critical from the not as critical. At the end of several articles, the reader will find a relevant table—What Not To Miss—a list of clinically significant signs and symptoms not to ignore, or conditions (differential diagnosis) that may masquerade as that discussed

Otolaryngol Clin N Am 44 (2011) xiii–xv
doi:10.1016/j.otc.2011.01.016
0030-6665/11/$ – see front matter

in the article but critically important that the practitioner should not overlook in the evaluation of the patient. Many articles in this issue start with a clinical scenario so the reader can recognize common presenting symptoms, demographic features, and factors in the medical history that will aid in making the diagnosis. In an Appendix, several authors have provided questionnaires for patients presenting with dizziness—you are free to download these questionnaires from www.oto.theclinics.com.

As noted, the issue is organized by age—the pediatric section begins with a review of vestibular embryology and physiology and moves toward a comprehensive discussion of methods—both bedside and in the vestibular lab—to evaluate the child with dizziness, or "clumsiness." The pediatric section concludes with an exploration of the differential diagnosis of dizziness and relevant findings. A review on dizziness in the adolescent points to migraine headache as a common cause, enumerates treatment strategies for migraine-associated vertigo, and offers guidelines for when to image the adolescent with dizziness.

The section regarding adult patients is more a compilation of the relevant diagnoses (mostly peripheral vestibular etiologies of dizziness), but the section starts with dizziness that can affect young adults—especially members of our Armed Forces serving overseas—traumatic brain injury/blast injury. This particular presentation also has relevance for patients in motor vehicle accidents and head injury patients and suggests that vestibular dysfunction is more common in these patients than was once appreciated. Medicolegal aspects of evaluation and management of dizzy patients are succinctly covered in "Evaluation of Dizziness in the Litigating Patient." The final article in this section, "Other Causes of Dizziness," provides a very thorough overview of unusual causes of dizziness in the adult population (eg, mal de debarquement).

Dizziness associated with advancing age is quite common and often multifactorial, as is highlighted in the article, "Dizziness in the Elderly." A comprehensive review of the posterior cerebral circulation, transient ischemic attacks, and posterior circulation stroke is presented in the article, "Vertebrobasilar Insufficiency." Older patients take more medicines, and these medicines can produce unintended symptoms (dizziness), especially with greater numbers of medications. No coverage of dizziness in the elderly is complete without an exposition of polypharmacy and medication effects. Other common diagnoses of dizziness in the elderly are thoughtfully reviewed along with a survey of new and old techniques to rehabilitate the older patient with dizziness or disequilibrium.

We acknowledge overlap among some of the articles, but repetition serves to affirm and reinforce important information. In addition, each article brings a unique perspective such that the reader will enjoy a compilation of information from the best and brightest minds currently practicing clinical care of the dizzy patient. Our hope is that the reader uses this issue of *Otolaryngology Clinics* both for adding to their own information on the dizzy patient as well as for a clinical reference when seeing patients with dizziness. Our ultimate hope is that the reader enjoys reading this issue as much as we enjoyed bringing it to fruition.

We gratefully acknowledge the authors of these articles. Their hard work, experience, and expertise have been invaluable in making this issue possible.

Bradley W. Kesser, MD
Division of Otology/Neurotology
Department of Otolaryngology–Head and Neck Surgery
University of Virginia Health System
Box 800713
Charlottesville, VA 22908-0713, USA

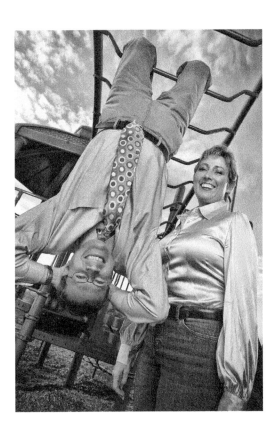

A. Tucker Gleason, PhD
Department of Otolaryngology–Head and Neck Surgery
Division of Audiology and Vestibular & Balance Center
University of Virginia
Charlottesville, VA 22908-0871, USA

E-mail addresses:
bwk2n@virginia.edu (B.W. Kesser)
atg2v@virginia.edu (A.T. Gleason)

Development of the Vestibular System and Balance Function: Differential Diagnosis in the Pediatric Population

Robert O'Reilly, MD[a,b],*, Chris Grindle, MD[b],
Emily F. Zwicky, AuD, CCC-A[c], Thierry Morlet, PhD[d]

KEYWORDS

- Vestibular maturation • Vestibulo-ocular reflex
- Vestibulospinal reflex • Vestibulocollic reflex
- Motor development • Differential diagnosis

Pediatric vestibular disorders are just beginning to be adequately recognized as an area of significant importance in the overall well-being of children. Mandates for universal newborn hearing screening have resulted in an early focus on auditory function in infants, facilitating early identification and management of children with auditory pathology. This approach has vastly improved outcomes for children and has resulted in a welcome increase in awareness that auditory and vestibular pathology frequently co-occur.

From the day we are born until we reach old age, we are profoundly reliant on our sense of balance for well-being and survival. Balance relies on complex interactions and central mediation of 3 important senses: vision, vestibular function, and proprioception. Structurally, the sensory systems related to balance are fully developed at

The authors have nothing to disclose.
[a] Departments of Pediatrics and Otolaryngology, Thomas Jefferson University Hospital, Gibbon Building, 111 South 11th Street, Philadelphia, PA 19107, USA
[b] Otolaryngology, Alfred I. duPont Hospital for Children, 1600 Rockland Road, Wilmington, DE 19803, USA
[c] Department of Pediatric Audiology, Alfred I. duPont Hospital for Children, 1600 Rockland Road, Wilmington, DE 19803, USA
[d] Auditory Physiology and Psychoacoustics Research Laboratory, Alfred I. duPont Hospital for Children, 1600 Rockland Road, Wilmington, DE 19803, USA
* Corresponding author. Otolaryngology, Alfred I. duPont Hospital for Children, 1600 Rockland Road, Wilmington, DE 19803.
E-mail address: roreilly@nemours.org

Otolaryngol Clin N Am 44 (2011) 251–271
doi:10.1016/j.otc.2011.01.001
0030-6665/11/$ – see front matter © 2011 Elsevier Inc. All rights reserved.

birth. From infancy, balance function continues to mature with sequential acquisition of motor milestones for head control, sitting, standing, and walking, and develops thereafter through experiential learning and adaptation until adolescence. Changes in balance function are most rapid and pronounced during infancy and preschool years when motor milestones needed for walking are realized, and as postural control and coordinated movements are refined. Nevertheless, changes in balance function continue to be evident as a function of aging throughout the human life span.[1]

OVERVIEW OF THE VESTIBULAR SYSTEM

The vestibular system includes 2 otolith organs (the saccule and utricle), which sense linear acceleration (ie, gravity and translational movements), and 3 semicircular canals, orthogonal with respect to each other, which are responsive to angular acceleration. Sensory hair cells are located in the maculae of the otolith organs, and in the ampullae of the semicircular canals. Hair cell activation resulting from endolymphatic fluid flow generates afferent impulses that are transmitted to bipolar cells of the vestibular nerve, whose cell bodies are located in the vestibular ganglia. The axons of bipolar cells pass through the internal auditory canal and reach the medulla, alongside the cochlear nerve. In the internal auditory canal, vestibular fibers are segregated into 2 distinct bundles forming superior and inferior branches of the nerve. The superior vestibular nerve supplies the superior and lateral semicircular canals as well as the utricle. The inferior vestibular nerve supplies the posterior canal and the saccule. The superior and inferior vestibular nerves join to form a common bundle, which enters the brainstem. These first-order neurons terminate in the vestibular nuclei in the floor of the fourth ventricle and do not cross the midline. The 4 major vestibular nuclei include the superior (or Bechterew), lateral (or Deiter), medial, and inferior (or descending) vestibular nuclei. From the vestibular nuclei, projections go to the cerebellum, motor nuclei of the extraocular muscles, antigravity muscles, and contralateral vestibular nuclei. The cortical representation of the vestibular system is at the level of the parietal and insular regions of the cortex.[2]

EMBRYOLOGY
Inner Ear

Ongoing research and technological advances have significantly improved our understanding of the cellular differentiation and morphogenesis of the human vestibular labyrinth.[3] The first stages of inner ear development begin as diffuse thickenings of surface ectoderm on either side of the embryonic (rhomboencephalon) hindbrain. During the third week of embryonic development, thickened surface ectoderm of the embryonic hindbrain begins to invaginate, forming the otic placodes.

During week 4, the otic placodes are surrounded by proliferating embryonic mesoderm, creating otic pits. The otic pits subsequently pinch off from the surface ectoderm to form the closed, rounded structures of the otic vesicles. The otic vesicles further differentiate into upper and lower portions, forming the vestibular apparatus and membranous cochlea, respectively. Different rates of growth among the canals, the vestibular aqueduct, the oval window, the round window, and the cochlea have been observed, which suggests that each part of the inner ear follows distinct trajectories during development.[4] The vestibular apparatus, located superiorly in relation to the cochlea, develops earlier and grows at a faster rate than the cochlea. The otic vesicle elongates and differentiates to form a dorsal utricular portion and a ventral saccular portion. The utricular portion becomes the semicircular canals and the utricle. The superior semicircular canal forms first, followed by the posterior, then lateral canal.

The saccular portion becomes the saccule and the cochlear duct. The communication between the saccule and membranous cochlea narrows to form the ductus reuniens.

The bony capsule that surrounds the membranous labyrinth forms rapidly from embryonic mesoderm over a period of approximately 5 weeks, between gestational weeks 19 and 23. Ossification of the otic capsule first occurs in the area of the cochlea and superior semicircular canal at approximately 19 weeks' gestation. Development appears to progress in an outward fashion from the areas surrounding the vestibule to the canal vertices, with the last area of encapsulation being the posterolateral area of the horizontal semicircular canal at approximately 21 to 23 weeks' gestation.[3] Current consensus is that the vestibule is adult-like in form and size by 25 weeks of gestation; however, recent findings suggest that some parts of the labyrinth reach final size only after birth. This seems to be the case for the internal aperture of the vestibular aqueduct, which is still growing and is smaller than adult size at 39 weeks.[4]

Maturation of Vestibular Receptors

Around the third week of gestation, sensory epithelia emerge from ectoderm in the cristae forming the semicircular canals, and in the maculae forming the otolith organs. By 7 weeks' gestation, small quantities of otoconia are present in the utricle. Thereafter, development proceeds quite rapidly, and within 1 week, greater amounts of otoconia are present in both the utricle and saccule, and cellular differentiation of the macular neural substrate is readily evident. At 7 to 12 weeks' gestation, the calcium content of the otoconia increases markedly in both the utricle and saccule; however, comparisons along the entire continuum of macular development reveal that the otoconia of the utricle appear to be more mature and varied in size and shape than saccular otoconia.[5] Vestibular hair cells first appear at approximately 7 weeks' gestation. Although not fully differentiated, the beginning of synapse formation in vestibular hair cells is observed in the human fetus at approximately 9 to 10 weeks' gestation. Differentiation of Type I and Type II hair cells begins between 11 and 13 weeks' gestation. In general, the morphologic sequence is from apex to base in the cristae and from the center to periphery in the maculae. Significant numbers of fully formed calyx nerve endings are observed at 20 weeks' gestation. The maturing ampullary cristae become active as early as the eighth or ninth week of fetal life.[6] Vestibular receptors become active by the 32nd week, at which time a fully developed Moro reflex can be elicited.[7] These observations suggest that vestibular afferents are mature and functional in early stages of human development.

Development of Vestibular Pathways

Vestibular ganglion cells are of various shapes until the 21st week of gestation and become uniform in shape around the 24th week of gestation when the development of the inner ear is complete. Morphometric studies show that ganglion cells grow until the 39th week, reaching maturity around the time of birth.[8] Neuronal connections between the labyrinths and the oculomotor nuclei in the brainstem occur between the 12th and 24th weeks of gestation. Myelination of the vestibular nerve begins around the 20th fetal week; it is the first cranial nerve to complete myelination.[9] The vestibular nuclear complex is functional at 21 weeks' gestation.

DEVELOPMENTAL REFLEXES

With maturation of physiologic processes and anatomic structures, certain developmental reflexes can be elicited at birth or soon thereafter. These reflexes are primitive in nature, usually disappear as the child matures, and primarily reflect the integrity of the brainstem and spinal cord.[10] Their persistence beyond the normally expected age of dissipation indicates delayed maturation or impaired nervous system function. Their asymmetry suggests either a central or a peripheral nervous system disorder.

The *Moro reflex* is elicited by holding the child supine and allowing the head to drop approximately 30° in relation to the trunk. Extension and abduction of the arms with fanning out of the fingers followed by adduction of the arms at the shoulder takes place as a normal response. This reflex normally disappears by the age of 5 to 6 months.

The *tonic neck reflex* is tested by turning the head of the child to one side while supine with the shoulders fixed. The arm and leg of the side toward which the head is turned will extend, while the arm and leg on the opposite side will flex. This reflex normally disappears by the age of 6 months.

The *head righting reflex* develops by the age of 4 to 6 months. To test this reflex, when the child's trunk is held 30° from vertical, a normally responding infant will tilt the head so as to remain vertical. At about age 5 months, the child will additionally move the lower limbs away from the side to which they have been tilted, thereby reflecting functional integration of visual, vestibular, and proprioceptive stimuli.[9]

The *parachute reaction* is elicited beyond the age of 5 months, when a sudden downward movement of a vertically held child causes the lower limbs to extend and abduct. This reflex is considered to represent visual-vestibular interaction[9] with the otoliths presumably involved.

The *doll's eye response* is found normally in full-term babies within 2 weeks of birth. When the baby (facing the examiner) is held at arm's length and rotated in one direction around the examiner, a deviation of the eyes and head opposite to the direction of the rotation is produced, representing vestibular activity. Due to an immature saccadic system at this stage, the fast component of a normal nystagmic response is not seen. Later, however, nystagmus is apparent with the fast component in the direction of rotation.[11]

DEVELOPMENT OF VESTIBULAR-INDUCED REFLEXES

Balance and equilibrium are maintained through a series of events triggered by sensory stimulation. Incoming sensory inputs received from the vestibular, visual, and somatosensory/proprioceptive systems are directed to the vestibular nuclei and cerebellum for processing and calibration. In response to afferent inputs, the vestibular nuclear complex creates direct and remarkably rapid efferent connections to muscles controlling the eyes, the neck, and the spinal cord. These motor outputs result in 3 categories of vestibular reflexes (vestibulo-ocular, vestibulospinal, and vestibulocollic), which allow us to maintain our balance and equilibrium. It is through examination of these reflexes that we are provided a window for uncovering vestibular dysfunction. Understanding how vestibular responses differ among infants, children, adolescents, and adults is crucial when attempting to evaluate and diagnose vestibular pathology.

Vestibulo-Ocular Reflex

The purpose of the vestibulo-ocular reflex (VOR) is to stabilize gaze and maintain clear vision when the body or head is in motion. Objects of visual interest are maintained on the fovea of the retina through inputs from the semicircular canals and otolith organs.

Data regarding VOR function in infants and children have been somewhat limited historically, due to technical difficulties inherent in achieving compliance and obtaining accurate recordings. The VOR is subject to alteration from a variety of nonvestibular influences, including subject attention and state of arousal, unintended ocular fixation due to light leaks, inadequate calibration, and insufficient head stabilization during testing. In several decades of research with children, a variety of techniques have been employed to explore and record the pediatric VOR (see article by the Valente in this publication). These methods include caloric stimulation, rotational stimulation (torsion swing), as well as passive whole body (en bloc) rotation techniques. Depending on the technique employed, parameters such as speed of the slow component in degrees of eye movement per second, amplitude of nystagmus beat, as well as latency and duration of response have been recorded.[12] Researchers using en bloc rotation techniques have explored factors such as gain (ratio of peak eye velocity to peak head velocity), phase (timing difference between head and eye velocities), symmetry (comparison of rightward and leftward eye velocities), and time constant of decay (time for the slow-phase eye velocity to decline by two-thirds of its maximum value).

The VOR is present at birth; however, its time constants are found to be approximately one-half of normal adult values in neonates aged 24 to 120 hours. Time constants appear to approach adult values by 2 months of age.[13] These differences are likely a reflection of immaturity of the visual pathways at birth, which suggests that maturation of the visual pathways is a necessary precursor for adequate calibration of the VOR and for competent function of the velocity storage mechanism necessary for stable vision. Reflexive slow component nystagmus of the VOR generated by vestibular stimulation is routinely observed at birth. However, the centrally mediated fast component, which returns and maintains the eyes within the physical confines of the orbits, is variably present.[14] Infants demonstrate inaccurate saccades, frequently requiring more than one saccade to reach the target. The saccadic system is immature at birth, continuing to develop up to the age of 2 years.[15] The speed of the slow component as well as the frequency of beats increase as a function of age until age 6 to 12 months, after which values reach a plateau and stabilize.[12] Smooth pursuit is also only possible at very low frequencies in this age group, due to foveal immaturity. A higher gain of the VOR response to sinusoidal rotation is observed in children compared to adults, and poorer suppression of the VOR response is seen due to immature visual-vestibular interaction. Gain and time constant parameters of the VOR in response to constant angular acceleration reveal that time constants increase, whereas VOR gain shows small but significant decreases as a function of age from 2 months to 11 years of age.[16] In a recent large longitudinal study, Casselbrant and colleagues[17] observed that in response to both sinusoidal and constant velocity rotations on an earth vertical axis, VOR gain increases linearly as a function of age from 3 to 9 years, although phase differences appeared to remain stable. These findings are in contrast to several other studies that have shown decreasing or stable VOR gain as a function of a child's increasing age.

In summary, the VOR goes through several developmental stages, with healthy responses developing by several months beyond full term.[18] Absence of the VOR by the age of 10 months should be considered an abnormal finding.[12,19] It is evident that regardless of the parameters explored, the prevailing constant across all studies of the pediatric VOR is that qualitative differences exist between the VOR functions of children and adults,[20–24] and that these differences seem to persist until pre-adolescence.

Vestibulospinal Reflex

Whether the body is stationary or in motion, continuous afferent signals from vision and vestibular inputs detect the body's orientation and relationship to gravity. These inputs combine with touch receptors on the skin as well as proprioceptors on the soles of the feet, the hands, joints, and torso to detect the body's contact with the environment. The sum of these inputs provides the information needed to generate the vestibulospinal reflex (VSR), which stabilizes the body and maintains postural control. VSR output signals travel along 3 major pathways, including the lateral, medial, and reticulospinal tracts. When activated, these tracts impact anterior horn cells of the spinal cord and generate myotatic deep tendon reflexes in the antigravity skeletal muscles of the limbs and trunk.

The VSR has more numerous and complex innervations than the VOR, but just as the VOR works to contract and relax paired ocular muscles, the VSR works similarly to create push-pull arrangements of agonist and antagonist muscle firing across the neural axis. A variety of diagnostic tests exploring aspects of VSR function have been developed for use with both children and adults. In general, when comparing the VSR function of children with adults, as noted by Rine,[25] the postural control of these groups varies significantly. As detailed later in this article, the vestibulospinal mechanism or effectiveness of the vestibular system in postural control continues to develop until at least 15 years of age.

Vestibulocollic Reflex

The vestibulocollic reflex (VCR) plays an important role in stabilizing vision by compensating for head movements when the body is in motion. Through patterned contractions of the neck muscles, the VCR minimizes bobbing of the head caused by vibrations transmitted from the heels as they strike the ground during walking and running. Thus, the VCR assists in stabilizing the head on the neck and in keeping the head still and level, especially during ambulation. During walking, vestibular signals caused by linear translations stimulate nerve receptors of the saccule. In response, the saccule transmits afferent signals along the inferior vestibular nerve and ganglion to the vestibular nuclear complex in the brainstem. From the vestibular nucleus, efferent signals are sent via the medial vestibulospinal tract and spinal accessory nerve to the neck muscles, including the sternocleidomastoid muscles—one of the long neck muscles extending from the thorax to the base of the skull behind the ear.

In the last decade, VCR function has become routinely evaluated through recordings of vestibular evoked myogenic potentials (VEMPs). VEMPs have become an increasingly popular clinical technique because, unlike other tests of vestibular function, information is provided regarding saccular and inferior vestibular nerve function. This is a significant benefit, because the otolith organs and superior and posterior semicircular canals may be more instrumental in locomotion and posture control than the horizontal semicircular canals, evaluated using the VOR.[26] In addition, the VEMP test is an objective measure that can be reliably recorded from surface electrodes in a wide variety of patients, including infants and young children. VEMPs are stimulated by high-intensity auditory stimuli that cause robust vibration of the ossicular chain and stimulate the saccule, resting in close proximity. Impulses traveling along the VEMP neural pathway stimulate the VCR, creating an efferent inhibitory release of the tonically contracted sternocleidomastoid muscle. VEMP recordings appear as biphasic electromyographic potentials, with an initial positive deflection at 13 milliseconds post stimulus onset (P13), and a negative deflection at 23 milliseconds (N23).

Studies recording VEMPs in preterm neonates, infants, and young children have confirmed the presence of VEMP responses in the pediatric population. These studies have pointed out differences between the VEMP responses of children and adults, suggesting maturational effects from preschool age through adolescence.[24,27]

BALANCE AND MOTOR DEVELOPMENT

Maintenance of postural balance requires an active sensorimotor control system. In adults, the sensory systems are well organized and act in a context-specific way.[28] Postural control involves sensory feedback,[29] and visual and proprioceptive inputs need to be integrated in order for the center of foot pressure to move in phase with the center of mass. In children the sensory systems are not completely developed, although their anatomic structures are mature early in life.[30] The proprioceptive, visual, and vestibular systems develop more slowly than automatic motor processes that mature early in childhood.[31] The importance of visual cues in maintaining static posture has been well demonstrated, particularly in children who are used to visually monitoring the body during posture.[32,33] Also important are cognitive functions for organization and integration of available sensory information, in both static and dynamic conditions, and this also has been well documented.[34] Hence, the selection of the appropriate balance strategy not only depends on environmental demands but is also a function of central nervous system maturation and experience.

In typically developing children, the growth of postural stability proceeds in a cephalocaudal fashion, with the infant achieving control of the head first, then the trunk, and finally postural stability in standing.[35,36] The newborn infant when held ventrally with a hand under the abdomen cannot hold up the head. By 6 weeks of age the head is held in the plane of the body, and above this level by 12 weeks. Head control allowing the baby to look around in a horizontal plane is achieved by 16 weeks of age, and by the 36th week, the infant is able to sit unsupported for a few minutes. By the age of 1 year the child is able to crawl on hands and knees, and stand up holding on to furniture. At about 15 to 16 months of age the child is able to start walking.[37]

The coordination of postural responses develops until at least 10[28,31] to 15 years of age.[24,26,38,39] In balance control, somatosensory inputs are given priority in adults, whereas children prefer visual inputs to vestibular information in achieving postural equilibrium.[40] Infants and young children (aged 4 months to 2 years) are dependent on the visual system to maintain balance.[41,42] At 3 to 6 years of age, children begin to use somatosensory information appropriately,[31,40,43,44] although some studies indicate that development continues until the age of 9 to 11 years.[45] In the case of intersensory conflict, the vestibular system acts as a referential function by suppressing input not congruent with vestibular information.[43] Adults may improve their postural control, even with misleading visual information, due to presumed mature vestibular function, whereas children by age 12 are still not able to select and process misleading visual information.[46] Among the 3 sensory inputs in children, the vestibular system seems to be the least effective in postural control,[40,47–49] and functional efficiency of the vestibular system in children 10 to 15 years old is still developing.[43,44,48] The ultimate development of several visual functions (eg, saccade latency, contrast sensitivity, and chromatic sensitivity) does not asymptote to adult level until about 12 years of age.[50] The visual influence on standing stability is reported to be established at adult levels around the same age of 15 years.[43,44] Adult-like postural stability due to complete maturation of the 3 sensory systems and the ability to resolve intersensory conflict situations can thus be assumed in adolescents around 15 years of age.[24,26,43,44,48,51]

In summary, vestibular function is present at birth, but continues to mature so that it is most responsive between 6 and 12 months of age. Subsequently, vestibular responses are gradually modulated by developing central inhibitory influences, cerebellar control, and central vestibular adaptation,[9,15,16] and reach adult-like values around 15 years of age.

INCIDENCE OF VESTIBULAR DISORDERS IN THE PEDIATRIC POPULATION

The general prevalence of pediatric vestibular dysfunction is estimated at between 8% and 18%, though the incidence of vertigo as a primary complaint in a review of hospital records was less than 1%.[52]

THE DIFFERENTIAL DIAGNOSIS
Definition

Children do not complain about vestibular dysfunction, and therefore the diagnosis relies on careful questioning of the child (if applicable) and parents, targeted imaging/testing, and an astute clinician to synthesize the findings into a cohesive diagnosis. Signs of abnormal balance development in children need further clarification to distinguish whether the problem rests primarily with the vestibular system, vestibular pathways, or with abnormalities in the visual, motor, or proprioceptive systems, which jointly contribute to the acquisition of motor milestones.

Patient History

Vertigo, defined as the subjective sensation of movement, can be difficult for many patients to describe, because the central vestibular projections to the cerebral cortex are diffuse. This challenge is even more apparent in the pediatric population, as patients do not have the breadth of experience or vocabulary to describe this sensation. As such, vestibular disorders in children can be difficult to recognize. Children with vestibular disorders are often written off as clumsy or uncoordinated and are thought to be normal, or dysfunction is misjudged to be secondary to behavioral abnormality. Children may present with complaints of abdominal pain, ataxia, headache, visual disturbances, hearing loss, otalgia, or otorrhea. On the other hand, children with vestibular disorders may have no complaints. In a study of 62 children with basilar skull fracture, 34% of whom had sensorineural hearing loss (SNHL), "few" of the children had vestibular complaints.[53]

It is frequently possible with a careful history, engaging both the child and the caregiver, to identify the likely cause of the balance disorder even in the most complex patients. A series of focused questions, based on the excellent work of Halmagyi,[54] will differentiate the nature of the pathology in most patients (**Table 1**).

Care should be given to note any signs and symptoms that may be related to vestibular dysfunction such as vertigo, oscillopsia, drop attacks without loss of consciousness, lateropulsion (veering off course while walking), and vegetative symptoms (nausea, emesis, malaise). Of particular importance in children is to determine if there is any history of delayed motor development (rolling over, sitting up, crawling, walking, or running), frequent falls, or learning disabilities that may result from poor dynamic visual acuity due to deficiency of the VOR.

"What does it feel like?"

This question is the first step in differentiating a true illusion of movement (vertigo) that indicates an abnormality in the vestibular end-organ or pathways from some other unrelated sensation such as a presyncopal feeling. This situation is particularly important in early teenage females who can develop orthostatic hypotension. One must elicit any evidence of anxiety with hyperventilation that will produce a lightheaded feeling. Vestibular disorders will almost always produce some sense of vertigo that is exacerbated by movement. Central vestibular pathway disorders tend to produce neither as large a degree of vegetative symptoms nor exacerbation by movement as peripheral disorders. Any change in sensorium, particularly with a history of seizure disorder, should prompt consideration of temporal lobe seizures.

Table 1
Clinical information regarding the history of the patient obtained from a series of focused questions

Question	Clinical Information
What does it feel like?	Is this vestibular/labyrinthine (vertigo) or something else (presyncope, syncope, seizure)
What other symptoms are associated with it?	Declining hearing after head trauma (EVA) Tinnitus, hearing loss (hydrops) Dysarthria, diplopia, paresthesias (vertebrobasilar disease) Cranial nerve weakness (skull base, intracranial lesions) Headache, paroxysmal torticollis (migraine, BRVC) Sweating, palpitations, dyspnea (orthostasis, panic attacks)
How long do the symptoms last and how many have occurred?	Seconds to minutes (BPPV) Hours (TIA, migrant, hydrops) Days to weeks (labyrinthitis, vestibular neuritis)
What makes it better or worse?	Vestibular generated vertigo always worse with movement Rolling, bending (BPPV) Valsalva (PLF)
What is the background history?	Otologic disease (PLF, labyrinthitis, BPPV) SNHL (syndromic/nonsyndromic/congenital vs acquired), ototoxic medications, congenital or acquired vestibular hypofunction Neuropathies (peripheral neuropathy) Vascular disease (congenital cardiopulmonary disease, von Hippel-Lindau with intracranial vascular lesions) Family history of neoplasms (NF-2, Gorlin syndrome, Costello syndrome) (acoustic neuroma, medulloblastoma) Anxiety/depression (panic attacks) Motion intolerance (migraine) Family history of balance disorders (periodic ataxias, migraine, hereditary vestibulopathy) Autoimmune disease (autoimmune inner ear disease) Seizure history (temporal lobe seizures) Ophthalmologic disease (oculomotor anomaly, amblyopia, disorders of acuity, depth perception)

Abbreviations: BPPV, benign paroxysmal positional vertigo; BRVC, benign recurrent vertigo of childhood; EVA, enlarged vestibular aqueduct; NF-2, neurofibromatosis Type II; PLF, perilymph fistula; SNHL, sensorineural hearing loss; TIA, transient ischemic attack.

"What other symptoms are associated with it?"

It is important to ascertain any evidence of aural symptoms (hearing loss, aural fullness, tinnitus, fluctuation in hearing) that might be related to a vestibulopathy. Any evidence of neurologic symptoms or cranial nerve weaknesses needs to be investigated. A headache history or history of paroxysmal torticollis is important in ascertaining if the patient suffers from migraine-related vertigo or benign recurrent vertigo of childhood. The clinician should also inquire about palpitations, dyspnea, feelings of anxiety, or motion sensitivity (eg, carsickness).

"How long do the symptoms typically last and how many have occurred?"

This is a key question that helps differentiate the nature of the vestibulopathy. Very brief, recurrent episodes generally indicate benign paroxysmal positional vertigo

(BPPV); this is important to consider in the setting of head trauma. Episodes lasting hours at a time may indicate attacks of hydrops, migraine, or posterior circulation compromise (which is extremely rare in children). One long episode generally indicates an insult to the vestibular apparatus such as vestibular neuritis or labyrinthitis. In contradistinction to adults, most children with a normal central nervous system will attain central compensation for this type of lesion much more rapidly (days vs weeks to months).

"What makes it worse or better?"

Onset with rolling over, bending over, or looking up is typical of posterior canal BPPV. Worsening of vertigo with Valsalva maneuver or straining may be seen with superior canal dehiscence (see article by Hegemann and Carey in this publication) or perilymph fistula, particularly in the context of head or ear trauma or in children with known middle or inner ear malformations.

"What is the background history?"

It is of vital importance to elicit any history of otologic disease or surgery (cochlear implant, chronic ear or cholesteatoma surgery), exposure to ototoxic medications, head or ear trauma, autoimmune diseases, seizure disorders, ophthalmologic disease, hearing loss of any type, vascular or cardiac disease, and family history of neoplasms, as these may guide the differential diagnosis and workup.

Physical Examination

The physical examination should include the standard ear, nose, and throat examination, and neurologic examination including cranial nerve examination, muscle strength, deep tendon reflexes, and cerebellar testing. In addition, tests of visual acuity and dynamic visual acuity should be considered. Next, the clinician should search for evidence of static and dynamic imbalance of vestibular function.

Static imbalance

In infants and young children who cannot cooperate with many parts of the examination, the presence of a functional VOR can be assessed by looking for per-rotatory and post-rotatory nystagmus while accelerating in a circle. The clinician sits on a rotating stool, occupies the child's gaze with an interesting object attached to the clinician, and accelerates briefly in alternating directions. With an intact VOR, fast-phase nystagmus toward the direction of acceleration can be observed. Older children are instructed to look at a finger or some interesting object that will hold their attention while the clinician searches for spontaneous or gaze-evoked nystagmus; the former indicates active asymmetry in vestibular function and the latter indicates a central nervous system disorder (**Fig. 1**). Spontaneous nystagmus is most easily seen when fixation is removed with Frenzel glasses (**Fig. 2**), which should be done in all cardinal positions of gaze, but not the extremes of gaze (>30°) to prevent physiologic nystagmus secondary to extraocular muscle elasticity. In patients recovering from an acute peripheral vestibular injury, the progression of central compensation can be observed as progress is made from third degree to first degree to no spontaneous nystagmus.

Vertical nystagmus indicates either a pontine lesion (up-beating nystagmus) or cranial-cervical junction lesion (down-beating nystagmus). The latter is very important to note in children because it may be seen in association with ataxia in children with large, compressive Chiari malformations. This appearance may be magnified by asking the patient to perform a Valsalva maneuver. Having the patient slightly hyperventilate may unmask the nystagmus produced by demyelinating lesions of the brain parenchyma or from eighth nerve compression. Tragal compression may produce the predominantly horizontal nystagmus seen in perilymph fistula, or vertical, rotatory

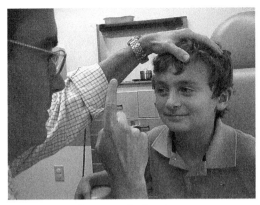

Fig. 1. Search for spontaneous and gaze-evoked nystagmus.

nystagmus seen in superior canal dehiscence. Neck rotation with the head stable is said to produce nystagmus related to "cervical vertigo."

Dynamic imbalance

Tests of dynamic imbalance include the "head-thrust maneuver" or "head impulse test." The patient is asked to fixate on a stationary target while the head is rapidly moved left, right, up, or down (**Fig. 3**). If the VOR is deficient, stationary gaze cannot be maintained and corrective saccades are evident. This test may be followed by a test to observe post-headshake nystagmus. With Frenzel glasses in place, the head is oscillated from side to side symmetrically and then stopped. Asymmetric vestibular function will lead to several easily observable beats of nystagmus, with the fast phase directed to the side of the intact horizontal semicircular canal. The Dix-Hallpike maneuver may be performed to search for evidence of BPPV (**Fig. 4**). Right, left, and center head hanging positions are tested; this can be followed by a particle repositioning maneuver if necessary (see article by Cho and White in this publication).

Vestibulospinal testing

The clinician can assess the Romberg and sharpened Romberg tests, and tests of past pointing. The Fukuda stepping test is easily performed by asking the child to march in place with the eyes closed while the examiner looks for abnormal rotation (**Fig. 5**).

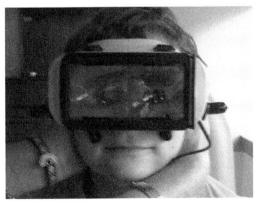

Fig. 2. Frenzel glasses (high diopter lenses) prevent fixation and aid in identification of nystagmus.

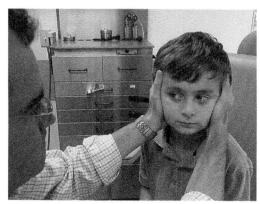

Fig. 3. Head-thrust maneuver tests the VOR.

Gait and gross motor assessment

Subjective evaluation of age-appropriate gait can be tested in the clinic to look for gait asymmetry and ataxia. Age-appropriate gross motor assessments are also available, such as the Peabody test of gross motor development (15 days to 71 months of age) and the Bruininks-Ostresky test of motor performance (4–21 years of age). These tests are important for completing the picture in children with imbalance, as hypotonia and delayed motor development will significantly affect balance performance.

CHARACTERISTICS OF VESTIBULAR DISORDERS IN THE PEDIATRIC POPULATION

To streamline the differential diagnosis of balance disorders in children, various investigators have subcategorized the disorders based on site of origin (ie, peripheral or central), frequency (ie, acute non-recurring, recurrent, or chronic), or non-vertiginous dizziness, disequilibrium, or ataxia.[55,56] Since balance is maintained by visual, proprioceptive, and vestibular systems and a dysfunction in any one of these areas could manifest as a balance disorder, it is understandable that the differential diagnosis would be broad. In a review of all pediatric patients who presented to the authors' clinics over a 4-year period with a complaint of vestibular dysfunction, patients could be broadly categorized into 3 groups. Peripheral vestibulopathy was found in 29.5%

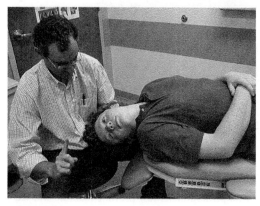

Fig. 4. Dix-Hallpike maneuver.

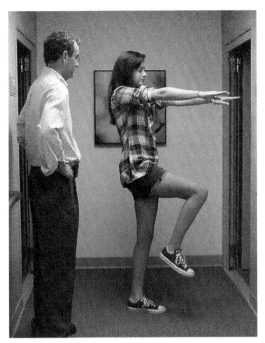

Fig. 5. Fukuda stepping test.

(39 of 132) of the patients, migraine/benign recurrent vertigo of childhood was found in 24.2% (32 of 132), and the remainder were divided into multiple groups, each comprising fewer than 10% of the total patient population. Diagnoses in this group included motor/developmental delay, traumatic brain injury, central nervous system structural lesion, behavioral disorders, idiopathic imbalance, neurodegenerative disease, encephalopathy, vascular lesions, peripheral neuropathy, and oculomotor disorders.

These findings are consistent with other large series that have examined pediatric vestibular dysfunction.[52,55–59]

Sensorineural hearing loss (SNHL) is reported to be associated with vestibular dysfunction in 20% to 70% of cases.[60] Evaluating children with profound SNHL, Cushing and colleagues[61] found a 50% incidence of horizontal semicircular canal dysfunction and a 38% incidence of saccular dysfunction. Identification of these concomitant vestibular impairments is of critical importance, as therapies can be tailored to adequately deal with multiple sensory deficiencies.

Otitis media can be a significant contributor to balance disorders in children. Otitis media is thought to be caused by pressure changes within the middle ear, or due to toxins secreted into the middle ear that leak into the inner ear and directly affect the labyrinth.[62,63] When tested, children with history of otitis media often have abnormalities present in electronystagmography and motor proficiency tests. Myringotomy with tympanostomy tube insertion has been reported to help balance disorders associated with otitis media.[64] In the case of chronic otitis media with cholesteatoma, there may be direct involvement/erosion of the vestibule or semicircular canals by the cholesteatoma. Typically this occurs in the horizontal semicircular canal. There may be erosion of bone, leading to a perilymph fistula or labyrinthitis. In some cases, vertigo or disequilibruim may be the presenting symptom of chronic otitis media with cholesteatoma. Children with otitis media with effusion rely more on vision than those without effusion. These children also demonstrate increased postural sway with moving visual scenes.[65]

Congenital vestibular hypofunction can be associated with syndromic or nonsyndromic causes. Usher syndrome is the most common autosomal recessive SNHL associated with vestibular dysfunction. There are 3 major types: Type I includes profound hearing loss, retinitis pigmentosa, and vestibular hypofunction; Type II has less hearing loss and normal vestibular function; and Type III is characterized by progressive SNHL and progressive vestibular dysfunction. It is important to differentiate among these types, as this can have profound effects on targeted therapy for patients with multiple sensory losses.

Pendred syndrome is another autosomal recessive cause of vestibular dysfunction. This syndrome is a constellation of Mondini malformation (incomplete partition of the cochlea) and enlarged vestibular aqueduct (EVA). Vestibular dysfunction may be present in up to one-third of cases.[66] Nonsyndromic, congenital malformations of the inner ear, such as Mondini malformation, Scheibe aplasia (cochleosaccular dysplasia), and EVA may have vestibular manifestations. Patients with CHARGE syndrome (coloboma, heart defects, choanal atresia, retardation of growth and development, genital anomalies, and ear abnormalities) have variable degrees of vestibular malformation, though almost all patients have congenital absence of the semicircular canals.

Benign paroxysmal positional vertigo (BPPV) is the most common cause of balance disorder in the adult population. This phenomenon of brief periods of fatigable vertigo associated with movement and preceded by a latent period is thought to arise from displaced otoconia within the semicircular canals or on the cupula of the semicircular canals (typically the posterior semicircular canal). This pathological condition is rare in children. For those children affected, there is often a history of antecedent trauma or vestibular neuritis. Symptoms typically resolve over time, but patients may benefit from canalith repositioning exercises.

Vestibular neuritis is presumed to result from viral infection of vestibular nerves or labyrinthine end-organ (see article by Goddard and Fayad in this publication). Children with vestibular neuritis experience severe, sudden onset of vertigo and spontaneous nystagmus without hearing loss. The onset of symptoms is typically abrupt and is caused by a sudden loss of vestibular function on the affected side. These symptoms may last for weeks to months, but in children, symptoms typically resolve completely by 2 to 4 weeks, possibly reflecting increased plasticity of central compensation in children.[67]

Ménière's disease is an idiopathic condition of the labyrinth associated with endolymphatic hydrops. The complete pathophysiology of Ménière's disease is poorly understood. The symptoms in children are the same as those in adults: tinnitus, fluctuating hearing loss (especially in low frequencies), and episodic vertigo. Ménière's disease is rare in children, responsible for fewer than 4% of children with balance disorders.[68] Because of its rarity in children, care must be taken to rule out other inner ear anomalies (EVA syndrome) and autoimmune inner ear disease that may present a "hydropic" clinical picture.

Congenital cytomegalovirus (CMV) infection is estimated to affect 0.4% to 2.3% of live births in the United States, and up to 90% of those are asymptomatic at birth. Eight to 15% of asymptomatic patients will present later in life with SNHL. Symptomatic CMV infection will lead to SNHL in 30% to 65% of patients. Vestibular insult can be expected in patients who are severely affected. The dual central nervous system and inner ear insults resulting from congenital CMV may be very difficult to rehabilitate.

Fluctuation and deterioration in hearing typically parallel spells of vertigo in this population.[69]

The surgical trauma of *cochlear implantation* can cause vestibular symptoms. Standard placement of the implant electrode array within the scala tympani of the cochlea is purported to cause alterations in normal inner ear fluid composition, inflammation, and fibrosis with hair cell loss.[70] Transient dizziness is common after cochlear implantation, but this typically resolves rapidly. It has been noted that up to 50% of cochlear implant candidates have preexisting vestibular deficits, and that those with normal vestibular function will have alteration of vestibular function after implantation.[71] This finding appears to be of limited consequence clinically in the majority of patients, as they achieve rapid vestibular compensation in the face of a normal central nervous system.

Trauma of the temporal bone can precipitate vertigo. Temporal bone fractures occur in approximately 10% of pediatric blunt head trauma.[66] Fractures can be longitudinal, that is, along the axis of the petrous bone (70%–80%), or transverse (20%–30%). Transverse is most likely to involve the otic capsule with resultant vestibular injury and SNHL.[55] In addition to injury from the trauma itself, the insult can predispose the patient to BPPV later in life.

Direct trauma to the tympanic membrane or middle ear may result in acquired perilymphatic fistulas. An example of this would be stapes subluxation from Q-tip injury to the tympanic membrane. The typical symptoms of perilymph fistula include hearing loss and vertigo, particularly after straining. In cases of suspected perilymph fistula, surgical repair may be considered to control vertigo symptoms when conservative management is unsuccessful.

Cogan syndrome is an autoimmune disorder that presents with nonsyphylitic interstitial keratitis, acute SNHL, and vestibulopathy. The hearing loss may be progressive. The timing and association of symptoms of Cogan syndrome can be highly variable, making diagnosis difficult.[72] Despite this, accurate and prompt diagnosis is essential, as high-dose steroids may help to limit the degree of SNHL and vestibulopathy.

Labyrinthitis is an acute inflammatory process of the labyrinth. Symptoms are typically both auditory and vestibular, and may range from minor to severe. Bacterial labyrinthitis is usually the result of bacterial invasion of the inner ear through the cochlear aqueduct in patients with bacterial meningitis. The labyrinth may also be infected from a middle ear source. Both medical and surgical intervention may be required to control this process, and the vestibular insult is often profound. In addition, several viruses, including mumps, measles, influenza, and Epstein-Barr, are known to cause labyrinthitis.

Congenital and acquired "third windows" of the labyrinth may result in vestibular symptoms through the "Tullio" effect. Semicircular canal dehiscence and EVA are readily diagnosed by appropriate imaging (computed tomography), and abnormally low VEMP thresholds with very large amplitude responses are characteristic.[73]

Unlike the typical presentation in adults of throbbing unilateral frontal pain, children often manifest *migraine* with other symptoms. Disequilibrium and vertigo are very common migraine equivalents. In the authors' series, migraine was the underlying diagnosis in 24.2% of patients. Vertigo and disequilibrium may precede headache; however, vertigo may occur in isolation separate from the headaches. The symptoms may be severe and may last for several hours. Patients may have associated nausea, vomiting, photophobia, phonophobia, and sensitivity to smells. Symptoms may be worsened by fatigue.[56]

Diagnosis of *migraine-related vertigo* requires careful and detailed history and physical examination. The otologic examination is normal, although there may be subtle abnormalities in audiometric and vestibular testing, including pathologic nystagmus during an acute attack[74] and reduced otoacoustic emission suppression.[75] However, audiometry is usually normal[76]; thus the lack of objective findings does not preclude the diagnosis. Imaging is often obtained to rule out any intracranial masses or lesions, and the findings on computed tomography and magnetic resonance imaging are normal. Migraine-related vertigo is most common in teenage females (see article by Taylor and Goodkin in this publication).

Benign paroxysmal vertigo of childhood (BPVC) is a unique migraine variant that was first described by Basser in 1964.[77] BPVC typically occurs in children 3 to 8 years old. Attacks are sudden in onset, may occur in any position (sitting, standing, moving, stationary), and are typically brief, lasting only a few seconds to minutes. The affected child may remain still, refusing to move, or may grab onto something for support, and nystagmus is often noted during the attack. There is often associated anxiety, pallor, nausea, sweating, and occasionally vomiting. No pain is associated with the event and there is no loss of consciousness. At the completion of the attack, the child usually resumes normal activity.[59] Physical examination and all imaging studies typically are normal. After a few years, the episodes of BPVC cease. It is reported that 43% of patients will have a positive family history of migraine. Children affected with BPVC may develop classic migraines later in life, reported at an incidence of 13%,[78] often many years after the cessation of the BPVC symptoms.[79]

Paroxysmal torticollis of infancy is considered in the same spectrum as BPVC, as a component of the periodic juvenile migraine disorders.[59] Paroxysmal torticollis consists of episodic head tilt, which may have associated nausea, vomiting, pallor, and agitation. The episodes are brief and self-limited, and may alternate from side to side. The symptoms typically resolve by 2 to 3 years of age.[55]

Basilar migraine is a particular variant of migraine that comprises 3% to 19% of childhood migraine. Vertigo may be particularly apparent in this form of migraine. These children present clinically with aura of vertigo, visual disturbances, or ataxia. Pain follows, but may be occipital in location, unlike the usual frontal or bitemporal pain of typical migraine.[80] The average age of onset is 7 years, and females are most affected.

Head trauma and *resultant traumatic brain injury or labyrinthine concussion* can result in a vestibulopathy. The reported incidence of dizziness after head trauma varies greatly through the literature, ranging from 15% to 78%. Nonetheless, it should be considered that even minor head trauma may result in vestibular pathology. Mechanisms for this include direct trauma to the eighth nerve complex and root entry zone at the brainstem or labyrinthine concussion. In the latter, there are several theories as to the cause of the injury to the vestibular end organ. There may be disruptions of the microcirculation of the vestibule with resultant hemorrhage and inflammation. The pressure wave itself may cause rupture of the membranous labyrinth.[81] Patients typically are affected immediately after the trauma. Children usually recover completely; however, rarely they may develop BPPV.[55]

Central nervous system (CNS) structural lesions are among the principal concerns when a child presents with new onset of vertigo. In the authors' series, CNS lesions accounted for 9.1% of patients with vertigo and dysequilibrium. Symptomatic malformations may include Chiari malformation with syrinx formation, spinocerebellar atrophy, arachnoid cyst of the posterior fossa, and delayed myelination disorders. Tumors of the posterior fossa may also contribute to balance dysfunction. The most common tumors of the posterior fossa in children are astrocytoma, medulloblastoma, ependymoma, and glioma. Rarely will dizziness be the only presenting symptom.[66] Cerebellopontine angle tumors are very rare in children, and if found, should prompt consideration of neurofibromatosis type II (bilateral CPA tumors). Concerns for a CNS structural lesion should be investigated with magnetic resonance imaging.

Various *behavioral and psychiatric disorders*, such as sensorimotor integration disorder, conversion disorder, anxiety, tic disorder, autism, or attention deficit/hyperactivity disorder, may have associated vestibular or balance complaints. Children who present with a nonorganic cause of their balance symptoms can be identified by a mismatch of symptoms with clinical findings, evidence of secondary gain by their symptoms, and possibly by nonphysiologic responses with evidence of malingering on objective vestibular testing. The importance of integrating the psychosocial history with the clinical picture cannot be overemphasized.[56]

Neurodegenerative disease (eg, familial ataxia) and encephalopathy result in imbalance from dysfunction of the central and sometimes peripheral vestibular pathways. The authors find that up to 7% of patients referred for disequilibrium carry these diagnoses (see article by Cherchi in this publication).

This article focuses at length on the factors that affect the vestibular system. It should be remembered that impaired vision, and inability to converge or fixate with binocular vision may result in a feeling of unsteadiness or vertigo. In addition, any peripheral neuropathy that impairs proprioception may also lead to these sensations.

REFERENCES

1. Sidebotham P. Balance through the ages of man. J Laryngol Otol 1988;3:203–8.
2. Brandt T, Glasauer S, Stephan T, et al. Visual-vestibular and visuovisual cortical interaction: new insights from fMRI and PET. Ann N Y Acad Sci 2002;956:230–41.
3. Jeffery N, Spoor F. Prenatal growth and development of the modern human labyrinth. J Anat 2004;204:71–92.
4. Richard C, Laroche N, Malaval L, et al. New insight into the bony labyrinth: a microcomputed tomography study. Auris Nasus Larynx 2010;37:155–61.
5. Wright CG, Hubbard DG. SEM observations on development of human otoconia during the first trimester of gestation. Acta Otolaryngol 1982;94(1/2):7–18.
6. Holt K. Movement and child development. Clinics in developmental medicine. No. 55. Philadelphia: Lippincott; 1975.
7. Schulte FJ, Linke I, Michaelis E, et al. Excitation, inhibition and impulse conduction in spinal motoneurones of preterm, term and small-for-dates newborn infants. In: Robinson RJ, editor. Brain and early behavior development in the fetus and infants. CASDS Study Group on Brain mechanisms or early behavioural development. New York: Academic Press; 1969. p. 87–114.
8. Kaga K, Sakurai H, Ogawa Y, et al. Morphological changes of vestibular ganglion cells in human fetuses and in pediatric patients. Int J Pediatr Otorhinolaryngol 2001;60:11–20.
9. Blayney AW. Vestibular disorders. In: Adams DA, Cinnamond MJ, editors, Paediatric otolaryngology, Scott-Brown's otolaryngology, vol. 6. 6th edition. Oxford (UK): Butterworth-Heinemann; 1997. p. 1–29.
10. Swaiman KF. Neurologic examination after the newborn period until two years of age. Pediatric neurology principles and practice. 3rd edition. St Louis (MO): Mosby; 1999. p. 31–53.
11. Eviatar L, Eviatar A, Naray L. Maturation of neurovestibular responses in infants. Dev Med Child Neurol 1974;16:435–46.
12. Eviatar L, Eviatar A. The normal nystagmic response of infants to caloric and perrotatory stimulation. Laryngoscope 1979;89:1036–44.

13. Weissman BM, Di Seenna AO, Leigh RJ. Maturation of the vestibulo-ocular reflex in normal infants during the first 2 months of life. Neurology 1989;39:534–8.
14. Cohen B. Origin of quick phases of nystagmus. In: Brodal A, Pompeiano O, editors. Basic aspects of central vestibular mechanisms. Amsterdam: Elsevier; 1972. p. 1–649.
15. Ornitz EM, Atwell CW, Walter DO, et al. The maturation of vestibular nystagmus in infancy and childhood. Acta Otolaryngol 1979;88:244–56.
16. Ornitz EM, Kaplan AR, Westlake JR. Development of the vestibulo-ocular reflex from infancy to adulthood. Acta Otolaryngol 1985;100:180–3.
17. Casselbrant ML, Mandel EM, Sparto P, et al. Longitudinal posturography and rotational testing in children three to nine years of age: normative data. Otolaryngol Head Neck Surg 2010;142:708–14.
18. Donat JFG, Donat JR, Swe Lay K. Changing response to caloric stimulation with gestational age in infants. Neurology 1980;30:776–8.
19. Fife TD, Tusa RJ, Furman JM, et al. Assessment: vestibular testing techniques in adults and children. Neurology 2000;55:1431–41.
20. Van der Laan FL, Oosterveld WJ. Age and vestibular function. Aerosp Med 1974; 45:540–7.
21. Mulch G, Petermann W. Influence of age on results of vestibular function tests. Review of literature and presentation of caloric test results. Ann Otol Rhinol Laryngol Suppl 1979;88:1–17.
22. Andrieu-Guitrancourt JA, Peron JM, Dehesdin D, et al. Normal vestibular responses to air caloric tests in children. Int J Pediatr Otorhinolaryngol 1981;3:245–50.
23. Staller SJ, Goin DW, Hildebrandt M. Pediatric vestibular evaluation with harmonic acceleration. J Otolaryngol Head Neck Surg 1986;95:471–6.
24. Valente M. Maturational effects of the vestibular system: a study of rotary chair, computerized dynamic posturography, and vestibular evoked myogenic potentials with children. J Am Acad Audiol 2007;18:461–81.
25. Rine RM. Management of the pediatric patient with vestibular hypofunction. In: Herdman S, editor. Vestibular rehabilitation. 3rd edition. Philadelphia: F.A. Davis Co; 2007. p. 360–75.
26. Shinjo Y, Jin Y, Kaga K. Assessment of vestibular function of infants and children with congenital and acquired deafness using ice-water caloric test, rotational chair test and vestibular-evoked myogenic potential recording. Acta Otolaryngol 2007;127:736–47.
27. Kelsch TA, Schaefer LA, Esquivel CR. Vestibular evoked myogenic potentials in young children: test parameters and normative data. Laryngoscope 2006;116: 895–900.
28. Shumway-Cook A, Woollacott MH. The growth of stability: postural control from a development perspective. J Mot Behav 1985;17:131–47.
29. Nashner LM, Stupert CL, Horak FB, et al. Organization of postural controls: an analysis of sensory and mechanical constraints. Prog Brain Res 1989;80:411–8.
30. Ornitz EM. Normal and pathological maturation of vestibular function in the human child. In: Romand R, editor. Development of auditory and vestibular systems. New York: Academic Press Inc; 1983. p. 479–536.
31. Forssberg H, Nashner LM. Ontogenetic development of postural control in man: adaptation to altered support and visual conditions during stance. J Neurosci 1982;2:545–52.
32. Wiener-Vacher SR, Toupet F, Narcy P. Canal and otolith vestibule-ocular reflexes to vertical and off vertical axis rotation in children learning to walk. Acta Otolaryngol 1996;116:657–65.

33. Bucci MP, Kapoula Z, Yang Q, et al. Speed-accuracy of saccades, vergence and combined eye movements in children with vertigo. Exp Brain Res 2004;157: 286–95.
34. Shumway-Cook A, Woollacott M. Attentional demands and postural control: the effect of sensory context. J Gerontol A Biol Sci Med Sci 2000;55:M10–6.
35. Bradley NS. Motor control: developmental aspects of motor control in skill acquisition. In: Campbell SK, editor. Physical therapy for children. Philadelphia: WB Saunders Co; 1997. p. 39–77.
36. Burleigh AL, Horak FB, Malouin F. Modification of postural responses and step initiation: evidence for goal-directed postural interactions. J Neurophysiol 1994; 72:2892–902.
37. Illingworth RS. The normal child. 8th edition. Edinburgh (UK): Churchill Livingstone; 1983.
38. Hatzitaki V, Zisi V, Kollias I, et al. Perceptual-motor contributions to static and dynamic balance control in children. J Mot Behav 2002;34(2):161–70.
39. Hsu YS, Kuan CC, Young YH. Assessing the development of balance function in children using stabilometry. Int J Pediatr Otorhinolaryngol 2009;73: 737–40.
40. Foudriat BA, Di Fabio RP, Anderson JH. Sensory organization of balance responses in children 3-6 years of age: a normative study with diagnosis implication. Int J Pediatr Otorhinolaryngol 1993;27:255–71.
41. Starkes J, Riach CL. The role of vision in the postural control of children. Clin Kinesiol 1990;44:72–7.
42. Woollacott MH, Debu B, Mowatt M. Neuromuscular control of posture in the infant and child: is vision dominant? J Mot Behav 1987;19:167–86.
43. Hirabayashi S, Iwasaki Y. Developmental perspective of sensory organization on postural control. Brain Dev 1995;17:111–3.
44. Steindl R, Kunz K, Schrott-Fischer A, et al. Effect of age and sex on maturation of sensory systems and balance control. Dev Med Child Neurol 2006;48:477–82.
45. Riach CI, Hayes KC. Maturation of postural sway in young children. Dev Med Child Neurol 1987;29:650–8.
46. Ionescu E, Morlet T, Froehlich P, et al. Vestibular assessment with Balance Quest: normative data for children and young adults. Int J Pediatr Otorhinolaryngol 2006; 70:1457–65.
47. Ferber-Viart C, Ionescu E, Morlet T, et al. Balance in healthy individuals assessed with Equitest: maturation and normative data for children and young adults. Int J Pediatr Otorhinolaryngol 2007;71:1041–6.
48. Cherng RJ, Chen JJ, Su FC. Vestibular system in performance of standing balance of children and young adults under altering sensory conditions. Percept Mot Skills 2001;92:1167–79.
49. Charpiot A, Tringali S, Ionescu E, et al. Vestibulo-ocular reflex and balance maturation in healthy children aged from six to twelve years. Audiol Neurootol 2010;15: 201–10.
50. Yang Q, Bucci MP, Kapoula Z. The latency of saccades, vergence, and combined eyes movements in children and in adults. Invest Ophthalmol Vis Sci 2002;43:2939–49.
51. Peterka RJ, Black FO. Age-related changes in human posture control. Sensory organization tests. J Vestib Res 1990;1:73–85.
52. Neimensivu R, Pyykko I, Wiener-Vacher S. Vertigo and balance problems in children—an epidemiologic study in Finland. Int J Pediatr Otorhinolaryngol 2006;70: 259–65.

53. Vartiainen E, Karjalainen S, Kärjä J. Vestibular disorders following head injury in children. Int J Pediatr Otorhinolaryngol 1985;9:135–41.
54. Halmagyi GH. History II. Patient with vertigo. In: Baloh RW, Halmagyi GH, editors. Disorders of the vestibular system. New York: Oxford University Press; 1996. p. 171–7.
55. Casselbrant ML, Mandel EM. Balance disorders in children. Neurol Clin 2005;23: 807–29.
56. Wiener-Vacher SR. Vestibular disorders in children. Int J Audiol 2008;47:578–83.
57. Balatsouras DG, Kaberis A, Assimakopoulos D. Etiology of vertigo in children. Int J Pediatr Otorhinolaryngol 2007;71:487–94.
58. Szirmai A. Vestibular disorders in childhood and adolescents. Eur Arch Otorhinolaryngol 2010;267:1801–4.
59. Niemensivu R, Pyykko I, Erna K. Vertigo and imbalance in children. Arch Otolaryngol Head Neck Surg 2005;131:996–1000.
60. Arnvig J. Vestibular function in deafness and severe hardness of hearing. Acta Otolaryngol 1955;45:283–8.
61. Cushing SL, Papsin BC, Rutka JA, et al. Evidence of vestibular and balance dysfunction in children with profound sensorineural hearing loss using cochlear implants. Laryngoscope 2008;118(10):1814–23.
62. Waldron M, Matthews J, Johnson I. The effect of otitis media with effusions on balance in children. Clin Otolaryngol Allied Sci 2004;29:318–20.
63. Choung YH, Park K, Moon SK, et al. Various causes and clinical characteristics in vertigo in children with normal eardrums. Int J Pediatr Otorhinolaryngol 2003;67: 889–94.
64. Golz A, Netzer A, Angel-Yeger B. Effects of middle ear effusion on the vestibular system in children. Otolaryngol Head Neck Surg 1998;119:695–9.
65. Casselbrant ML, Redfern MS, Furman JM, et al. Visual induced postural sway in children with and without otitis media. Ann Otol Rhinol Laryngol 1998;107:401–5.
66. Luxon L, Pagarkar W. The dizzy child. In: Graham JM, Scadding GK, Bull PD, editors. Pediatric ENT. Berlin (Heidelberg): Springer; 2008. p. 459–78.
67. Taborelli G, Melagrana A, D'Agostino R. Vestibular neuronitis in children: study of medium and long term follow-up. Int J Pediatr Otorhinolaryngol 2000;54:117–21.
68. Akagi H, Yuen K, Maeda Y. Ménière's disease in childhood. Int J Pediatr Otorhinolaryngol 2001;61:259–64.
69. Pryor SP, Demmler GJ, Madeo AC, et al. Investigation of the role of congenital cytomegalovirus infection in the etiology of enlarged vestibular aqueducts. Arch Otolaryngol Head Neck Surg 2005;131:388–92.
70. Buchman CA, Joy J, Hodges A, et al. Vestibular effects of cochlear implantation. Laryngoscope 2004;114:1–22.
71. Jacot E, Van Den Abbeele T, Wiener-Vacher S. Vestibular impairments pre- and post-cochlear implant in children. Int J Pediatr Otorhinolaryngol 2009;73:209–17.
72. Migliori G, Battisti E, Pari M, et al. A shifty diagnosis: Cogan's syndrome. A case report and review of the literature. Acta Otorhinolaryngol Ital 2009;29:108–13.
73. Mikulec AA, McKenna MJ, Ramsey MJ, et al. Superior semicircular canal dehiscence presenting as conductive hearing loss without vertigo. Otol Neurotol 2004; 25(2):121–9.
74. von Brevern M, Zeise D. Acute migrainous vertigo: clinical and oculographic findings. Brain 2005;128:365–74.
75. Murdin L, Premachandra P, Davies R. Sensory dysmodulation in vestibular migraine: an otoacoustic emission suppression study. Laryngoscope 2010;120: 1632–6.

76. Battista RA. Audiometric findings of patients with migraine-associated dizziness. Otol Neurotol 2004;25:987–92.
77. Basser LS. Benign paroxysmal vertigo of childhood. (A variety of vestibular neuronitis). Brain 1964;87:141–52.
78. Ralli G, Atturo F, deFilippis C. Idiopathic benign paroxysmal vertigo in children, a migraine precursor. Int J Pediatr Otorhinolaryngol 2009;73:S16–8.
79. Lempert T, Neuhauser H. Migrainous vertigo. Neurol Clin 2005;23:715–30.
80. Lewis D. Pediatric migraine. Neurol Clin 2009;27:481–501.
81. Fitzgerald D. Head trauma: hearing loss and dizziness. J Trauma 1996;40(3):488–96.

Assessment Techniques for Vestibular Evaluation in Pediatric Patients

L. Maureen Valente, PhD[a,b,*]

KEYWORDS

- Pediatric vestibular evaluation • Videonystagmography
- Video-oculography • Rotary chair testing
- Computerized dynamic posturography
- Vestibular evoked myogenic potentials

The area of pediatric vestibular evaluation has become popular in audiology and otolaryngology clinics in recent years. As early identification of hearing impairment has unfolded, so too has early identification of vestibular disorders. With regard to both audiology and otolaryngology, the earlier the identification, the earlier remediation strategies can be implemented. Researchers and clinicians have contributed valuable information related to vestibular disorders in the pediatric population. There has been a paucity of both clinical and research work related to vestibular evaluation techniques useful for young children. This review focuses on adaptation of adult vestibular evaluation techniques for use with pediatric patients, beginning with the medical/physical examination and progressing through major tests of vestibular function. An important concept recurring throughout is that the use of pediatric normative data is crucial, so that results obtained after testing a pediatric patient are not compared with adult normative data.

HISTORY AND THE MEDICAL EVALUATION

Many clinicians who perform vestibular evaluations have remarked that the case history is one of the most important diagnostic tools available when evaluating a dizzy patient. Although the author firmly believes that this premise also holds true with

The author has nothing to disclose.
[a] Program in Audiology and Communication Sciences, Washington University School of Medicine, 660 South Euclid Avenue, Campus Box 8042, St Louis, MO 63110, USA
[b] Department of Otolaryngology, Washington University School of Medicine, 660 South Euclid Avenue, St Louis, MO 63110, USA
* Corresponding author. Program in Audiology and Communication Sciences, Washington University School of Medicine, 660 South Euclid Avenue, Campus Box 8042, St Louis, MO 63110.
E-mail address: ValenteL@wustl.edu

Otolaryngol Clin N Am 44 (2011) 273–290
doi:10.1016/j.otc.2011.01.002
0030-6665/11/$ – see front matter © 2011 Elsevier Inc. All rights reserved.

oto.theclinics.com

pediatric patients, a need exists within the profession for development of a reliable case history instrument. On searching the literature regarding vestibular evaluation in children, one may view several different bodies of work. On one hand, Physical Therapy and Occupational Therapy studies document evaluation and remediation techniques utilized with such disorders as autism, motor delay, learning disability, and behavioral disorders.[1–7] While fascinating, these evaluative tools are very different from those discovered within the Audiology and Otolaryngology bodies of literature. Many studies within this latter group link vestibular disorders to such entities as migraine syndrome, benign recurrent vertigo of childhood, otitis media, and sensorineural hearing loss.[8–13] Additional research is needed regarding other syndromes associated with childhood dizziness including CHARGE association, Cogan syndrome, and Usher syndrome, among others.[14–16] As evaluative tools and remediation strategies are also variable among disciplines, greater understanding of other disciplines and greater degree of collaboration are worthy goals.

Many challenges exist with regard to vestibular evaluation of children. For example, pediatric patients may not be able to thoroughly describe dizziness and other symptoms, necessitating the development of appropriate checklists and parent questionnaires. Another challenge related to vestibular evaluation is that the cost of many pieces of technologically advanced equipment is prohibitive, regardless of patient age. This article highlights adaptation of adult screening techniques for pediatric patients, and describes the relative ease of performance of these tests in an office setting with minimal equipment.

PHYSICAL EXAMINATION

Within an office setting, the clinician may begin by checking for any spontaneous and/or gaze-evoked nystagmus that may be present. One simple method is to have the child look straight ahead, if able to follow such verbal commands, and then to follow an examiner's finger as it moves to the right and left and in upward and downward directions. Mental alerting is important with regard to many vestibular measures, and must be geared to the child's age and capabilities. In this case and especially in viewing spontaneous nystagmus, informal conversation and establishing rapport should suffice. It may be possible to use Frenzel lenses for magnification and alleviation of visual fixation suppression, depending on the child's age. At this point the clinician may also briefly check to determine that the eyes are moving conjugately.

As the clinician approaches a dynamic evaluation, consideration may be given to testing "head-shake nystagmus" (HSN). According to Fife and colleagues,[17] the vestibulo-ocular reflex (VOR) should be readily observable by the age of 9 to 12 months in typically developing infants. Visualization may be enhanced via Frenzel lenses, electro-oculography (EOG), or infrared video. As with adults, the child's head may be gently rotated back and forth in a rhythmic, horizontal manner. Theoretically, symmetric vestibular function will not induce symptoms, although some children may not be in a developmental position to verbalize the presence of such symptoms. HSN will not be seen in patients with symmetric peripheral vestibular function, although it may be observed in the presence of a vestibular asymmetry. HSN screening may be advantageous in situations where bithermal caloric irrigations and/or rotary chair testing may not be feasible. If the child is able to perform these tests, HSN screening may provide complementary information by incorporating higher frequencies of head motion.

Head-thrust testing (HTT) may also be performed with young children as part of a medical/physical workup. This procedure is based on the VOR, which as previously mentioned should be observable by the age of 9 to12 months in typically developing children. The examiner gently rotates the child's head by approximately 30° in the yaw plane, while asking the child to focus on the examiner's nose. One may creatively devise placement of colorful stickers or cartoon characters to facilitate such testing. The examiner incorporates a brief and rapid head thrust back to center, making certain that visual fixation is maintained. Any "catch-up" saccade may indicate a disorder of the ipsilateral semicircular canal. **Figs. 1** and **2** display the successful demonstration of HTT with a 4-year-old child.

Children may also be evaluated via dynamic visual acuity (DVA) techniques, with modification of the typical Snellen Eye Chart for this population. Familiar to most, this chart is highly utilized during eye examinations as the patient reads smaller and smaller lines of various letter "E" configurations. For example, child-friendly characters could be easily substituted for the more traditional ones. With this procedure, a baseline is obtained in the form of the smallest line of characters that the child can discern from a calibrated distance. The child again attempts to read the smallest line of figures during back and forth rotation of the head, approximating 1 to 2 Hz. On reading, a loss of one line may be considered insignificant whereas a loss of 3 lines or more may indicate a VOR deficiency. Advances in computerized technology may facilitate this evaluation. The clinician may also perform rudimentary oculomotor tasks, such as checking rapid saccadic eye movement and smoothness of pursuit, by following an examiner's finger or other sinusoidal maneuver.

Although children rarely demonstrate the true benign paroxysmal positional vertigo (BPPV) that is prevalent in adults (see article by Cho and White in this publication), they may experience positional vertigo and/or sudden vertiginous episodes. Positioning and positional testing can be successfully performed with children. With all procedures, establishing rapport with the child is critical, and the child's comfort level may be increased by being seated on a parent's lap and/or having a parent present. The traditional Dix-Hallpike maneuver involves rapidly taking the patient from a seated to a lying-back position. The clinician assists the patient in turning the head to the right or left and lying back, and then the procedure is repeated as the patient lies back while turning the head to the opposite side. As Hallpike testing is very time-efficient and noninvasive, it may be performed with children along with more traditional positional testing. It is important for the child to be able to understand instructions and to receive continual reassurance, in that the room environment may be darkened. Typical

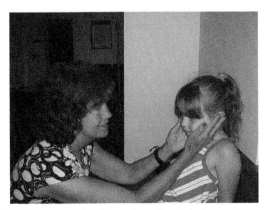

Fig. 1. Example of clinician preparing to perform head-shake nystagmus testing/screening with a 4-year-old child.

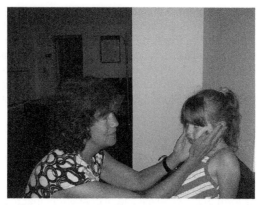

Fig. 2. Example of clinician preparing to perform head-thrust testing/screening with a 4-year-old child.

positions may be similar to those performed with adults: supine, head right, head left, right lateral, and left lateral. As the clinician searches for the presence of nystagmus, it is also important to supplement this information with any subjective symptoms that the child may report.

Finally, during the physical examination, the clinician may ask the child to perform various types of standing balance tasks for screening postural stability. An example is the Romberg maneuver, for which the child stands with feet together and sway is noted with eyes both open and closed. A variation is the tandem Romberg, whereby such stability is evaluated in a heel-to-toe format. **Fig. 3** depicts the author as she performs the tandem Romberg maneuver with a 4-year-old patient.

Examiners may ask the child to march in place with eyes closed to determine straightness versus deviation of walking path and/or may also encourage the child to walk forward in a heel-to-toe pattern. With the latter, cerebellar dysfunction may be suspected if difficulties arise.[18,19] Other cerebellar signs may include slurred

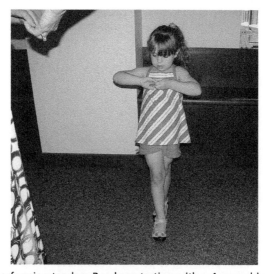

Fig. 3. Clinician performing tandem Romberg testing with a 4-year-old child.

speech, upper or lower extremity dysfunction, ataxia, muscle incoordination, tremors, and abnormalities noted on oculomotor tasks.

VIDEO-OCULOGRAPHY

Video-oculography (VOG) has replaced EOG in most clinics, with the advent of infrared cameras mounted in eye goggles to replace electrodes for recording eye movements. An example of such eye goggles is seen in **Fig. 4**, with the clinician making use of the smallest size possible for evaluation of the pediatric patient.

This vestibular evaluation procedure is actually a battery of tests that assists the clinician in determining whether dizziness is of central or peripheral origin. If peripheral, components of the test battery may help determine the affected side of the deficit. Components of this test battery include testing for spontaneous nystagmus and gaze nystagmus, performing various oculomotor tests, measuring positioning and positional nystagmus, and performing bithermal caloric irrigations. Several investigators have effectively described some of the adaptations of adult VOG techniques that may be used with children.[20]

As the parent makes certain that the child is optimally prepared for vestibular evaluation, it is important that certain medications (such as those for cough or cold) be withheld for 24 to 48 hours. As some aspects of the test battery may induce nausea, it is important that the child eat only lightly prior to the appointment. VOG may be performed in a darkened room so that visual fixation of nystagmus does not occur; therefore, children may feel more comfortable when a parent is present in the examining room. During calibration, a light bar is utilized with adult patients, and the patient is asked to look at targets appearing to the left and right of center gaze. Children's attention may be maximized if asked to focus on interesting cartoon characters that illuminate in place of the lights. Various oculomotor tests may also be performed using the light bar: measurement of saccades or rapid eye movements, optokinetic testing (following lights that induce the slow and then fast phase of nystagmic eye movements), and sinusoidal tracking that should result in smooth pursuit eye movements.

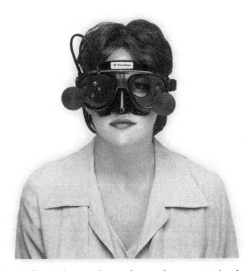

Fig. 4. Goggles utilized for video-oculography and computerized rotary chair testing. (*Courtesy of* Micromedical Technologies, Inc; with permission.)

With all of these oculomotor tests, interesting cartoon characters may replace the traditional light bar used with adults. Just as with audiometry, the clinician may wish to employ an assortment of novel stimuli (cartoon characters in this case) to regain attention, should habituation take place.

Measurement of spontaneous nystagmus, addressed in a previous section, may be more formally measured as an initial component of the VOG test battery. The child is asked to sit quietly as the clinician records eye movements while the child looks at a target and while vision is compromised (ie, in complete darkness). Nystagmus is not elicited in any way, and the audiologist exercises care in making certain that mental alerting measures appropriate for the individual child are carried out. Gaze nystagmus may also be measured with a light bar displaying interesting cartoons, or the clinician may ask the child to "look at the lightning bugs" if a traditional light bar is utilized. In this manner, it is feasible to measure gaze nystagmus in right, left, upward, and downward positions. Standard positioning and positional tests previously described also may be performed in the pediatric vestibular laboratory. The clinician may use discretion regarding expanding the test battery to include right and left lateral, as well as other positions. As with the office examination, it is important to check for the presence of nystagmus and to recognize subjective report of symptoms.

Adaptations of positioning and positional testing with children include establishing excellent rapport, having a parent present, and ensuring that the child is comfortable at all times. The clinician should be conscious of allaying fears at all times, especially if the testing session progresses within a darkened room. Hearing-impaired children may need special modifications, such as making certain hearing devices are in place and/or providing signs with written instructions when necessary. Children who communicate via sign language may be effectively tasked by asking them to sign stories or words to familiar children's songs.[11] The clinician may think of additional creative modifications that may be implemented with children demonstrating other types of disability. Bithermal caloric irrigation, considered a "gold standard" in evaluating the status of each ear independently, is arguably the most challenging to implement with a pediatric patient. In this author's experience, this section of the test battery may efficiently be performed by the developmental age of 5 to 6 years (although much variability exists among children). The clinician irrigates each ear with warm and cool water or air, stimulating the vestibular system and recording slow-phase eye movement velocity of each subsequent response. Small children may not tolerate this stimulating irrigation or lying still for several minutes as the post-irrigation nystagmic response is recorded and measured. Children may be fearful of the irrigation equipment and procedure, and also of becoming dizzy or experiencing the sensation of movement following stimulation. **Fig. 5** displays state-of-the art VOG equipment that may be easily adapted for children, including the goggles, light bar, and computerized recording equipment.

Adaptations are numerous, including selection of open loop water, closed loop water, or air irrigation systems. Some clinicians have experienced success with closed loop or air systems, whereas others have found that children enjoy a water and "bath-like" analogy. Many pediatric evaluative techniques approach a screening as opposed to thorough diagnostic evaluation, and this aspect may be no exception. The clinician, for example, may choose to perform 2 instead of 4 irrigations as success is achieved in obtaining some type of reliable measure for each ear. Although there may be equipment challenges in doing so, it also may be possible to perform bilateral simultaneous irrigations to diminish test time, number of irrigations, and negative post-irrigation patient response. Mental alerting during bithermal caloric irrigations is critical, through use of previously described pediatric techniques. It is also very important to calm fears

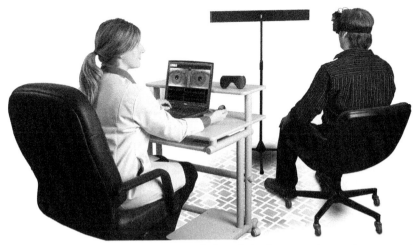

Fig. 5. Video-oculography equipment, including light bar, goggles, and computerized console for test performance and data analysis. (*Courtesy of* Micromedical Technologies, Inc; with permission.)

and to view the actual recording of the nystagmus, in addition to viewing computer calculations following each irrigation. **Fig. 6** demonstrates the image of an eye projected on a computer screen, so that the clinician may supplement computerized data analysis with subjective viewing of the eye movement recordings.

Along with advances in computerized technology, additional vestibular laboratory procedures have been developed for adults and can be adapted for use with children: computerized rotary chair (CRC), computerized dynamic posturography (CDP), and

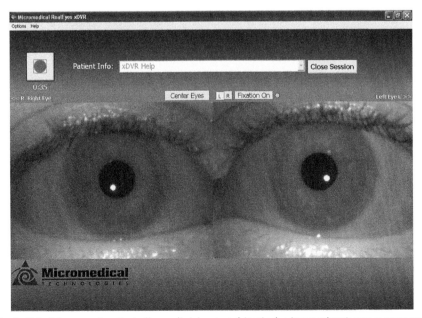

Fig. 6. Television monitor that allows clinician to subjectively view patient's eye movements. (*Courtesy of* Micromedical Technologies, Inc; with permission.)

vestibular evoked myogenic potentials (VEMPs). Adaptation of these techniques has been very valuable with children, especially in view of the challenges faced in performing aspects of the VOG test battery with very young children.

COMPUTERIZED ROTARY CHAIR (CRC)

Use of CRC serves to complement the vestibular evaluation battery with adult patients. Advantages of CRC include clarification of questionable VOG results and assessment of the VOR at multiple test frequencies. **Fig. 7** shows an example of currently available CRC equipment that may easily be adapted for patients across the life span.

Precursors to CRC testing with pediatric patients included evaluation of per-rotatory and post-rotatory nystagmus as part of the physical examination.[21,22] In evaluating the VOR resulting from rotational stimulation, it was common for the clinician to evaluate parameters such as frequency and amplitude of nystagmic beats, as well as duration of nystagmic activity. Cyr and colleagues[23,24] were among the first investigators to evaluate and clinically use CRC techniques with pediatric patients, in both pediatric and full-term infants. These investigators painted their darkened enclosure to resemble a spaceship, piped in familiar children's songs for mental alerting purposes, and seated the children on parents' laps. Techniques approached a screening, in that examiners successfully evaluated the VOR at 0.08 Hz. Staller and colleagues[25] also successfully performed CRC techniques with very young children, advocating the importance of testing sinusoidal harmonic acceleration (SHA) at more than one test frequency whenever possible; this is because the vestibular system is not linear, and varying responses may be noted at different test frequencies. In addition to obtaining computerized measurements following rotation, investigators have stressed the importance of viewing the VOR via infrared camera and TV monitor.

As demonstrated, SHA appears to be the most popular subtest performed with pediatric patients. In 2007, Valente[26] performed SHA at 0.08 Hz and 0.50 Hz with two age groups of typically developing children: pre-schoolers and pre-adolescents. In successfully evaluating children via previously mentioned modification of adult techniques, Valente also noted that most children readily adapt to "ride-like"

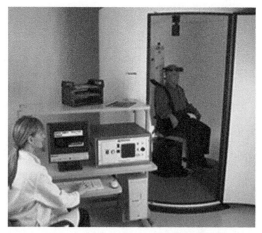

Fig. 7. Computerized rotary chair equipment that may be utilized across the life span: clinician begins to prepare patient for testing. (*Courtesy of* Micromedical Technologies, Inc; with permission.)

techniques. Appropriate mental alerting is implemented, and chair restraints may be either adapted or foregone for the smaller patient. It is important for the examiner to be in continual contact with the child via a talk-back system, and the door may be opened between subtests. As with adult patients, parameters of gain, phase, and symmetry of the resulting VOR may be accurately measured. Gain is a measure that refers to the reflex strength and may be defined as slow-phase eye velocity divided by chair (ie, head) velocity. The phase measure refers to timing of the response, specifically of head movement, as compared with compensatory eye movement. When phase is less than zero, eye velocity "lags" head velocity, and when phase is greater than zero, eye velocity "leads" head velocity.[27] Symmetry helps the examiner compare contribution of the right ear versus contribution of the left ear toward the total response. These primary measures must be reliable, which may present challenges with small children, and may also vary as a function of frequency. It is critical for the clinician and researcher to gather normative data as a function of age within their own facility.

Although Valente's study did not find significant differences in gain, phase, or symmetry measures between the two previously described groups of children, children's gain measures were significantly higher at 0.08 Hz and 0.5 Hz than adult normative data. She further reported successfully performing step velocity (SV) testing with pre-school and adolescent children. SV testing is an additional CRC subtest whereby the patient is rotated in one direction at approximately 100° per second. The clinician observes and records the building of nystagmic activity while the chair accelerates toward a constant velocity, at which time the nystagmus begins to fade. This per-rotatory nystagmus, which beats in the same direction as rotation (eg, right beating nystagmus during clockwise rotation), may be measured via either clockwise or counterclockwise rotation directions, with vestibular time constants (in seconds) measured for each rotation. A vestibular time constant is defined as the amount of time necessary for the per-rotatory nystagmus response to diminish to 37% of its original intensity. The time constant is compared with normative data to assist with differential diagnosis.[27] On sudden stopping of the chair, post-rotatory nystagmus will occur, which beats in the direction opposite to the stimulating rotation (eg, left beating nystagmus following clockwise rotation). A post-rotation vestibular time constant may also be measured as the nystagmus begins to diminish, and is also defined as the amount of time required for the nystagmus to diminish to 37% of its original strength. Although SV testing may be performed efficiently on many young children, it is important to be certain of adequate head restraint so that the most reliable measures possible can be obtained.

Cyr and colleagues[20,24] demonstrated the efficacy of performing optokinetic testing with children, using CRC enclosures. Children tend to automatically follow lights or stripes, and the enclosure allows the clinician to fill the visual field with eliciting stimuli so that visual fixation does not interfere with test findings. The clinician may also adequately assess visual fixation skills through use of CRC equipment and accompanying stimuli.

CRC involves numerous other subtests, such as assessment of visual vestibular interactions (VVOR and VFX) and dynamic subjective visual vertical (SVV) testing. With the former, the patient views stripes or a single visual target projected on the enclosure wall as the chair rotates. The patient tracks these stimuli through integration of the VOR and the visual pursuit systems. With the latter, patients adjust a luminous line in darkness to indicate their perception of an upright earth-vertical position. Deviations from true earth-vertical are measured in degrees, and individuals with otolith injury may show alteration in judgment of vertical positioning. Although CRC and other vestibular evaluation measures have gained popularity with children, especially before and after cochlear implantation,[28–30] much research and clinical work are still needed regarding the performance of all subtests with pediatric populations.

In summary, with some adaptation of adult techniques, CRC may serve as a highly successful assessment tool to use with children, particularly important when caloric irrigations may not be tolerated by the child. Main adaptations include a more "child-friendly" enclosure, asking the child to be seated on a parent's lap, and making certain that mental alerting techniques are appropriate for a pediatric patient. The test may serve as more of a screening than a diagnostic evaluation, particularly if the entire frequency range cannot be tested because of limited attention span. If a limited frequency range is implemented, it is important to represent low-, medium-, and high-frequency ranges whenever possible. As the clinician evaluates computerized measurements, it is also critical to view the actual nystagmic activity projected on the video monitor. The major protocols of CRC testing (SHA, SV, visual vestibular interactions, and SVV) may be successfully performed with many children, especially if appropriate head restraints are implemented. More research is needed regarding test-retest reliability and obtaining the most accurate possible measures. Obtaining additional normative data for children is crucial, as are additional studies regarding differential diagnosis and anticipated findings with various disorders and syndromes (see article by McCaslin and colleagues in this publication).

COMPUTERIZED DYNAMIC POSTUROGRAPHY

CDP has been clinically useful over recent years in assessing functional balance and relative contributions of visual, proprioceptive, and vestibular cues. The patient is asked to stand on a platform with safety harnesses in place and faces a visual surround. Sensors within the platform plate measure the force exerted by the feet on displacement of the patient's center of gravity.[31] CDP equipment is shown in **Fig. 8.**

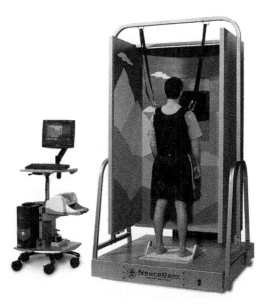

Fig. 8. NeuroCom Balance Manager System utilized for computerized dynamic posturography. (*Courtesy of* NeuroCom International, Inc; with permission.)

Perhaps the most commonly implemented subtest is the sensory organization test (SOT). This test is composed of 6 conditions that become progressively more difficult, whereby the patient must maintain the best balance possible despite compromising visual and/or proprioceptive cues. There are 3 trials of each condition for reliability purposes; although equipment and protocols may vary, each trial lasts approximately 20 seconds. Scores are reported out of a maximum score of 100, which would indicate perfect balance and absence of sway. In addition to scores reported for each condition, there is also a composite score that represents all scores, with heavier weighting on those conditions that rely more heavily on the use of vestibular cues alone. A description of the 6 SOT conditions is tabulated as follows:

	Platform	Visual Surround
Condition 1	Stable	Stable—eyes open
Condition 2	Stable	Stable—eyes closed
Condition 3	Stable	Sway-referenced—eyes open
Condition 4	Sway-referenced	Stable—eyes open
Condition 5	Sway-referenced	Stable—eyes closed
Condition 6	Sway-referenced	Sway-referenced—eyes open

In 1996, DiFabio and Foudriat[32] reported that a child as young as 3 years may be tested using CDP techniques, although performance increases as the child ages. Hirabayashi and Iwasaki[33] conducted a CDP study with a large number of children, reporting that the proprioceptive system matures by approximately 4 years of age and the visual system by 15 years of age. These investigators believed that the vestibular system is the last to mature and that many children have not reached maturity by 15 years. Shimizu and colleagues[34] found that CDP performance varied greatly between pediatric and adult populations when studying the performance of children aged 6 through 13 years. Cyr and colleagues[20,24] felt that CDP should be performed with children when parents report a history of imbalance, "clumsiness," neurologic impairment, or suspected organic disease. More recently, Rine and colleagues[35,36] performed SOT measures on children from 3 through 7 years of age. These investigators concluded that CDP testing provides useful measures of all systems involved and important information related to their maturation. In 2007, Valente[26] compared SOT findings with preschool and pre-adolescent children, with further comparisons of pediatric findings to adult normative data. Of importance, she reported that younger children performed significantly poorer than older children on all 6 conditions. Further, both age groups of children performed significantly poorer on all SOT conditions than adults. These points reiterate that pediatric results should be compared with pediatric normative data, that one should obtain normative data in one's own clinic for all measures, and that special adaptations should be made for testing children.

When performing CDP with pediatric patients, the smallest harness may be utilized for safety. With all subjects, height and weight should be ascertained to ensure proper platform and sensor calibration, as well as to ensure accuracy of measures. The clinician should consult the manufacturer's equipment manual to determine the smallest weight recommended for proper measurement. As with any pediatric assessment tool, the clinician should establish excellent rapport and calm fears, although many children feel that CDP is "ride-like." Parents may be present, and positive reinforcement appropriate for the individual child is always in order. As the child faces the visual surround, the clinician may consider arranging a more interesting or "child-friendly" visual stimulus. For example, the visual surround could display interesting cartoon characters, a nursery rhyme, or other familiar landscape, or even photos of the child. The creative clinician may also devise other means to maintain attention, such as an interesting video or video game. Three trials of the 6 SOT conditions may tax the attention span of a small child, even though each trial is a mere 20 seconds in length. At the risk of compromising reliability, the examiner may forego all 3 trials; future research may explore validity of results if the clinician were to forego earlier conditions and only test more difficult conditions when fatigue is present.

The motor control test (MCT) is a second CDP subtest whereby the platform experiences unexpected perturbations—small, medium, and large in degree—in both forward and backward directions. Latencies in milliseconds are measured from the start of the platform translation to the force exerted by the feet as the patient attempts to maintain balance.[31] As previously mentioned, perturbations are proportional to the height of the patient and so are smaller with a child than with an adult. This test is quick and efficient to use with children, although some children may fear the unexpected platform movement. Valente[26] found that pediatric results are comparable to those obtained with adults, although there is a need for additional pediatric normative data. With both SOT and MCT, a learning curve may be seen from trial to trial.

A third subtest of CDP is the adaptation test, whereby the platform also moves unexpectedly as the toes progress from facing forward to an upward ("toes up") position and from facing forward to a downward ("toes down") position. The patient's ability to regain balance on such disruption is measured, along with how well the patient adapts to change from trial to trial. There is a paucity of both clinical and research work related to the adaptation test in children.

As an additional adaptation of adult techniques for children, it may be helpful for children to receive a sticker or other tangible reward following completion of each subtest trial. CDP provides much valuable information for the clinician, in addition to the subtest scores, and much of this information is unexplored with children. For example, there are strategy scores that provide helpful information about correct utilization of ankle, hip, and step strategies for maintaining balance. Information may be gained regarding how well a patient integrates visual, vestibular, and proprioceptive cues and whether there is an overdependence on one modality. There are measures that help determine if a patient is equally distributing weight on the right and left sides of the body. Although remediation is beyond the scope of this article, it is clear that this wealth of information may provide great benefit in cases when remediation is in order. Directions for future research are many, including development of equipment and test procedures for younger and younger children. Investigations regarding anticipated results with various childhood disorders and syndromes would be a welcome addition to the body of literature. Further adaptations of techniques for use with children and further establishment of pediatric normative data for all aspects of all subtests are also in order.

VESTIBULAR EVOKED MYOGENIC POTENTIALS

VEMPs have gained much popularity over the past few decades, as their use has transitioned from animal to human studies and then toward clinical vestibular evaluation. VEMPs are quick and efficient to perform and are objective to interpret. Their debut within the vestibular evaluation arena was a welcome one, in that most existing vestibular test procedures focus on function of the horizontal semicircular canals. Clinicians have had few assessment tools at their disposal with which to measure the function of otolithic structures, the utricle and the saccule. Via evidence-based principles, investigators[37,38] pinpointed that these auditory stimulus-driven evoked potentials arise from the saccule; some subjects with severe to profound sensorineural hearing loss demonstrate normal VEMP tracings. To the contrary, some patients with normal hearing sensitivity and disorder of the inferior branch of the vestibular nerve have abnormal or absent VEMP tracings. Although VEMP tracings have been measured from many parts of the body, eliciting the cervical VEMP (cVEMP) involves placement of electrodes in the following manner: ground on the forehead, noninverting electrodes on each contracted sternocleidomastoid muscle (SCM), and inverting electrodes on each sternum or sternoclavicular juncture. **Fig. 9** demonstrates standard electrode placement for cVEMP testing, in this case with a 4-year-old child.

Standard auditory brainstem response (ABR) equipment may be adapted for elicitation of VEMPs using insert earphones.[39] When the auditory stimulus is presented in an air-conducted fashion, the afferent auditory pathway involves stimulation of the saccule, eighth nerve, and vestibular nuclei.[40] Efferent pathways travel to motoneurons of the neck muscles, including those of the SCM. Current VEMP elicitation techniques were originally described by Colebatch and colleagues,[41] and current research involves enhancing the clinician's test administration and interpretation. Several techniques to maintain adequate SCM contraction may can be utilized. One such method is for the patient to turn the heads to the right or left to elicit muscle contraction while remaining in a seated position. Some examiners may have the patient gently push the head against an object to create resistance so that the SCM may be optimally contracted. Other examiners may ask patients to lie in a supine position and raise their heads to contract the SCM in either a chin-to-chest position or head turned to right or left position.

The actual VEMP tracing may be observed via a 2-channel recording, often depicting a 25-millisecond pre-stimulus baseline of raw electromyographic (EMG) activity followed by a tracing that highlights a positive peak (P1) and a negative peak (N1). A VEMP tracing obtained on a 6-year-old patient is shown in **Fig. 10**.

Interpreting the VEMP, the audiologist first observes wave morphology to ensure that the waveform displays the proper pattern and that waves P1 and N1 are easily discernible. The audiologist compares the patient's P1 and N1 latencies in milliseconds to clinic-specific normative data for that particular age group. Research has

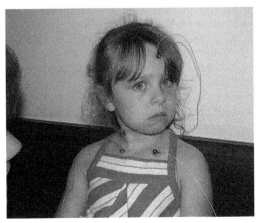

Fig. 9. Electrode placement for vestibular evoked myogenic potential testing.

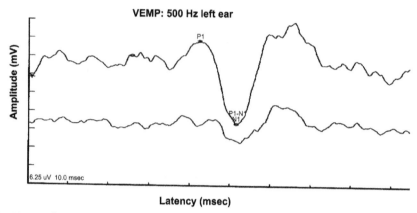

Fig. 10. Vestibular evoked myogenic potential tracing obtained with a 6-year-old patient.

shown that there is a relationship between auditory tone-burst stimulus frequency and latency of P1 and N1 waveforms.[39] That is, higher frequency stimuli typically elicit waveforms with earlier latencies, whereas lower frequency stimuli may elicit waveforms that display later latencies. Another important parameter to use in VEMP interpretation is the P1-N1 amplitude, labeled in microvolts and described as the distance from the height of P1 to the depth of N1. This parameter has proved to be challenging to measure and interpret for two major reasons. First, the P1-N1 amplitude is directly related to the tonic level of neck contraction and this may vary from patient to patient. Second, this amplitude measure is also positively correlated with the intensity level of the acoustic stimulus.

Investigators have reported important ways to control for variability, including incorporating additional electrodes and computer software so that the patient may monitor neck contraction levels to meet specific visual targets displayed on a computer screen.[39] Clinicians may also calculate a normalized amplitude measure, dividing raw amplitude by the average amplitude of pre-stimulus EMG baseline activity. With regard to the amplitude measure, some clinicians calculate an asymmetry ratio, defined as the difference between amplitudes of unaffected and affected sides divided by the amplitude sum of both sides. Via these calculations, a smaller number indicates greater symmetry while a larger number indicates greater asymmetry. Each laboratory has difference levels that are felt to be significant, and many clinics consider this difference to be 30% to 40% or greater. Minor and colleagues[42] have also reported great clinical utility in the VEMP threshold measure, especially in diagnosing superior canal dehiscence (SCD) (see article by Hegemann and Carey in this publication). This threshold measure is generally defined as the lowest level of auditory intensity that elicits a discernible VEMP tracing. In cases of SCD, the VEMP threshold on the affected side is much lower than that for the unaffected side. Again, a large asymmetry in thresholds between the ears would be noted.

The efficiency and objectivity of VEMP testing facilitate its use with pediatric patients. In 2005, Sheykholeslami and colleagues[43] studied a group of typically developing neonates and a group of neonates exhibiting "clinical findings." These investigators reported that VEMP tracings, readily obtained with this population, demonstrated morphology similar to that of adults; they noted shorter latencies of the N1 peak, and greater amplitude variability with children as compared with adults. In 2006, Kelsch and colleagues[44] concurred that VEMP testing is easily accomplished with children from ages 3 through 11 years, and found shorter initial peak latencies than those occurring with adults. Valente[26] studied samples of preschool and adolescent children in 2007, finding shorter P1 and N1 latencies with children as compared to adult subjects. Valente readily measured VEMPs in children with the use of 500-Hz tone-burst and click stimuli, and suggested that VEMP testing in children may also approach a screening rather than diagnostic assessment. Further, she reported that testing with both stimuli may prove redundant if children have a very limited attention span, although it is always crucial to replicate each waveform. Her most robust waveforms were obtained through use of lower-frequency tone-burst stimuli.

As adult techniques are modified for children, the clinician may find that pediatric patients do not view VEMP testing as "fun" or "ride-like" as with other vestibular evaluation measures already discussed. The clinician may refer to electrodes as "stickers," promising a "prettier and more fun" sticker on completion of the test. This author has attempted to use EMG-monitoring software with young children to ensure adequate SCM contraction, finding challenges related to the need to place multiple electrodes on a small neck and finding some electrodes to be very heavy and cumbersome. EMG-monitoring software is being developed for use with children, and one may creatively devise avenues for maintaining attention and helping children maintain adequate SCM contraction using child-friendly computer screen visual targets. The child may be seated on a parent's lap for testing and will require much positive reinforcement as with other test techniques. It may be beneficial for the child to turn the head 90° to contract the SCM and focus on a wall-mounted sticker or cartoon character. The parent may also provide hand, shoulder, and upper body resistance in order to steady the child and help create resistance during data collection. Pediatric insert earphones are readily available for presentation of acoustic stimuli, and most children readily adapt to these transducers. Although protocols vary, some examiners present 128 stimulus sweeps for obtaining a VEMP tracing; many find that interpretable tracings are obtained following 64 stimulus sweeps, and this adaptation may be advantageous when testing children. In the event of limited time and attention span, the clinician may also choose to obtain bilateral tracings as opposed to testing in a monaural fashion.

SUMMARY

Adult vestibular techniques may be adapted for children, and many children should undergo vestibular evaluation. The audiologist may be only one member of the team, with other members including the otolaryngologist, neurologist, psychologist, pediatrician educators, physical therapist, parents, and others. The audiologist bears in mind that the scope of practice is very broad and that other evaluative measures may be performed with a particular child: thorough audiologic evaluation, electrophysiologic measures, hearing aid evaluation, cochlear implant assessments, and various (re)habilitative strategies.

There are many pre-evaluation measures that the physician and the audiologist may obtain before performing more formal assessment. Examples include gait and balance screenings, observation of spontaneous nystagmus and gaze-evoked nystagmus, oculomotor testing, HTT, and others. With creativity and warm interpersonal skills, these measures may easily be performed with many pediatric patients. Video-oculography (VOG) has been performed successfully with adults and older children for many years, and this equipment is readily available in most clinics. Adaptations have been described, such as substitution of cartoon characters for lights when performing oculomotor testing. Challenges presented when attempting to perform VOG with children include positional testing and especially the successful performance of bithermal caloric irrigations. Newer technologies, such as those involved with development of CRC and CDP, may be more easily adapted for vestibular evaluation in pediatric patients. Adaptation of adult techniques, such as child-friendly mental alerting measures with CRC testing and a more child-friendly visual surround with CDP testing, have been highly successful. Finally, VEMPs commonly performed with adult patients may successfully be obtained with children, applying adaptations such as seating the child on a parent's lap, maintaining head and body position via parental support, and focusing on child-friendly cartoon characters.

It is important to adapt adult techniques for use with young children, as well as to obtain pediatric normative data. It is imperative that results obtained following the evaluation of a child not be compared with adult normative data. Future areas of research are many. Studies regarding anticipated findings with various CRC and CDP subtests are needed, especially as related to differential diagnosis with children. CDP appears to provide the clinician with much useful information that may be applied toward rehabilitation. Additional studies will explore best rehabilitative practice with pediatric patients, with additional collaboration of all team members involved in diagnostic and treatment processes. Additional VEMP studies will explore optimal stimulus and recording parameters for air-conducted and bone-conducted stimulus presentation, types of tracings obtained via presentation of various auditory stimuli, and expected results with various disorders and syndromes. More adequate monitoring procedures of EMG activity and neck contraction are recommended, as well as investigations related to measuring the VEMP from alternative anatomic sites. Through additional data gathering, clinicians will gain greater understanding of which children should be tested and referred for treatment, as well as optimum evaluation and rehabilitation strategies and techniques. As with hearing impairment, the earlier a pediatric vestibular disorder is identified, the earlier remediation can be initiated.

ACKNOWLEDGMENTS

The author thanks the editors for the invitation to participate and for their very helpful suggestions, which serve to strengthen this article. She would like to thank Joel Goebel MD, Medical Director of the Dizziness and Balance Center, Department of Otolaryngology at Washington University School of Medicine in St Louis. Dr Goebel's ongoing support, sharing of resources, and imparting of vast knowledge, as well as that of Belinda Sinks AuD, are most appreciated. The author is very grateful to Ms René Miller and to Ms Ava Miller for creating photo opportunities that serve to enhance the written text of this article.

REFERENCES

1. Ayers AJ. Learning disabilities and the vestibular system. J Learn Disabil 1978; 11(1):18–29.
2. Ottenbacher K, Watson PJ, Short MA. Association between nystagmus hyporesponsivity and behavioral problems in learning-disabled children. Am J Occup Ther 1979;33(5):317–22.
3. Ottenbacher K. Excessive postrotary nystagmus duration in learning-disabled children. Am J Occup Ther 1980;34(1):40–4.
4. Polatajko HJ. A critical look at vestibular dysfunction in learning-disabled children. Dev Med Child Neurol 1985;27:283–92.

5. Shumway-Cook A, Horak F, Black FO. A critical examination of vestibular function in motor-impaired learning-disabled children. Int J Pediatr Otorhinolaryngol 1987; 14:21–30.
6. Horak FB, Shumway-Cook A, Crowe TK, et al. Vestibular function and motor proficiency of children with impaired hearing, or with learning disability and motor impairments. Dev Med Child Neurol 1988;30:64–79.
7. Crowe TK, Horak FB. Motor proficiency associated with vestibular deficits in children with hearing impairments. Phys Ther 1988;68(10):1493–9.
8. Casslebrandt ML, Furman JM, Mandel EM, et al. Past history of otitis media and balance in four-year-old children. Laryngoscope 2000;110:773–8.
9. Mira E, Piacentino G, Lanzi G, et al. Benign paroxysmal vertigo in childhood. Acta Otolaryngol Suppl 1984;406:271–4.
10. Mira E, Piacentino G, Lanzi G, et al. Benign paroxysmal vertigo in childhood: a migraine equivalent. ORL J Otorhinolaryngol Relat Spec 1984;46(20):97–104.
11. Brookhouser PE, Cyr DB, Beauchaine KA. Vestibular findings in the deaf and hard of hearing. Otolaryngol Head Neck Surg 1982;90:773–7.
12. Cyr DG, Brookhouser PE, Beauchaine KA. Language and learning skills of hearing-impaired children: vestibular evaluation. ASHA Monogr 1986;23:21–3.
13. Huygen PL, van Rijn PM, Cremers CW, et al. The vestibulo-ocular reflex in pupils at a Dutch school for the hearing-impaired: findings related to acquired causes. Int J Pediatr Otorhinolaryngol 1993;25:39–47.
14. Wiener-Vacher SR, Amanou L, Denise P, et al. Vestibular function in children with the CHARGE association. Arch Otolaryngol Head Neck Surg 1999;125:342–7.
15. Ndiaye IC, Rassi SJ, Wiener-Vacher SR. Cochleovestibular impairment in pediatric Cogan's syndrome. Pediatrics 2002;109(2):1–7.
16. Fishman GA, Kumar A, Joseph ME, et al. Usher's syndrome: ophthalmic and neuro-otologic findings suggesting genetic heterogeneity. Arch Ophthalmol 1983;101:1367–74.
17. Fife TD, Tusa RJ, Furman JM, et al. Assessment: vestibular testing techniques in adults and children. Neurology 2000;55:1431–41.
18. Desmond A. Vestibular function: evaluation and treatment. New York: Thieme Medical Publishers; 2004. p. 52–9.
19. McFeely WJ, Bojrab DI. Performing the physical exam: posture and gait tests. In: Goebel JA, editor. Practical management of the dizzy patient. Philadelphia: Lippincott, Williams and Wilkins; 2001. p. 107–11.
20. Cyr DG. The vestibular system: pediatric considerations. Sem Hear 1983;4(1):33–45.
21. Eviatar L, Eviatar A. Neurovestibular examination of infants and children. Adv Otorhinolaryngol 1978;23:169–91.
22. Eviatar L, Eviatar A. The normal nystagmic response of infants to caloric and perrotatory stimulation. Laryngoscope 1979;89:1036–45.
23. Cyr DG. Vestibular testing in children. Ann Otol Rhinol Laryngol 1980;89:63–9.
24. Cyr DG, Brookhouser PE, Valente M, et al. Vestibular evaluation of infants and preschool children. Otolaryngol Head Neck Surg 1985;93(4):463–8.
25. Staller SJ, Goin DW, Hildebrandt M. Pediatric vestibular evaluation with harmonic acceleration. Otolaryngol Head Neck Surg 1986;95(4):471–6.
26. Valente LM. Maturational effects of the vestibular system: a study of rotary chair, computerized dynamic posturography, and vestibular evoked potentials with children. J Am Acad Audiol 2007;18(6):461–81.
27. Goebel JA, Hanson JM. Vestibular physiology. In: Hughes GB, Pensak ML, editors. Clinical otology. 2nd edition. New York: Thieme Medical Publishers; 1997. p. 43–52.

28. Licamelli G, Zhou G, Kenna MA. Disturbance of vestibular function attributable to cochlear implantation in children. Laryngoscope 2009;119(4):740–5.

29. Cushy SL, Papsin BC, Rutka JA, et al. Vestibular end organ and balance deficits after meningitis and cochlear implantation with children. Otol Neurotol 2009;30: 488–95.

30. Jacot E, Van Den Abbele T, Debri HR, et al. Vestibular impairment pre- and post-cochlear implant. Int J Pediatr Otorhinolaryngol 2010;74(1):105.

31. Nashner LM. Computerized dynamic posturography. In: Goebel JA, editor. Practical management of the dizzy patient. Philadelphia: Lippincott, Williams and Wilkins; 2001. p. 143–70.

32. DiFabio RP, Foudriat BA. Responsiveness and reliability of a pediatric strategy score for balance. Physiother Res Int 1996;1(3):180–94.

33. Hirabayashi S, Iwasaki Y. Developmental perspective of sensory organization on postural control. Brain Dev 1995;17(2):111–3.

34. Shimizu K, Asai M, Takata S, et al. The development of equilibrium function in childhood. In: Taguchi K, Igarashi M, Mori S, editors. Vestibular and neural front. New York: Elsevier Science BV; 1994. p. 183–6.

35. Rine RM, Rubish K, Feeney C. Measurement of sensory system effectiveness and maturational changes in postural control in young children. Pediatr Phys Ther 1998;10:16–22.

36. Rine RM, Cornwall G, Gan K, et al. Evidence of progressive delay of motor development in children with sensorineural hearing loss and concurrent vestibular dysfunction. Percept Mot Skills 2000;90:1101–12.

37. Halmagyi GM, Colebatch JG. Vestibular evoked myogenic potentials in the sternocleidomastoid muscle are not of lateral canal origin. Acta Otolaryngol Suppl 1995;520(1):1–3.

38. Murofishi T, Halmagyi GM, Yavor RA, et al. Absent vestibular evoked myogenic potentials in vestibular neurolabyrinthitis: an indicator of vestibular nerve involvement? Arch Otolaryngol Head Neck Surg 1996;122(8):845–8.

39. Akin FW, Murnane OD. Vestibular evoked myogenic potentials: preliminary report. J Am Acad Audiol 2001;12(9):445–52.

40. Halmagyi GM, Curthoys LS. Otolith function tests. In: Herdman SJ, editor. Vestibular rehabilitation. Philadelphia: FA David; 2000. p. 196–214.

41. Colebatch JG, Halmagyi GM, Skuse NF. Myogenic potentials generated by click-evoked vestibulocollic reflex. J Neurol Neurosurg Psychiatry 1994;57(2):190–7.

42. Minor LB, Cremer PD, Carey JP, et al. Symptoms and signs in superior canal dehiscence syndrome. Ann N Y Acad Sci 2001;942:445–52.

43. Sheykholeslami K, Megerian CA, Arnold JE, et al. Vestibular evoked myogenic potentials in infancy and early childhood. Laryngoscope 2005;115(8):1440–4.

44. Kelsch TA, Schaefer LA, Esquivel CR. Vestibular evoked myogenic potentials in young children: test parameters and normative data. Laryngoscope 2006; 116(6):895–900.

The Predominant Forms of Vertigo in Children and Their Associated Findings on Balance Function Testing

Devin L. McCaslin, PhD*, Gary P. Jacobson, PhD,
Jill M. Gruenwald, AuD

KEYWORDS
- Benign paroxysmal vertigo of childhood
- Migraine-associated vertigo • Electronystagmography
- Trauma • Vestibular neuritis • Otitis media
- Auditory neuropathy • Vestibular

There are many disorders that can cause dizziness in the pediatric population.[1–5] In 1999, Russell and Abu-Arafeh[6] published an epidemiologic study showing that 15% of school-age children had experienced at least one episode of vertigo in the previous year. Numerous investigators have also reported the most common disorders causing vertigo and imbalance in children in their clinics.[5–9] Even though these reports originate from different clinics and regions of the world, there is surprisingly good agreement regarding the primary causes of dizziness in the pediatric population. Regardless of this fact, children suffering from vertigo and imbalance have received less attention in the literature than their adult counterparts, most likely due to the difficulty that young children have in describing their symptoms, coupled with the challenges that exist for clinicians who work through the differential diagnostic process with children. Despite these limitations, it is now known that the most common disorders that cause dizziness in children may manifest themselves as abnormalities on quantitative balance function testing (ie, rotational testing, electronystagmography [ENG], and vestibular evoked myogenic potential testing). The purpose of this brief report is to describe techniques for determining which children may benefit from

Division of Audiology, Department of Hearing and Speech Sciences, Vanderbilt Bill Wilkerson Center, Hearing and Speech Sciences, Vanderbilt University Medical Center, 1215 21st Avenue South - MCE Suite 9302, Nashville, TN 37232-8025, USA
* Corresponding author.
E-mail address: devin.mccaslin@vanderbilt.edu

Otolaryngol Clin N Am 44 (2011) 291–307
doi:10.1016/j.otc.2011.01.003
0030-6665/11/$ – see front matter © 2011 Elsevier Inc. All rights reserved.

quantitative balance function testing and what the reported findings are for the 5 most common disorders accounting for vertigo and imbalance in children.

BACKGROUND: CHILDREN WITH VERTIGO

Assessment of the vestibular system in the pediatric population is gaining interest for several reasons. First, determining the integrity of the vestibular system can assist physicians in the diagnosis of the impairment and in defining the most appropriate course of treatment. Second, some children with dizziness/vertigo have serious health problems, and vestibular system assessment can help identify patients whose dizziness/vertigo stems from a significant neurologic impairment (eg, a brain tumor). However, unlike in adults, episodic vertigo occurs rarely in children. Further, dizziness in children can manifest itself in many forms.[10] For example, a child with an acute vestibular system impairment may present with many of the same symptoms as adults (eg, vomiting, nystagmus, hearing loss, or ataxia). As with adults, children with vestibular disorders may also present with a loss of vestibular function that is progressive or chronic, thereby affecting the development of postural control.[11] Identifying whether the pediatric dizziness is of vestibular origin requires a team approach beginning with an assessment by a physician. During this initial visit a detailed case history should be obtained along with a comprehensive neurologic and otologic examination. Following these examinations, if neurologic impairments can be excluded, quantitative balance function testing may help identify both peripheral and central vestibular system impairments.

Although dizziness and vertigo do occur in children, few dizziness clinics have expressed an interest in this population. One explanation for this is the challenge of extracting clinical and laboratory information from children. According to Wiener-Vacher,[8] children often cannot report vertiginous symptoms due to their inability to verbalize any abnormal sensations they are experiencing. Vestibular disorders in young children often are dismissed by professionals and caregivers alike, and the symptoms are consequently attributed to behavioral problems (eg, finding ways to attract attention) or simply being "clumsy." In addition, diseases that affect the vestibular system in adults have a different prevalence than the pediatric population. For example, benign paroxysmal positional vertigo (BPPV) is quoted as the most common form of vertigo in adults.[12–14] Its prevalence has been estimated at 2.4% in the general adult population.[15] In children, BPPV has been reported to occur in up to 6% of those presenting with symptoms of dizziness.[9,16,17] This finding means the provider must approach the diagnosis of childhood dizziness/vertigo with a very different background of knowledge. Finally, while there continues to be interest in the development of techniques for assessing the vestibular system in adults, the same energy has not been devoted to adapting these techniques for application to children. One of the pioneers in the assessment of vestibular function in the pediatric population was Dr David Cyr of the Boys Town Institute. Much of his work in the 1980s focused on adapting existing adult protocols for use in children.[18,19] Many of these adaptations are still in use today. While interest in the assessment of the vestibular system in children has led manufacturers to develop both age-adjusted pupil tracking algorithms and age-appropriate visual targets, the majority of manufacturers at the time of this report do not offer videonystagmography goggles that are small and lightweight enough to accommodate small children. Having equipment that allows for the accurate assessment of children is critical because many of the disorders causing dizziness and vertigo in children have a vestibular origin. While the clinical utility of quantitative balance function testing in children is well documented, continued research in and development of balance assessment techniques will further our understanding of pediatric dizziness/vertigo.

DIFFERENTIAL DIAGNOSIS

The medical diagnosis of the patient with vestibular dysfunction is the responsibility of the otolaryngologist, otologist, neurotologist, or otoneurologist. The differential diagnostic process is more complex in children than adults, due to several reasons. First, symptoms of dizziness can manifest differently in children than in adults. Also, young children have limited verbal skills, and often the clinician must rely on the caregiver's observations for the case history. Accordingly, determining which pediatric patients should receive vestibular testing can be difficult. In this regard, several investigators have designed structured case histories to be used for the evaluation of children reporting dizziness.[7,20–22] One example set forth by Ravid and colleagues[21] consists of a set of structured questions (**Fig. 1**; also in the Appendix of this issue) coupled with a computer algorithm designed to aid in the differential diagnosis of the dizzy child (**Fig. 2**).

To validate the effectiveness of the questionnaire, Ravid and colleagues[21] performed a retrospective analysis of data collected from all children presenting with dizziness to their clinic over a 2-year period. The structured questionnaire was pitted against the computer algorithm and both of those against the final diagnosis. A total of 62 medical records were reviewed and in 57 (92%) of the patients, the questionnaire-derived diagnoses matched the medical record diagnoses. For 52 patients (84%) the result of the computer-assisted algorithm was identical to the diagnosis given to the patient as stated in the medical record. In a similar vein,

Nature of Symptoms

Vertigo	☐ Yes	☐ No	Dizziness	☐ Yes	☐ No
Acute	☐ Yes	☐ No	Chronic	☐ Yes	☐ No
Paroxysmal	☐ Yes	☐ No	Continuous	☐ Yes	☐ No
Hearing loss	☐ Yes	☐ No			
Age, years	☐ >5	☐ ≤5			
Change of symptoms with head position	☐ Yes	☐ No			

Associated symptoms

Headache	☐ Yes	☐ No
Fever	☐ Yes	☐ No
Vomiting	☐ Yes	☐ No
Anxiety	☐ Yes	☐ No
Depression	☐ Yes	☐ No
Change in consciousness	☐ Yes	☐ No
Head trauma	☐ Yes	☐ No
Drugs	☐ Yes	☐ No

Family medical history

Hearing loss	☐ Yes	☐ No
Migraine	☐ Yes	☐ No
Seizures	☐ Yes	☐ No
Neurologic examination	☐ Normal	☐ Abnormal
Physical examination	☐ Normal	☐ Abnormal

Fig. 1. A structured questionnaire for differential diagnosis in children presented by Ravid and colleagues (2003). (*From* Ravid S, Bienkowski R, Eviatar L. A simplified diagnostic approach to dizziness in children. Pediatr Neurol 2003;29:318; with permission.)

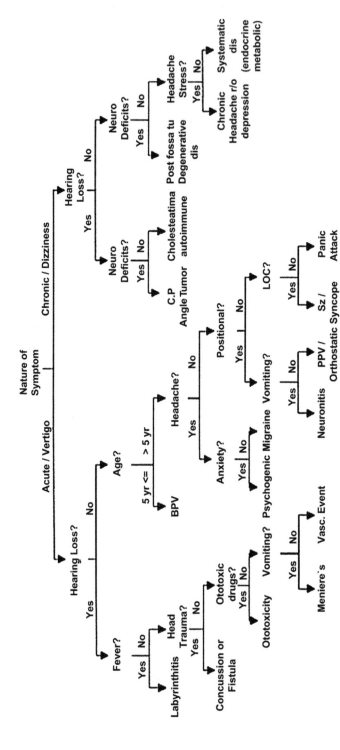

Fig. 2. A computer algorithm for differential diagnosis of dizziness in children as presented by Ravid, Bienkowski, and Eviatar (2003). PPV, paroxysmal positional vertigo; r/o, rule out, C-P, cerebellopontine; dis, disease; Vasc, vascular; LOC, loss of consciousness. (*From* Ravid S, Bienkowski R, Eviatar L. A simplified diagnostic approach to dizziness in children. Pediatr Neurol 2003;29:318; with permission.)

Niemensivu and colleagues[22] evaluated a structured case history for the diagnosis of dizzy children. Included in the sample were 24 vertiginous children with a history of episodic vertigo of unknown etiology. These children were age-matched and gender-matched, and underwent an otoneurologic examination, audiometry, and ENG. The most common disorders identified using this approach were otitis media–related vertigo, migraine-associated dizziness (MAD), and benign paroxysmal vertigo of childhood (BPVC).

In the authors' experience, using a structured case history coupled with a decision tree has worked well in identifying those patients who will benefit from vestibular testing. For instance, if the algorithm suggests the patient may have labyrinthitis, then quantitative testing can be ordered to determine whether the child has a peripheral impairment, whether it is unilateral or bilateral, if unilateral, how severe, and whether the child is compensating centrally for the impairment. Conversely, if a child presents with chronic dizziness, no hearing loss, and specific neurologic deficits, balance function testing would most likely not be indicated, and other issues would need to be ruled out (eg, degenerative disease or posterior fossa tumor) using different techniques (ie, imaging). This information is useful to both the physician and the pediatric physical therapist for prescribing treatment. This approach also streamlines the differential diagnostic process, and affords the physician the ability to be selective in determining which tests will be beneficial to the diagnosis and which will not.

THE MOST COMMON DISORDERS

Migraine headache, BPVC, and otitis media are commonly reported in the literature as associated with dizziness/vertigo in children. Trauma and vestibular neuritis also are cited as common causes of dizziness in children. Of note, all of these disorders can result in patients having abnormal findings on balance function testing. This fact reinforces the importance of having vestibular testing adapted for use with children, as well as pediatric normative response data available in the vestibular clinic. Two recent studies illustrate this argument well. First, a recent report by Szirmai[5] evaluated vestibular function in children (ie, younger than age 14 years, N = 66) and adolescents (ie, age 14–18 years, N = 79). Szirmai reported that migrainous vertigo (MV) was the most common disorder causing dizziness in the younger children, followed by extravestibular disease, and then labyrinthitis. Only 36% of the patients in this cohort demonstrated normal vestibular system function. In the group of adolescents, extravestibular disease was the most common cause of vertigo followed by migraine. Only 39% of the adolescents demonstrated normal vestibular results.

Another recent report by Wiener-Vacher[8] reviewed the most common vestibular disorders in more than 2000 children over a 14-year period. Patient records were examined retrospectively to determine the most common diagnoses in children presenting with dizziness and vertigo. Consistent with many earlier reports, the most commonly diagnosed vestibular disease was MV, which was responsible for nearly 25% of cases. BPVC represented 20% of the diagnoses. Cranial trauma and ophthalmological disorders each accounted for 10% of the dizziness cases. In this cohort, vestibular neuritis (5%) and posterior fossa tumors (<1%) were less often encountered.

Table 1 is a summary of findings from a series of studies each describing the most frequent causes of pediatric dizziness/vertigo. The characteristics of these disorders and diseases (ie, pathophysiology and balance function test findings) are now described.

Table 1
Summary of studies

		Total	%	Balatsouras et al,[9] 2007	Bower & Cotton,[10] 1995	Choung et al,[16] 2003	D'Agostino,[23] 1997	Erbek et al,[17] 2006	Ravid et al,[21] 2003	Riina et al,[3] 2005	Weisleder & Fife,[24] 2001	Wiener-Vacher,[8] 2008
Total subjects		687	%	54	34	55	282	50	62	119	31	>2000
Migraine	n (%)	116	16.89	11 (20.4)	4 (11.8)	17 (30.9)	15 (5.4)	17 (34)	24 (39)	17 (14.3)	11 (35.5)	25%
BPVC	n (%)	133	19.36	9 (16.7)	5 (14.7)	14 (25.5)	60 (21)	6 (12)	10 (16)	23 (19.3)	6 (19.4)	20%
Otitis media	n (%)	22	3.20	5 (9.2)	5 (14.7)	x		x		12 (10.1)		
Viral infection	n (%)	98	14.26	15 (27.7)	4 (11.8)	1 (1.8)	53 (18.8)	2 (4)	9 (14)	14 (11.8)		5%
Trauma	n (%)	103	14.99	3 (5.5)	3 (8.8)	4 (7.3)	85 (30.3)		2 (3)	6 (5)		10%

Literature reports of the most common causes of vertigo/dizziness in children. Some studies excluded children with otitis media (denoted with x).

Abbreviation: BPVC, benign paroxysmal vertigo of childhood.

MIGRAINE-ASSOCIATED VERTIGO IN CHILDREN

As mentioned previously, the most common diagnosis in children with vertigo and dizziness is migraine headache (ie, migraine equivalent), although the temporal relationship has been reported to be variable. That is, headache may precede, follow, or occur simultaneously with dizziness/vertigo, and often there are accompanying symptoms such as nausea and/or photophobia. However, the features can also be different from those seen in adults.[25] In children, migraines often are localized to the frontal or periorbital region, last less than 2 hours, and may not manifest themselves as the typical throbbing pain often described by adults.[24] Approximately 20% of children with migraine have associated dizziness. There are 3 commonly reported migraine variants that can produce abnormal findings on quantitative vestibular system testing[26]: basilar migraine (BM), MV, and BPVC.[27,28] BM occurs in about 3% to 19% of children with migraine and usually occurs at age 7 years.[25] Many migraines present with an aura consisting of different sensory sensations (eg, olfactory, visual, or vestibular). BM has been described in the literature as presenting with an aura consisting of audio-vestibular manifestations such as tinnitus, loss of hearing, acute imbalance, and vertigo.[29] Usually pediatric patients with BM demonstrate normal neurologic examinations. According to Eggers,[30] only a very small proportion of patients with MV meet the criteria for BM.

Etiology and Pathophysiology of Migraine

The pathophysiology of dizziness/vertigo in these migraine variants is currently unresolved. In basilar migraine, the root cause has been suggested to be asymmetric activation of brainstem vestibular nuclei or defective Ca^{2+} channels that are shared by the brain and the inner ear.[27,31] MV is considered by most its own entity, and like BM, its pathophysiology is still not completely understood. Investigators have set forth hypotheses, which include cortical spreading depression affecting the parietoinsular vestibular cortex and changes in activity between the parietal cortex and the vestibular nuclei.[32–34]

Balance Function Findings in Children with Migraine

Laboratory findings in patients with MV can consist of both central and peripheral impairment, and have been well documented in adults. In 1991 Olsson[35] evaluated 50 patients with BM, 49 of whom demonstrated abnormal ocular motor testing. When caloric test findings are combined across studies, the frequency with which unilateral impairments were observed ranged from 8% to 60% of patients.[32–36] Marcelli and colleagues[37] reported vestibular findings in 22 children diagnosed with migraine. Of this sample, 73% of the participants with MV demonstrated either peripheral or central vestibular abnormalities. The vestibular manifestations varied and included spontaneous-positional nystagmus, post head-shaking nystagmus, BPPV, vibration-induced nystagmus, absence of vestibular evoked myogenic potentials (VEMPs), and unilateral or bilateral caloric reductions. Vestibular system testing has been demonstrated to provide useful information in the differential diagnosis of children with migraine, especially in those children in whom the headaches are associated with vertigo or dizziness.

BENIGN PAROXYSMAL VERTIGO OF CHILDHOOD

BPVC was initially reported by Basser in 1964, describing the clinical presentation of BPVC in 17 children aged 4 years or younger.[38] Primary symptoms included episodic attacks of vertigo lasting from seconds to minutes, resulting in the child being unable to stand without support. Additional symptoms included nystagmus, tinnitus, pallor, diaphoresis, and vomiting. BPVC is a pediatric migraine equivalent recognized by the International Headache Society (IHS) classification system.[39] There is no loss of consciousness during attacks of BPVC, and complete recovery follows an attack. A child who is capable will describe a sensation of spinning. The age of onset of BPVC has been reported to typically occur before 4 years of age and is rarely seen after 8 years.[38] In an epidemiologic study by Russell and Abu-Arafeh,[6] 2% of school-age children met the criteria for BPVC (ie, at least 3 transient episodes of the sensation of rotation, either of the child or of the surrounding environment, severe enough to interfere with normal activity, and not associated with loss of consciousness or any neurologic auditory abnormality).

Etiology and Pathophysiology of Benign Paroxysmal Vertigo of Childhood

While the pathophysiology of BPVC is currently unknown, there is strong supporting evidence that BPVC is a migraine headache variant. Many children with BPVC will go on to develop migraine later in life.[6,40–44] At present, the etiology of BPVC remains unknown but there is mounting evidence suggesting that in many cases it is vascular in origin.[31,38,45,46] For example, episodic vasospasm could result in ischemia to the inner ear culminating in an end-organ impairment and vertigo. A proposed central mechanism that has been postulated to be responsible is interruption in blood flow to the vestibular nuclei and associated pathways.[45] Regardless of the etiology, the variable nature of laboratory findings makes diagnosing this disorder difficult. At present, the diagnosis of BPVC is primarily dependent on a reliable and characteristic history.

Balance Function Findings in Children with Benign Paroxysmal Vertigo of Childhood

There has been great variability in the quantitative vestibular test results obtained from patients with BPVC. Several studies have reported that children with BPVC commonly present with significant bithermal caloric asymmetry.[38,47,48] However, other investigators have found no such relationship.[49,50] Mierzwinski and colleagues[51] evaluated 124 children with vertigo, 13 of whom presented with characteristics commonly associated with BPVC. Results showed that of this subset of 13 patients, normal ENG test results occurred for 5 patients. In addition, 1 patient was found to have a significant unilateral weakness, and the other 7 patients had either central vestibular impairments or a mixture of peripheral and central vestibular system impairments.

TRAUMA

Head trauma in young children is common. The Centers for Disease Control and Prevention have reported that children 0 to 14 years of age comprise approximately 500,000 emergency department visits for traumatic brain injury each year.[52] Children suffering from head injuries as a result of trauma can present with headache, cognitive impairment, changes in personality, and sleep disturbance. Dizziness/vertigo is also a common symptom for a significan number of children presenting with trauma.

Etiology and Pathophysiology of Trauma

Head trauma is frequently subcategorized as blunt head trauma or penetrating head trauma. Blunt head injuries, including whiplash injuries, can lead to dizziness through fracture of the temporal bone or labyrinthine concussion.[53,54] In cases of a fracture or concussion where the labyrinth or vestibular nerve is affected, children can experience severe vertigo with nystagmus and nausea, indicating unilateral loss of function in the peripheral vestibular system (ie, end-organ or vestibular nerve). Penetrating head injuries have been reported to cause vertigo secondary to perilymph fistula.[55] As in adults, pediatric BPPV secondary to head trauma can also occur.[17]

Balance Function Findings in Children with Trauma

Vestibular and audiologic test results in children suffering from trauma-induced vertigo have been rarely reported. The few studies that have included quantitative balance function testing in the diagnostic approach for trauma show mixed results. For example, Choung and colleagues[16] described test results in 55 pediatric patients with vertigo, 4 of whom were diagnosed with vertigo due to trauma. Whereas all 4 patients demonstrated normal caloric examinations, they demonstrated abnormalities during rotational testing. Any abnormality of phase, gain, or symmetry was considered an abnormal result, though specifics were not given as to which parameters were abnormal. Perilymph fistula should be suspected in cases of head trauma where the child presents with dizziness and/or hearing loss. One example was reported by Kojima and colleagues.[56] The investigators described vestibular manifestations in an 11-year old boy who suffered a penetrating injury while rock-climbing. During the child's physical examination 2 weeks after injury, he demonstrated horizontal nystagmus, hearing loss, and significant positional nystagmus. The presence of perilymph fistula was confirmed during exploratory surgery. Surgical intervention repaired the perilymph fistula, and though the boy's vertigo resolved, his hearing did not recover. In this regard, Neuenschwander and colleagues[57] and Kim and colleagues[55] described cases of ataxia and/or vertigo following penetrating and blunt head injuries in children. Three of the 5 case studies resulted in diagnoses of perilymph fistula, 1 with dehiscence of the oval window, and 1 ossicular chain injury without surgical evidence for fistula. All case studies demonstrated hearing impairment, 4 of these being sensorineural in origin and 1 conductive in origin. Spontaneous nystagmus was observed in 3 of the 5 cases.

In one of the most comprehensive studies describing the effect of blunt head injuries in children, Vartiainen and colleagues[58] described findings in 199 children. The investigators compared 61 children treated for acute blunt head injury with 59 age-matched controls. An additional 138 children with previous diagnosis of blunt head trauma were invited for examination to determine post-traumatic findings in the long term. A total of 39 patients (19.6%) had sustained a skull fracture. The results of this study are summarized in **Table 2**.

Spontaneous and/or positional nystagmus was defined by a maximum slow-phase velocity that was 7°/s or greater. Abnormal smooth pursuit and failure of fixation suppression for a minimum of 2 caloric irrigations were considered central ENG findings. The investigators also studied subjective vestibular disturbances in their patients. Of the 61 patients with acute head injury, only 1 (2%) complained of vertigo. Of 138 patients examined more than 12 months after head injury, 2 patients (1%) described vertigo. The investigators hypothesized that while objective vestibular lesions are common in children with head injuries, children rarely express subjective symptoms; this also may be attributable to children's ability to compensate quickly for unilateral vestibular system disturbance.[58]

Surprisingly, reports describing findings on quantitative balance function testing in children post trauma are rare, with the exception of the large-scale study by Vartiainen and colleagues.[58] Often, children who have sustained head trauma are referred for a hearing evaluation. If a child has incurred a hearing loss, quantitative vestibular testing may be indicated as well. In particular, sensorineural hearing loss is often a sentinel symptom of a fracture to the temporal bone or the presence of a perilymph fistula. Children presenting with audio-vestibular signs (eg, ataxia, vertigo, hearing

Table 2 Summary of study of blunt head trauma	Blunt Trauma (n = 61, Caloric Testing Performed on 41)		Blunt Trauma (n = 138, Caloric Testing Performed on 113)
	Immediately Following Trauma	6–12 Months Post-Trauma	2–8 Years Post-Trauma
Spontaneous and/or positional nystagmus	21 (46%)	8 (17%)	22 (18%)
Central ENG finding	20 (43%)	10 (24%)	14 (12%)
Caloric abnormality (performed in 154 of 190 total patients)	40 (21%)	13 (7%)	11 (6%)

Summary of large-scale study by Vartiainen and colleagues[58] describing findings in 199 children with blunt head traumas at different intervals post injury. Results are presented in n (%) format.

loss, or tinnitus) should be considered candidates for both a hearing evaluation and vestibular assessment.

VESTIBULAR NEURITIS

Vestibular neuritis in adults presents as a sudden onset of rotary vertigo and vomiting lasting for several days to weeks (see article by Goddard and Fayad in this publication). Children suffering from an attack of vestibular neuritis often present with the same symptoms as their adult counterparts.[9,10,16,17,23,59–62]

Etiology and Pathophysiology of Vestibular Neuritis

While the cause of vestibular neuritis is somewhat controversial, many investigators have suggested that vestibular neuritis is viral in origin, though bacterial and other types of infections have also been suggested.[63–65] It has also been suggested that unknown factors may contribute to reactivation of a latent virus (eg, herpes zoster oticus), resulting in inflammation of the nerve and potentially causing cell damage.[65,66]

Balance Function Findings in Children with Vestibular Neuritis

Vestibular neuritis is uncommon in children. However, there have been published accounts in which findings of quantitative vestibular assessments are reported. The caloric examination is the gold standard for documenting the side and degree of peripheral vestibular impairment, and can provide information regarding the integrity of the lateral semicircular canals and/or superior vestibular nerves. The clinical utility of the caloric examination for measuring the peripheral function in children with vestibular neuritis is documented. One such study conducted by Balatsouras and colleagues[9] evaluated 54 children with dizziness, 15 of whom received a final diagnosis of viral infection. Peripheral ENG findings were documented in 13 of these children, and were defined as the presence of spontaneous nystagmus, directional preponderance, and/or caloric weakness. The remaining 2 children demonstrated a combination of peripheral findings in addition to one or more of the following central findings: saccadic pursuit, gaze-evoked nystagmus, spontaneous central nystagmus, positional central nystagmus, or impaired fixation suppression during caloric testing. In 3 separate reports, 5 children diagnosed with vestibular neuritis demonstrated significant caloric weakness.[16,17,62] Other studies of caloric function in children have also supported its role in quantifying vestibular impairment in cases of vestibular neuritis. Bower and Cotton[10] reported their findings for 3 children with vestibular neuritis. One of the patients demonstrated a significant caloric weakness. Melagrana and colleagues[61] reported their findings from 72 children with unilateral sensorineural hearing loss of possible viral origin. Of this sample, 20 children (28%) displayed a significant unilateral vestibular weakness during caloric examination. In addition, either spontaneous or positional nystagmus was found in 53% of this sample.

Rotational testing can also be a useful tool in assessing children with suspected vestibular neuritis. Choung and colleagues[16] reported the results of positional, rotational, and caloric testing in 55 children with the chief complaint of vertigo or dizziness, one of whom was diagnosed with vestibular neuritis. This lone patient demonstrated unilateral caloric weakness and no significant positional nystagmus. In addition, abnormal gain, phase, or symmetry (not specified by the investigators) of the vestibulo-ocular reflex (VOR) during rotational testing was observed, with normal VOR fixation, further suggesting a peripheral origin of the dizziness.

Other investigators have described the characteristics of children with vestibular neuritis during the physical examination and bedside testing. In a review of 282 children with vertigo by D'Agostino and colleagues,[23] 50 children were diagnosed with labyrinthitis, 2 with vestibular neuritis, and 1 with cochleo-vestibular neuritis. The two patients with diagnosed vestibular neuritis demonstrated spontaneous nystagmus and positive Romberg sign, and one demonstrated "moderate" positional nystagmus. In separate case studies of children with vestibular neuritis, Ergul and colleagues[59] and Zanolli and colleagues[62] described findings from bedside testing. In both cases the children presented with vestibular spontaneous nystagmus, a positive head-thrust test in the direction of the suspected impairment, and positive Romberg sign.

One must be careful not to rely on vestibular testing alone to diagnose vestibular neuritis but rather consider it a part of the entire evaluation. In a recent study, Goudakos and colleagues[67] evaluated adult patients with vestibular neuritis. When caloric responses were analyzed, 90% of patients continued to present with a significant vestibular system weakness after 1 month. When patients were evaluated 6 months after symptom onset, 80% of patients continued to have abnormal caloric findings. In this regard, Eviatar and Eviatar[60] identified 5 of 50 children in their cohort with vestibular neuritis. Each of these children had an acute onset of vertigo and nausea without impairment of hearing following an upper respiratory infection and mild earache. Vestibular testing was completed 2 weeks after onset, and 2 of the 5 children demonstrated directional preponderance on caloric stimulation with no caloric weakness. The remaining 3 children demonstrated normal vestibular examinations, implying spontaneous recovery.

The majority of studies to date have used caloric testing and bedside testing to describe impairments in the vestibular system believed to be due to viral origin. Further investigations centered on the clinical utility of tests such as the cervical and ocular VEMPs for assessing pediatric dizziness will certainly be done in the coming years. There is also a paucity of data describing the effects of central nervous system compensation in children and how this can affect quantitative vestibular testing. While these data are available in adults, it is currently unknown how the rate of recovery is different in children with vestibular neuritis.[68]

OTITIS MEDIA

Otitis media and middle ear effusion are frequently quoted as one of the most common causes of vestibular complaints in children.[2,7,10,69,70] The reported symptoms are typically complaints of "unsteadiness" and "clumsiness" rather than true vertigo.

Etiology and Pathophysiology of Otitis Media

Different theories have been proposed as to how middle ear pathologies can affect the vestibular labyrinth. Golz and colleagues[71] postulated that toxins present in middle ear fluid enter the inner ear fluid and cause serous labyrinthitis. Other researchers have proposed that pressure changes in the middle ear cause displacements of the round and oval windows, leading to secondary movement of labyrinthine fluids.[72,73] Although the etiology remains unclear, many research studies have focused on how otitis media with effusion (OME) affects children's balance.[70,71,74–77]

Balance Function Findings in Children with Otitis Media

The traditional vestibular test battery can be difficult to perform in the pediatric OME population. Conductive hearing loss frequently accompanies OME and confounds air-conducted VEMP testing. In addition, OME is prevalent in very young children who may not tolerate caloric or rotational testing. The study by Golz and colleagues[71] used ENG to compare 136 children with OME history and 74 children without middle ear history. Neither study group showed abnormalities during optokinetic or pursuit testing. However, 42 children with OME (31%) demonstrated spontaneous nystagmus, and 24 (17.5%) showed positional nystagmus consistent with BPPV. Thirteen children showed both spontaneous and positional nystagmus. Therefore, 79 children with OME (58%) had abnormal ENG findings compared with 3 children (4%) in the control group. In line with this study, Koyuncu and colleagues[76] evaluated spontaneous and positional nystagmus in 30 children with OME and 15 matched controls. Spontaneous nystagmus of greater than 7°/s was observed in 1 child with OME, and positional nystagmus was observed in 10 children with OME. The control group demonstrated no abnormalities on ENG testing. The study group was then reevaluated 1 month following myringotomy and tube insertion. No spontaneous or positional nystagmus was observed postoperatively.

Rotational testing was performed on 40 children with a history of OME and compared with 31 children with no significant history.[78] Three stimuli were used: 0.02-Hz rotation at 50°/s, 0.1-Hz rotation at 50°/s, and 0.1-Hz rotation at 150°/s. The study group showed significantly poorer gain than controls during the latter test, with comparable phase and symmetry. These same 71 children were also

---

"What not to miss"

Auditory neuropathy (AN) or auditory neuropathy spectrum disorder (ANSD) is a term that describes a condition consisting of a distinct collection of auditory abnormalities.

The ANSD pattern is commonly composed of abnormal results from tests assessing the function of the vestibulo-cochlear nerve and normal findings from tests that evaluate the function of the cochlear outer hair cells.

However, it is not only hearing loss that distinguishes AN patients from their normal counterparts. Recently, evidence has been emerging that this group of patients with "auditory neuropathy" may also demonstrate "vestibular neuropathy."

At present there are very few studies examining vestibular function in patients with confirmed AN; however, there is mounting evidence that these patients demonstrate abnormal findings on balance function testing as well.[79–81]

It has been suggested that the vestibular branch of the vestibulo-cochlear nerve is also impaired in cases of AN.[79–82]

evaluated using computerized dynamic posturography, with no significant differences observed between groups. The posturography findings of the study are contradicted by findings in other research articles. Casselbrant and colleagues[70] showed higher velocity of sway in a group with OME. Jones and colleagues[75] showed that body sway was more pronounced in children with secretory otitis media as compared with a control group. Finally, a study of 20 children with OME before and after tube insertion by Waldron and colleagues[77] showed poorer results on sway posturography preoperatively versus postoperatively. Although the origin of balance dysfunction related to middle ear pathology may be debated, it is certain that more research is needed to evaluate vestibular function and delay in children with OME.

SUMMARY

In children with vertigo and imbalance a thorough physical and neurotological examination is required. Tools such as the structured case history approach presented in this report can assist the clinician in the determination of who does and who does not require quantitative vestibular testing. The 5 most common disorders affecting pediatric balance all may result in abnormal results on quantitative vestibular testing. Vestibular tests assess function and are inexpensive when compared with neuroimaging tests, which often are ordered as part of the assessment of the dizzy child (eg, magnetic resonance imaging and computed tomography). However, as this review illustrates, there are currently no clear patterns in results from vestibular testing that can be expected from any of the 5 most common disorders causing dizziness/vertigo in children. There are several reasons for this. First, the balance function results that have been reported in various impairments causing dizziness in children all have different criteria for what is determined to be normal, as well as different methodology (eg, air vs water caloric stimulation). What is abnormal for one laboratory may not be for another. Second, there is most certainly variability in the criteria for diagnosis between dizziness centers. Finally, children are difficult to assess, as discussed earlier in this article. For additional information regarding pediatric vestibular test techniques, the reader is referred to the article by Valente in this publication. Often a child will not complete an entire test or will not be cooperative. Nonetheless, it is most critical to document whether a vestibular impairment exists in a child. Vestibular system impairment in children can lead to motor incoordination and visual disturbances that can slow normal locomotor development. In order for appropriate rehabilitative therapy to be prescribed, the presence or absence of vestibular system impairment should be documented to guide management and treatment. It is undisputed that large-scale studies using the same methods and criteria need to be completed in children with dizziness. The resurgence of interest in pediatric balance function testing will surely lead to new techniques and research studies that will advance understanding of how to better manage and treat this challenging population.

REFERENCES

1. Fried MP. The evaluation of dizziness in children. Laryngoscope 1980;90(9): 1548–60.
2. Busis SN. Dizziness in children. Pediatr Ann 1988;17:648.
3. Riina N, Ilmari P, Kentala E. Vertigo and imbalance in children. Arch Otolaryngol Head Neck Surg 2005;131:996–1000.
4. Tusa RJ, Saada AA, Niparko JR. Dizziness in childhood. J Neurol 1994;9(3): 261–74.

5. Szirmai A. Vestibular disorders in childhood and adolscents. Eur Arch Otorhino-laryngol 2010;267(11):1801–4.
6. Russell G, Abu-Arafeh I. Paroxysmal vertigo in children—an epidemiological study. Int J Pediatr Otorhinolaryngol 1999;49(Suppl 1):S105–7.
7. Blayney AW, Colman BH. Dizziness in children. Clin Otolaryngol 1984;9(2):77–85.
8. Wiener-Vacher SR. Vestibular disorders in children. Int J Audiol 2008;47:578–83.
9. Balatsouras DG, Kaberos A, Assimakopoulos D, et al. Etiology of vertigo in children. Int J Pediatr Otorhinolaryngol 2007;71:487–94.
10. Bower CM, Cotton RT. The spectrum of vertigo in children. Arch Otolaryngol Head Neck Surg 1995;121:911–5.
11. Eviatar L, Miranda S, Eviatar A, et al. Development of nystagmus in response to vestibular stimulation in infants. Ann Neurol 1978;5:508–14.
12. von Brevern M, Radtke A, Lezius F, et al. Epidemiology of benign paroxysmal positional vertigo: a population based study. J Neurol Neurosurg Psychiatry 2007;78(7):710–5.
13. Furman JM, Cass SP. Benign paroxysmal positional vertigo. N Engl J Med 1999;341(21):1590–6.
14. Johkura K, Momoo T, Kuroiwa Y. Positional nystagmus in patients with chronic dizziness. J Neurol Neurosurg Psychiatry 2008;79(12):1324–6.
15. Fife TD. Benign paroxysmal positional vertigo. Semin Neurol 2009;29(5):500–8.
16. Choung Y, Park K, Moon S, et al. Various causes and clinical characteristics in vertigo in children with normal eardrums. Int J Pediatr Otorhinolaryngol 2003;67:889–94.
17. Erbek SH, Erbek SS, Yilmaz I, et al. Vertigo in childhood: a clinical experience. Int J Pediatr Otorhinolaryngol 2006;70:1547–54.
18. Cyr DG. Vestibular testing in children. Ann Otol Rhinol Laryngol 1980;89:63–9.
19. Cyr DG. The vestibular system: pediatric considerations. Semin Hear 1983;4(1):33–45.
20. Eviatar L. Dizziness in children. Otolaryngol Clin North Am 1994;27(3):557–71.
21. Ravid S, Bienkowski R, Eviatar L. A simplified diagnostic approach to dizziness in children. Pediatr Neurol 2003;29(4):317–20.
22. Niemensivu R, Kentala E, Weiner-Vacher S, et al. Evaluation of vertiginous children. Eur Arch Otorhinolaryngol 2007;264:1129–35.
23. D'Agostino R, Tarantino V, Melagrana A, et al. Otoneurologic evaluation of child vertigo. Int J Pediatr Otorhinolaryngol 1997;40:133–9.
24. Weisleder P, Fife T. Dizziness and headache: a common association in children and adolescents. J Child Neurol 2001;16:727–30.
25. Lewis DW. Pediatric migraine. Neurol Clin 2009;27(2):481–501.
26. Prensky AR, Sommer D. Diagnosis and treatment of migraine in children. Neurology 1979;29(4):506–10.
27. Cass SP, Furman JM, Ankerstierne K, et al. Migraine-related vestibulopathy. Ann Otol Rhinol Laryngol 1997;106(3):182–9.
28. Lewis DW, Middlebrook MT, Mehallick L, et al. Pediatric headaches: what do the children want? Headache 1996;36(4):224–30.
29. Johnson GD. Medical management of migraine-related dizziness and vertigo. Laryngoscope 1998;108:1–28.
30. Eggers SD. Migraine-related vertigo: diagnosis and treatment. Curr Neurol Neurosci Rep 2006;6(2):106–15.
31. Baloh RW, Honrubia V. Childhood onset of benign positional vertigo. Neurology 1998;50(5):1494–6.

32. Dieterich M, Brandt T. Episodic vertigo related to migraine (90 cases): vestibular migraine? J Neurol 1999;246(10):883–92.
33. Cutrer FM, Baloh RW. Migraine-associated dizziness. Headache 1992;32(6): 300–4.
34. Furman JM, Sparto PJ, Soso M, et al. Vestibular function in migraine-related dizziness: a pilot study. J Vestib Res 2005;15(5–6):327–32.
35. Olsson JF. Neurotologic findings in basilar migraine. Laryngoscope 1991; 101(1 Pt 2 Suppl 52):1–41.
36. Kayan A, Hood JD. Neuro-otological manifestations of migraine. Brain 1984; 107(4):1123–42.
37. Marcelli V, Furia T, Marciano E. Vestibular pathways involvement in children with migraine: a neuro-otological study. Headache 2010;50(1):71–6.
38. Basser LS. Benign paroxysmal vertigo of childhood. (A variety of vestibular neuronitis). Brain 1964;87:141–52.
39. Olesen J. The classification and diagnosis of headache disorders. Neurol Clin 1990;8(4):793–9.
40. Fenichel GM. Migraine as a cause of benign paroxysmal vertigo of childhood. J Pediatr 1967;71(1):114–5.
41. Herraiz C, Calvin FJ, Tapia MC, et al. The migraine: benign paroxysmal vertigo of childhood complex. Int Tinnitus J 1999;5(1):50–2.
42. Mira E, Piacentino G, Lani G, et al. Benign paroxysmal vertigo in childhood. Diagnostic significance of vestibular examination and headache provocation tests. Acta Otolaryngol Suppl 1984;406:271–4.
43. Lanzi G, Balottin U, Borgatti R. A prospective study of juvenile migraine with aura. Headache 1994;34(5):275–8.
44. Moretti G, Manzoni GC, Caffarra P, et al. "Benign recurrent vertigo" and its connection with migraine. Headache 1980;20(6):344–6.
45. Finkelhor BK, Harker LA. Benign paroxysmal vertigo of childhood. Laryngoscope 1987;97(10):1161–3.
46. Slater R. Benign recurrent vertigo. J Neurol Neurosurg Psychiatry 1979;42(4):363–7.
47. Dunn DW, Snyder CH. Benign paroxysmal vertigo of childhood. Am J Dis Child 1976;130(10):1099–100.
48. Koenigsberger MR, Chutorian AM, Gold AP, et al. Benign paroxysmal vertigo of childhood. Neurology 1968;18(3):301–2.
49. Eeg-Olofsson O, Odkvist L, Lindskog U, et al. Benign paroxysmal vertigo in childhood. Acta Otolaryngol 1982;93(3–4):283–9.
50. Lanzi G, Balottin U, Fazzi E, et al. Benign paroxysmal vertigo in childhood: a longitudinal study. Headache 1986;26(10):494–7.
51. Mierzwinski J, Polak M, Dalke K, et al. Benign paroxysmal vertigo of childhood. Otolaryngol Pol 2007;61(3):307–10.
52. Faul M, Xu L, Wald MM, et al. Traumatic brain injury in the United States: emergency department visits, hospitalizations, and deaths. Atlanta (GA): Centers for Disease Control and Prevention, National Center for Injury Prevention and Control; 2010.
53. Moller C. Balance disorders in children. In: Luxon L, Furman JM, Martini A, et al, editors. Textbook of audiological medicine: clinical aspects of hearing and balance. London: Martin Dunitz; 2003. p. 861–8.
54. Eviatar L, Bergrtraum M, Randel RM. Post-traumatic vertigo in children: a diagnostic approach. Pediatr Neurol 1986;2(2):61–6.
55. Kim SH, Kazahaya K, Handler SD. Traumatic perilymphatic fistulas in children: etiology, diagnosis and management. Int J Pediatr Otorhinolaryngol 2001;60:147–53.

56. Kojima H, Tanaka Y, Mori E, et al. Penetrating vestibular injury due to a twig entering via the external auditory meatus. Am J Otolaryngol 2006;27: 418–21.

57. Neuenschwander MC, Deutsch ES, Cornetta A, et al. Penetrating middle ear trauma: a report of 2 cases. Ear Hear 2005;84(1):32–5.

58. Vartiainen E, Karjalainen S, Karja J. Vestibular disorders following head injury in children. Int J Pediatr Otorhinolaryngol 1985;9:135–41.

59. Ergul Y, Ekici B, Tastan Y, et al. Vestibular neuritis caused by enteroviral infection. Pediatr Neurol 2006;34:45–6.

60. Eviatar L, Eviatar A. Vertigo in children: differential diagnosis and treatment. Pediatrics 1977;59:833–8.

61. Melagrana A, Tarantino V, D'Agostino R, et al. Electronystagmography findings in child unilateral sensorineural hearing loss of probable viral origin. Int J Pediatr Otorhinolaryngol 1998;42:239–46.

62. Zanolli R, Zazzi M, Muraca MC, et al. A child with vestibular neuritis. Is adenovirus implicated? Brain Dev 2006;28:410–2.

63. Bartual-Pastor J. Vestibular neuritis: etiopathogenesis. Rev Laryngol Otol Rhinol (Bord) 2005;126(4):279–81.

64. Davis LE. Viruses and vestibular neuritis: review of human and animal studies. Acta Otolaryngol Suppl 1993;503:70–3.

65. Strupp M, Brandt T. Vestibular neuritis. Semin Neurol 2009;29(5):509–19.

66. Baloh RW. Clinical practice. Vestibular neuritis. N Engl J Med 2003;348(11): 1027–32.

67. Goudakos JK, Markou KD, Franco-Vidal V, et al. Corticosteroids in the treatment of vestibular neuritis: a systematic review and meta-analysis. Otol Neurotol 2010; 31(2):183–9.

68. Choi KD, Oh SY, Kim HJ, et al. Recovery of vestibular imbalances after vestibular neuritis. Laryngoscope 2007;117(7):1307–12.

69. Balkany TJ, Finkel RS. The dizzy child. Ear Hear 1986;7(3):138–42.

70. Casselbrant ML, Furman JM, Rubenstein E, et al. Effect of otitis media on the vestibular system in children. Ann Otol Rhinol Laryngol 1995;104(8):620–4.

71. Golz A, Netzer A, Angel-Yeger B, et al. Effects of middle ear effusion on the vestibular system in children. Otolaryngol Head Neck Surg 1998;119(6):695–9.

72. Carlborg BI, Konradsson KS, Carlborg AH, et al. Pressure transfer between the perilymph and the cerebrospinal fluid compartments in cats. Am J Otol 1992; 13(1):41–8.

73. Suzuki M, Kitano H, Yazawa Y, et al. Involvement of round and oval windows in the vestibular response to pressure changes in the middle ear of guinea pigs. Acta Otolaryngol 1998;118(5):712–6.

74. Golz A, Angel-Yeger B, Parush S. Evaluation of balance disturbances in children with middle ear effusion. Int J Pediatr Otorhinolaryngol 1998;43:21–6.

75. Jones NS, Radomskij P, Prichard AJ, et al. Imbalance and chronic secretory otitis media in children: effect of myringotomy and insertion of ventilation tubes on body sway. Ann Otol Rhinol Laryngol 1990;99(6):477–81.

76. Koyuncu M, Saka MM, Tanyeri Y, et al. Effects of otitis media with effusion on the vestibular system in children. Otolaryngol Head Neck Surg 1999;120(1): 117–21.

77. Waldron MN, Matthews JN, Johnson IJ. The effect of otitis media with effusions on balance in children. Clin Otolaryngol Allied Sci 2004;29(4):318–20.

78. Casselbrant ML, Furman JM, Mandel EM, et al. Past history of otitis media and balance in four-year-old children. Laryngoscope 2000;110(5):773–8.

79. Fujikawa S, Starr A. Vestibular neuropathy accompanying auditory and peripheral neuropathies. Arch Otolaryngol Head Neck Surg 2000;126(12):1453–6.
80. Akdogan O, Selcuk A, Ozcan I, et al. Vestibular nerve functions in children with auditory neuropathy. Int J Pediatr Otorhinolaryngol 2008;72(3):415–9.
81. Sheykholeslami K, Megerian CA, Arnold JE, et al. Vestibular evoked myogenic potentials in infancy and early childhood. Laryngoscope 2005;115(8):1440–4.
82. Sazgar AA, Yazdani N, Rezazadeh N, et al. Vestibular evoked myogenic potential (VEMP) in patients with auditory neuropathy: auditory neuropathy or audiovestibular neuropathy? Acta Otolaryngol 2010;130(10):1130–4.

Dizziness and Vertigo in the Adolescent

Jennie Taylor, MD[a], Howard P. Goodkin, MD, PhD[a,b],*

KEYWORDS

- Vertigo • Dizziness • Adolescence • Brain development
- Episodic ataxia • Migraine • Chronic daily headache • POTS

KEY POINTS

- For those few adolescents who seek outpatient evaluation for these complaints, the majority are diagnosed with migraine headaches.
- In addition to migraine headache, the differential diagnosis in this age group includes episodic ataxia type II; chronic daily headaches; postural orthostatic tachycardia; intracranial mass lesions; psychiatric disorders (eg, depression or somatoform disorders); and rarely vestibular disorders, including viral labyrinthitis and Ménière's disease.
- Evaluation and, in the majority of cases, diagnosis is based on careful history and physical examination with neuroimaging performed for all adolescents with a history of trauma, an abnormal neurologic examination, persistent headaches, or indication of central lesion on vestibular testing.

M.C. is a 16-year-old girl presenting with a complaint of frequent episodes of dizziness that started when she was 13 years of age. The events are characterized by a feeling that she describes as "losing track of her body in space." The events are brief and last only 1 to 2 seconds. There is no associated change in vision, palpitations, or sweating. Although she does have a sensation of falling, she has not fallen. The events occur multiple times per week and are more frequent around the time of her menses or just before the onset of a headache, which she describes as a prolonged, severe throbbing pain with associated nausea and vomiting that resolve with sleep. The dizziness can occur both at rest and with activity and in any position. It is not triggered by head position.

Disclosures: Dr Taylor has no financial relationships to disclose.

Dr Goodkin has served as a consultant to MedImmune, Inc within the last 3 years and he receives funding from the NIH for projects not related to this work.

[a] Department of Neurology, University of Virginia Health Systems, PO Box 800394, Charlottesville, VA 22908, USA

[b] Department of Pediatrics, University of Virginia Health Systems, PO Box 800394, Charlottesville, VA 22908, USA

* Corresponding author.

E-mail address: hpg9v@virginia.edu

Her past medical history is otherwise benign. She has not required hospital admission or surgeries. She is not taking any medications. She denies the use of alcohol, tobacco, or illicit drugs; however, she notes that many of her friends have experimented with marijuana. Her review of systems is positive for significant stress regarding grades at school. She is active in several extracurricular activities. She describes much frustration with her parents for not allowing her more freedoms after she was caught attempting to shoplift when she was 13 years old. Her sleep patterns are erratic, and she does not think that she is sleeping well. Her mother has a diagnosis of migraine headaches. There is a maternal aunt who died in her twenties secondary to an astrocytoma and distant paternal cousin who died in his forties of a brain tumor.

Her general and neurologic examination is unremarkable. Because of the patient's and family's anxiety regarding the family history, an MRI of the brain was obtained, which is unremarkable.

Following the appointment, she is started on a low dose of amitriptyline at night, which results in a marked reduction in the frequency of her dizziness and headaches.

THE ADOLESCENT BRAIN

Adolescence, the developmental transition between the dependency of childhood and the independency of adulthood, encompasses the approximate time period between 12 and 18 years of age. Behavior during this developmental stage is frequently characterized by risk taking, impulsivity, and poor choices. The indestructible attitude of the adolescent, which can be met by negative consequences, promotes experimentation of adult practices, development of self-esteem, and eventually social acceptance.[1]

Although the brain reaches 90% of its adult size by 6 years of age, pruning (resulting in decreasing synaptic density) and cortical thinning occur throughout childhood and adolescence. The volume of white matter increases up to about 20 years of age as the result of ongoing myelination of white matter tracts. One of the last regions to undergo both of these maturational processes is the prefrontal cortex, the region of the brain that participates in executive, attention, and regulatory functions.[2]

Adolescence represents a unique time period of brain development marked by changes in both anatomic connectivity and functional activation. Recently, Casey and colleagues[1] suggested that the differential developmental trajectories of the limbic system and subcortical structures (eg, basal ganglia) as compared with the prefrontal cortex could, in part, explain the impulsivity and risk-taking behavior that occur during adolescence. In their model, earlier maturation of the limbic system and subcortical structures during adolescence drives adolescent behavior. As the connections of the prefrontal cortex mature, the influence of the limbic system and subcortical structures is reduced and the prefrontal cortex dominates, resulting in an improved ability to suppress impulses and greater emphasis on goal-driven choices. Their model is supported by recent demonstrations of an exaggerated response of the nucleus accumbens in the adolescent as compared to the adult and child in a task that manipulated reward values[1,3] and the correlation of the development of fiber tracts between the prefrontal cortex and basal ganglia with performance on a go/no-go task, a measure of inhibitory control.[4]

Vertigo represents the inappropriate sense or hallucination of motion and is related to dysfunction of the vestibular system. Although morphologic development of the vestibular system is complete by term gestation,[5] studies of the development of postural balance suggest that functional maturation of the vestibular system is ongoing during childhood and adolescence. (See article by O'Reilly and colleagues in this publication.) For example, Steindl and colleagues[6] used the Sensory Organization Test to measure postural stability in 140 children aged 3.5 to 16 years without known peripheral or central vestibular, proprioceptive, or visual disorders or medications that could affect balance. They observed increasing maturation of the vestibular afferent system up to 16 years of age. However, in contrast to a prior study[7] that suggested that vestibular development was not complete by 16 years of age, Steindl and colleagues[6] observed reduced vestibular influence on postural control in adults as compared with the 15- to 16-year-old age groups. Cumberworth and colleagues[8] suggested that the late functional development of the vestibular system as compared with the somatosensory and visual control of balance may explain differential rates of motion sickness in children and adolescents as compared with adults.

VERTIGO AND DIZZINESS IN THE ADOLESCENT

Vertigo and dizziness are not synonymous with each other, although they are often used interchangeably. Individuals with vertigo will often complain of a rotational or room-spinning sensation. They may feel as though they are on a carousel or bobbing in a boat. Nausea and vomiting are often associated complaints. True vertigo implies an equilibrium disturbance associated with the dysfunction of either the central or peripheral vestibular system. In contrast, dizziness may be used by patients to describe a distorted perception of the environment[9] associated with etiologies that range from true vertigo to presyncope to somatoform disorders. The majority of adults who presented to emergency departments (ED) in the United States between 1993 and 2005 with a chief complaint of dizziness did not have a vestibular disorder and were diagnosed with cardiovascular, neurologic, or metabolic/toxic illnesses.[10]

Complaints of dizziness and vertigo are common in the general population, occurring more frequently in women and those older than 60 years.[11] In a review of National Hospital Ambulatory Medical Care Survey data of persons who presented to the ED with a chief complaint that included vertigo/dizziness or the final diagnosis of a vestibular disorder, 16- to 19-year-old patients represented the smallest fraction.[10] In contrast, population-based studies suggest that episodic vertigo and dizziness may be more common during adolescence than suggested by the ED data. Russell and Abu-Arafeh[12] provided a screening questionnaire to 2165 children ranging in age from 5 to 15 years who attended school in the city of Aberdeen, Scotland. Of the children surveyed, 314 (14%) reported at least 1 episode of dizziness in the previous year and 92 children (4%) reported 3 or more episodes of dizziness. Although complaints of dizziness occurred at all ages in this study, it was more common in adolescents, with a peak onset at 12 years of age. More recently, Niemensivu and colleagues,[13] based on prospective polling of children and adolescents ranging in age from 1 to 15 years, found that 8% (75 of 938) experienced an episode of vertigo or dizziness at some point during their life, predominantly between 11 to 15 years of age. These studies and future studies that attempt to define the true prevalence of vertigo and dizziness during childhood and adolescence have multiple potential cofounders including the difficulty young children and adolescents may have in accurately describing their symptoms, the complaint may resolve quickly and thus be disregarded by the adolescent or their family, the family may disregard the complaint, and the vertigo or dizziness may be reported by the adolescent or family as clumsiness.[14]

Vertigo and dizziness during adolescence can be the presenting symptom, or more typically, are part of a complex of symptoms in a wide range of disorders that includes viral illnesses and intracranial tumors (**Box 1**). In a hospital-based study, Fried[15] reviewed the medical records of all admissions to the Boston City Hospital for the

---

Box 1
Common etiologies for vertigo and dizziness in adolescents

- Most common

  Migraine

  Migraine equivalent with benign paroxysmal vertigo of childhood being much more common in children than adolescents

  Psychogenic

  Viral infections or otitis media

- Common

  Chronic daily headache

  Trauma

  Postural orthostatic tachycardia syndrome

- Less common

  Intracranial tumor

  Epilepsy

  Meniere's disease

  Benign paroxysmal positional vertigo

  Vestibular neuritis

  Demyelinating disease

12-month period that spanned July 1976 to June 1977. The majority of adolescents admitted for dizziness during this time period had experienced a concussion (4 of 9). In contrast, retrospective reviews of outpatient medical records of adolescents evaluated in either neurology or otolaryngology clinics[13,14,16–18] consistently report migraine headaches and benign paroxysmal vertigo of childhood (BPVC) as the most common causes of vertigo and dizziness in adolescents and children. For example, Weisleder and Fife[19] reviewed the charts of 31 children and adolescents ranging in age from 6 to 17 years who were referred for vestibular testing at a tertiary care center over a 6-year period. The majority (n = 11; 35%) were diagnosed with vestibular migraine. Other diagnoses included benign paroxysmal vertigo of childhood (n = 6; 20%), anxiety attacks (n = 3; 10%), Ménière's disease (n = 2), idiopathic sudden-onset sensorineural hearing loss (n = 1), familial vertigo/ataxia syndrome (episodic ataxia type II, n = 1), and malingering (n = 1).

In addition to migraine headaches, these clinic-based studies have consistently observed a high incidence of depression and somatoform disorders among children and adolescents evaluated in these specialty clinics for complaints of vertigo or dizziness. For example, Ketola and colleagues[20] reported that psychogenic vertigo accounted for 8% (9 of 119) of children and adolescents with the chief complaint of vertigo who were evaluated at the Otolaryngologic Clinic of Helsinki University Central Hospital between the years of 2000 and 2004. Following psychiatric consultation, 3 children (aged 10 to almost 13 years) were diagnosed with depression; 1 adolescent (age 13.5 years) was diagnosed with a combination of conversion disorder, hyperventilation, and depression; 1 adolescent (age 15.6 years) was diagnosed with psychotic episode and depression; and the other 4 children (aged 9–11 years) were diagnosed with psychogenic headache, obsessive-compulsive disorder, panic disorder, and conversion disorder, respectively. Compared with those children and adolescents who were identified as having an organic cause for the vertigo, this group of children and adolescents had more frequent attacks or a complaint of constant vertigo, were more likely to suffer from school absenteeism, and were more likely to have dysfunctional relationships at school or at home. In addition, Emiroglu and colleagues[21] found that 29 (93.5%) of 31 subjects who presented to a pediatric neurology clinic for complaints of dizziness, headache, or fainting met criteria of the *Diagnostic and Statistical Manual of Mental Disorders (DSM-IV)* for a psychiatric comorbidity, even when the primary diagnosis was migraine headache.

Not all cases of vertigo and dizziness in the adolescent are likely to be referred for specialty clinic evaluation. Therefore, multiple causes of dizziness are likely to be underreported in neurology and otolaryngology clinic-based studies of vertigo and dizziness in the adolescent. For example, complaints of vertigo or dizziness in the setting of concussion is likely to be principally managed by the pediatrician[22]; the child with dizziness in the setting of syncope or presyncope may be managed by the pediatrician or is more likely to be referred to a cardiologist than to a neurologist or to an otolaryngologist for further management, and the child with a brain tumor is most likely to be managed by the oncologist and neurosurgeon.

DIAGNOSIS AND TREATMENT OF SPECIFIC CAUSES OF VERTIGO IN THE ADOLESCENT
Migraine

Upwards of 30% of adolescent girls experience migraine headaches[23,24]; and along with variants, migraines are the most common episodic disorder of childhood with an estimated prevalence of 5% to 10%.[25] Migraine and benign paroxysmal vertigo of childhood, considered by many to be a migraine variant in younger children,[26] account for 50% to 75% of children who present to specialty clinics with vertigo and normal eardrums; migraine frequency increases and BPVC frequency decreases with age[16,17] (see article by McCaslin and colleagues in this publication).

The vertigo associated with migraine may precede the headache (aura), may be part of the headache itself, or may not be temporally related to the headache in up to 60% of individuals.[17] Furthermore, vertigo is a well-established manifestation of basilar migraines, which also have associated complaints of ataxia, dysarthria, tinnitus, and visual changes. The vertigo associated with these headaches is often brief and frequently accompanied by nausea and vomiting.[19]

The pathophysiology of vertigo in migraines is poorly understood. Unilateral neuronal instability of the peripheral vestibular nerve, idiopathic asymmetric activation of the brainstem vestibular nuclei, and vasospasm causing transient ischemia of the labyrinth or central vestibular pathways have all been suggested.[19] Electronystagmography is often abnormal and demonstrates central findings in adults and children with basilar migraines, even between attacks[14,27] (see article by Cherchi and Hain in this publication).

Before making the diagnosis of migraine headache in the adolescent who is being evaluated for complaints of headache and vertigo, episodic ataxia type 2 (EA-2; previously known as familial cerebellar ataxia without myokymia, hereditary paroxysmal cerebellar ataxia, periodic vestibulocerebellar ataxia, and acetazolamide-responsive episodic ataxia) should be considered (see article by Cherchi in this publication). This rare autosomal dominant disorder is the result of a spectrum of mutations that affect *CACNA1A*,[28] the gene that encodes the α1A subunit of P/Q type calcium channels ($Ca_V2.1$) located on chromosome 19p. Missense mutations of this same gene are linked to familial hemiplegic migraine,[29] and a CAG expansion of exon 47 has been linked to spinocerebellar ataxia type 6.[30] EA-2 is characterized by episodic attacks that last from hours to days and can be precipitated by stress or exercise as well as caffeine and alcohol. Many features of the attack can overlap those of migraine headache: headache, which is typically occipital in location,[31] vertigo, nausea, and vomiting. Indeed, most people with EA-2 also meet the International Headache Society's diagnostic criteria for migraine.[32] Distinguishing features during the attack are the presence of concurrent ataxia and nystagmus as well as the strong family history consistent with autosomal dominant inheritance. During the attack, dysarthria, diplopia, tinnitus, dystonia, and hemiplegia may also be present. Onset is typically before the 20 years of age with a range from 2 to 61 years.[31,33,34] Of interest, a large percentage of individuals with EA-2 develop ataxia and nystagmus in the interictal periods, and atrophy of the cerebellar vermis has been observed on MRI.[35] An important reason to recognize this syndrome early is that acetazolamide has been shown to be effective in reducing the frequency of attacks[36] that are typically rare but have been reported as often as 4 times per week.[37]

Treatment of migraine headaches is divided into abortive and prophylactic therapies. For those with vertigo as the manifestation of their migraine without significant headache, management with antimotion sickness medications, such as scopolamine, has been proposed to provide symptomatic relief.[38] The American Academy of Neurology (AAN) guidelines for acute treatment of migraines in children and adolescents report level A evidence for sumatriptan nasal.[39] Nonsteroidals, triptans, or indomethacin should be used in place of medications with caffeine, barbiturates, or opiates as these are less likely to cause medication overuse.[40] Dihydroergotamine, intravenous valproate, or steroids have also been used for the abortive treatment of severe migraine headaches that have not responded to other outpatient treatments.[40–42]

If the migraines are frequent or disabling (ie, affecting school performance) then a prophylactic agent should be considered. Calcium channel blockers, beta-blockers, antiepiletpics, such as topirimate and valproate, or tricyclic antidepressants (eg, amitriptyline) have all been shown to be efficacious as migraine prophylaxis,[14] although the AAN guidelines report insufficient evidence to make formal recommendations for the adolescent.[39] One month at a therapeutic dose, if tolerated, should be attempted before altering therapy.

CHRONIC DAILY HEADACHES

In contrast to people with migraine headaches who will often describe true vertigo, a more general sense of dizziness is a common complaint of adolescents with chronic daily headache. Chronic daily headaches are defined as headaches lasting longer than 4 hours per day, for more than 15 days per month, for longer than 3 months without underlying pathology.[43] Prevalence studies estimate that 2% to 4% of adolescent girls and 0.8% to 2.0% of adolescent boys[44,45] suffer from chronic daily headache. A total of 75% of these patients have a history of episodic migraines, and the other 25% have suffered a recent viral illness or minor head trauma.[40] Diffuse weakness, unsteadiness, and visual changes frequently characterized as blurry vision in both eyes are common associated symptoms. The dizziness often worsens with changes in position, especially when getting out of bed in the morning, and syncope or near syncope can occur. Mood disorders are almost uniformly seen in adolescents who suffer from chronic daily headaches, and treating one may not always alleviate the other (ie, treatments for chronic daily headaches likely will not work if the mood disorder goes untreated).[40]

Indeed, chronic daily headaches are often more difficult to treat than episodic migraine headaches, and comorbidities, such as sleep disturbances, mood disorders, and medication overuse, make them even more challenging. Headaches may take weeks to months to improve. Patient (and parent) frustrations are common and can be confounding. Like migraine headaches, treatment is also divided between abortive and prophylactic medications,[40] with even less evidence of efficacy in the adolescent population. Amitriptyline has demonstrated safety and efficacy as a prophylactic agent in the treatment of chronic daily headaches in children, although higher doses may be needed than for migraine prevention.[40,46] Amitriptyline is also helpful in improving sleep onset, which is a common comorbidity. Cardiac side effects, such as prolongation of the QT interval, weight gain, and sedation, should be closely monitored.[40] Fluoxetine is the only selective serotonin reuptake inhibitor approved for the treatment of mood disorders in children, and may be an effective prophylactic treatment for chronic daily headaches.[47] However, for adolescents who take this medication, there is an increased risk of suicidal thoughts and suicidal attempts, and caution should be used when it is combined with tricyclics, as they are both metabolized through the same pathways leading to higher drug levels and more serious side effects, including the risk of serotonin syndrome.[40]

Nonpharmacologic methods should be included in treatment of both migraine headaches and chronic daily headaches. Headache diaries to help determine triggers are invaluable. Psychological consultation for biofeedback and treatment of underlying mood disorders,[48] and physical therapy evaluation for reintroduction of physical activity are helpful adjunctive treatments. Awareness of seasonal variations and effects on school performance also need to be addressed.[40]

POSTURAL ORTHOSTATIC TACHYCARDIA SYNDROME

Although postural orthostatic tachycardia syndrome (POTS) was not identified as a common cause of vertigo or dizziness in the specialty clinic-based studies previously cited, the majority of persons with this disorder do complain of dizziness.[49] This disorder of orthostatic intolerance affects mainly young women and is characterized by multiple complaints, including dizziness, headache, and fatigue as well as nausea, palpitations, diaphoresis, tachypnea, and diffuse weakness that occurs upon standing and is relieved by sitting or lying down.

Onset is often in the early teen years, can be preceded by an illness, and may have a monophasic or relapsing-remitting course.[50] Adolescents within 1 to 3 years of their growth spurt, who are unable to return to normal activity after suffering a minor illness or injury that may be prolonged and lead to a period of immobility, seem susceptible to POTS. When they attempt to return to normal activity, they become symptomatic when trying to stand upright.[51]

The etiologic cause of POTS is poorly understood. It is diagnosed more frequently in patients with hyperextensible joints and cellular matrix protein disorders (eg, Ehlers-Danlos) suggesting an abnormality in smooth muscle response to the autonomic nervous system.[52,53] The coincidence with puberty in adolescent girls suggests a hormonal influence, and at least 1 gene mutation in norepinephrine transport protein deficiency also implicates a genetic component.[51,54] As chronic fatigue is a frequent comorbidity in patients with POTS, chronic infections with viruses, such as Epstein-Barr virus and enterovirus, have been proposed as triggering events,[55] and antibodies to ganglionic acetylcholine receptors suggest an autoimmune cause.[56]

The differential diagnosis of those that present with autonomic dysfunction suggestive of POTS includes undiagnosed diabetes, autoimmune disorders (systemic lupus erythematosus or Sjögren syndrome), eating disorders with volume depletion, anemia, paraneoplastic syndromes, and medication effects.[57] Evaluation should include basic laboratory testing, a neurology consultation with electroencephalography to rule out seizures, and a cardiology consultation to evaluate for arrhythmias.[51]

The pathophysiological mechanism of POTS is likely related to improper interactions between carotid baroreceptors and chemoreceptors leading to reduced blood flow to the brain and the brain's ability to cope with changes in respiratory rate. When changing from a supine or sitting position to standing, there is an immediate decrease in venous return to the heart from the downward shift of blood in the legs. Under normal physiology, this is compensated for by an increase in heart rate and blood pressure. Blood is then redistributed to the vital organs by splanchnic and peripheral vasoconstriction, leading to normalization of blood distribution and therefore heart rate and blood pressure. Patients who suffer from POTS, however, are not able to achieve adequate venous return despite physiologic increases in heart rate. Therefore, their heart rate continues to increase without the appropriate elevation in blood pressure.[51,58]

Treatment is first geared toward the idea that patients with POTS suffer from relative hypovolemia with recommendations to drink at least 2 L of water daily. Studies have shown that 24-hour urine sodium excretion of less than 100 mEq is indicative of dehydration[56]; whereas, greater than 170 mEq should be satisfactory to adequately compensate for the hypovolemic state.[59] Aside from drinking more water, these patients also benefit from increased salt intake, which repletes their intravascular volume. Recommended intake is greater than 200 mEq of sodium daily, which, if unable to be accomplished by salting foods, can be supplemented with salt tablets.[51,57]

Beta-blockers can be used to minimize the acceleration in heart rate with the change in position and inappropriate relaxation of blood vessels. One study reported that more than 90% of subjects felt better after starting a low-dose beta-blocker,[60] although they should be closely monitored after starting treatment because overdosing can lead to fatigue.[57] Alpha-1 agonists, such as midodrine, increase peripheral vascular resistance and may be beneficial. However, frequent dosing is needed and compliance may be an issue when treating adolescent patients.[57] Supine hypertension is a significant side effect, and doses should be avoided before prolonged recumbency such as sleep.[51]

Synthetic mineralocorticoids, such as fludrocortisone, act on the distal renal tubules to enhance sodium reuptake and expand intravascular volume and have been used as adjuvant treatment in POTS. Little evidence, however, is present to support its efficacy in adolescents.[51,58,61]

OTHER CAUSES OF VERTIGO OR DIZZINESS IN THE ADOLESCENT

Viral labyrinthitis may be the cause of vertigo in up to 20% of children younger than 16 years.[14] Epilepsy is a rare cause of vertigo in children and adolescents and is often associated with altered awareness. Ménière's disease, vertigo typically accompanied by unilateral hearing loss and tinnitus, is also a rare cause of vertigo in this age group.[14] Benign paroxysmal positional vertigo, Meniere's disease, and otitis media are addressed in other articles (see articles by Cho and White, Semaan and Megerian, and McCaslin and colleagues in this publication).

CAUSES OF VERTIGO OR DIZZINESS IN THE ADOLESCENT REQUIRING HEAD IMAGING

Adolescents who complain of dizziness or vertigo should undergo extensive neurologic and neurotologic evaluation to assure the absence of intracranial masses or other treatable causes.[17] Despite extensive evaluation, a proportion of individuals are not diagnosed with a specific etiologic cause for their complaints.[14,16,17,19]

With their propensity for risk-taking behavior, adolescents commonly suffer head trauma and concussion. Those adolescents with a recent history of head trauma and new onset vertigo (with or without headache) should be imaged to assess for the presence of skull fracture. Although CT is superior to MRI in detecting fractures, MRI should be considered in this patient population to assess for intracranial abnormalities that may not be apparent on CT, such as diffuse axonal injury that can occur after high-speed collisions.[62] Magnetic resonance angiography may also be helpful in the setting of trauma to evaluate for the presence of cervical artery dissection. Even in the absence of a visualized fracture on CT, microscopic hemorrhages in the labyrinth, known as labyrinthine concussions, may be implicated as a cause of vertigo.[63]

Intracranial mass lesions (eg, demyelinating plaques and neoplasms) are an uncommon cause of vertigo and dizziness in the adolescent. In one series of 87 subjects aged between 0 and 16 years, a new neuroimaging abnormality accounted for vertigo in only 25% of cases; 38% had old abnormalities that were not attributed to the cause of vertigo, and 57% had normal neuroimaging. For those subjects who complained of vertigo alone without a history of trauma, neuroimaging did not contribute to the diagnosis.[62] For those with an abnormality, the neurologic examination (usually a cranial nerve deficit) was abnormal in more than 80%, and the other 20% of subjects had new-onset intense headache. Abnormalities seen in those subjects older than 12 years included skull fractures, benign brain tumors, demyelinating disease, and shunt malfunctions.[62] Although uncommon, cerebellar or brainstem tumors (medulloblastomas being the most common, but also astrocytomas, ependymomas, and hemangioblastomas) are also in the differential diagnosis for adolescents who present with vertigo. These patients also usually complain of headaches and signs of increased intracranial pressure, such as papilledema, cranial

---

Box 2
What not to miss: red flags to consider brain imaging in the adolescent with a complaint of vertigo or dizziness

- History

    Head trauma with new-onset vertigo with or without headache

    Associated complaints of double vision, difficulty swallowing, slurred speech, changes in vision, facial numbness: all concerning for cranial nerve deficits

    Difficulty with coordination

    New-onset severe headache

    Progressive symptoms of vertigo

    Episodes of loss of consciousness

    Altered mental status

    History of intracranial abnormality

- Examination

    Papilledema

    Cranial nerve deficits

    Weakness or ataxia

    Sensory deficits

deficits, and gait ataxia, observed on neurologic examination should prompt further evaluation with neuroimaging. Patients of all ages with vestibular schwannomas (acoustic neuromas) rarely report true vertigo, but the combination of imbalance and unilateral sensorineural hearing loss and tinnitus warrant further investigation.[14] Neuroimaging should be seriously considered in all adolescents with a history of trauma, an abnormal neurologic examination, persistent headaches (**Box 2**),[62] and in those whose vestibular testing is concerning for a central lesion.[14]

In those adolescents who have normal examinations and the clinical suspicion for a mass lesion is low, MRI can still be useful in providing families with significant reassurance. It relays to them that their child's complaints are being taken seriously and may go far in strengthening the doctor-patient relationship. As discussed, the cause of dizziness in adolescents is often entwined with an underlying psychological disorder, and parents may be more receptive to pursuing these diagnoses if other causes, especially intracranial mass lesions, have been thoroughly evaluated and excluded.

SUMMARY

Dizziness is an uncommon complaint in adolescent patients. Migraine headache is the most common cause of dizziness in adolescents but must be differentiated from episodic ataxia type II, chronic daily headaches, and postural orthostatic tachycardia syndrome. Other less common causes include vestibular neuritis, Meniere's disease, head trauma or traumatic brain injury, intracranial mass lesions, and psychogenic causes. Evaluation is primarily geared toward careful history and physical examination. Primary vestibular disorders are rare in adolescents, and treatment of the more common causes of dizziness in the adolescent may involve some trial and error. Imaging is indicated for new onset of neurologic deficit, change in mental status, or severe headache.

REFERENCES

1. Casey BJ, Getz S, Galvan A. The adolescent brain. Dev Rev 2008;28:62–77.
2. Toga AW, Thompson PM, Sowell ER. Mapping brain maturation. Trends Neurosci 2006;29:148–59.
3. Galvan A, Hare TA, Parra CE, et al. Earlier development of the accumbens relative to orbitofrontal cortex might underlie risk-taking behavior in adolescents. J Neurosci 2006;26:6885–92.
4. Liston C, Watts R, Tottenham N, et al. Frontostriatal microstructure modulates efficient recruitment of cognitive control. Cereb Cortex 2005;16:553–60.
5. Blayney AW, Colman BH. Dizziness in childhood. Clin Otolaryngol 1984;9:77–85.
6. Steindl R, Kunz K, Schrott-Fischer A, et al. Effect of age and sex on maturation of sensory systems and balance control. Dev Med Child Neurol 2006;48:477–82.
7. Hirabayashi S, Iwasaki Y. Developmental perspective of sensory organization on postural control. Brain Dev 1995;17:111–3.
8. Cumberworth VL, Patel NN, Rogers W, et al. The maturation of balance in children. J Laryngol Otol 2007;121:449–54.
9. Eviatar L. Dizziness in children. Pediatr Otol 1994;27(3):557–71.
10. Newman-Toker DE, Hsieh YH, Camargo CA, et al. Spectrum of dizziness visits to the US emergency departments: cross-sectional analysis from a nationally representative sample. Mayo Clin Proc 2008;83:765–75.
11. Neuhauser HK, von Brevern M, Radtke A, et al. Epidemiology of vestibular vertigo: a neurotologic survey of the general population. Neurology 2005;65: 898–904.

12. Russell G, Abu-Arafeh I. Paroxysmal vertigo in children – an epidemiological study. Int J Pediatr Otorhinolaryngol 1999;45:S105–7.
13. Neimensivu R, Pyykko I, Wiener-Vacher SR, et al. Vertigo and balance problems in children – an epidemiological study in Finland. Int J Pediatr Otorhinolaryngol 2006;70:259–65.
14. Balatsouras DG, Kaberos A, Assimakopoulos D, et al. Etiology of vertigo in children. Int J Pediatr Otorhinolaryngol 2007;71:487–94.
15. Fried MP. The evaluation of dizziness in children. Laryngoscope 1980;90: 1548–60.
16. Choung YH, Park K, Moon SK, et al. Various causes and clinical characteristics in vertigo in children with normal eardrums. Int J Pediatr Otorhinolaryngol 2003;67: 889–94.
17. Erbek SH, Erbek SS, Yilmaz I, et al. Vertigo in childhood: a clinical experience. Int J Pediatr Otorhinolaryngol 2006;70:1547–54.
18. Szirmai A. Vestibular disorders in childhood and adolescents. Eur Arch Otorhinolaryngol 2010;267(11):1801–4.
19. Weisleder P, Fife TD. Dizziness and headache: a common association in children and adolescents. J Child Neurol 2001;16:727–30.
20. Ketola S, Niemensivu R, Henttonen A, et al. Somatoform disorders in vertiginous children and adolescents. Int J Pediatr Otorhinolaryngol 2009;73: 933–6.
21. Emiroğlu FN, Kurul S, Akay A, et al. Assessment of child neurology outpatients with headache, dizziness, and fainting. J Child Neurol 2004;19(5):332–6.
22. Kaye AJ, Gallagher R, Callahan JM, et al. Mild traumatic brain injury in the pediatric population: the role of the pediatrician in routine follow-up. J Trauma 2010; 68:1396–400.
23. Abu-Arafeh I, Russell G. Prevalence of headache and migraine in schoolchildren. BMJ 1994;309:765–9.
24. Aromaa M, Sillanpaa ML, Rautava P. Childhood headache at school entry: a controlled clinical study. Neurology 1998;50:1729–36.
25. Parker C. Complicated migraine syndromes and migraine variants. Pediatr Ann 1997;26:417–21.
26. Mira E, Piacentino G, Lanzi G. Benign paroxysmal vertigo in childhood: a migraine equivalent. ORL J Otorhinolaryngol Relat Spec 1984;46:97–104.
27. Dieterich M, Brandt T. Episodic vertigo related to migraine (90 cases): vestibular migraine? J Neurol 1999;246:883–92.
28. Jen J, Kim GW, Baloh RW. Clinical spectrum of episodic ataxia type 2. Neurology 2004;62:17–22.
29. Ducros A, Denier C, Joutel A, et al. The clinical spectrum of familial hemiplegic migraine associated with mutations in a neuronal calcium channel. N Engl J Med 2001;345:17–24.
30. Zhuchenko O, Baily J, Bonnen P, et al. Autosomal dominant cerebellar ataxia (SCA6) associated with small polyglutamine expansions in the alpha 1A-voltage-dependent calcium channel. Nat Genet 1997;15:62–9.
31. Baloh RW, Yue Q, Furman JM, et al. Familial episodic ataxia: clinical heterogeneity in four families linked to chromosome 19p. Ann Neurol 1997;41:8–16.
32. Olsen J. Migraine classification and diagnosis. International Headache Society criteria. Neurology 1994;44:S6–10.
33. Farmer TW, Mustian VM. Vestibulocerebellar ataxia. Arch Neurol 1963;8:471–80.
34. Imbrici P, Eunson LH, Graves TD, et al. Late-onset episodic ataxia type 2 due to an in-frame insertion in CACNAIA. Neurology 2005;27:944–6.

35. Vighetto A, Froment JC, Trillet M, et al. Magnetic resonance imaging in familial paroxysmal ataxia. Arch Neurol 1988;45:547–9.
36. Griggs RC, Moxley RT 3rd, Lafrance RA, et al. Hereditary paroxysmal ataxia: response to acetazolamide. Neurology 1978;28:1259–64.
37. Von Brederlow B, Hahn AF, Koopman WJ, et al. Mapping the gene for acetazol-amide responsive hereditary paroxysmal cerebellar ataxia to chromosome 19p. Hum Mol Genet 1995;4:279–84.
38. Cass SP, Furman JM, Ankerstjerne K, et al. Migraine related vestibulopathy. Ann Otol Rhinol Laryngol 1997;106:182–9.
39. Lewis D, Ashwal S, Hershey A, et al. Practice parameter: pharmacological treatment of migraine headache in children and adolescents. Report of the American Academy of Neurology Quality Standards Subcommittee and the Practice Committee of the Child Neurology Society. Neurology 2004;63:2215–24.
40. Mack KJ. Episodic and chronic migraine in children. Semin Neurol 2006;26: 226–31. Neuhauser HK, Lempert T. Vertigo: epidemiologic aspects. Semin Neurol 2009;29:473–81.
41. Raskin NH. Repetitive intravenous ergotamine therapy for the treatment of intractable migraine. Neurology 1986;34:497–502.
42. Schwartz TH, Karpitskiy VV, Sohn RS. Intravenous valproate sodium in the treatment of daily headache. Headache 2002;42:519–22.
43. Headache Classification Subcommittee of the International Headache Society. International classification of headache disorders (ICHD-II). Cephalalgia 2004; 24(Suppl 1):23–136.
44. Wang SJ, Fuh JL, Lu SR, et al. Chronic daily headache in adolescents: prevalence, impact, and medication overuse. Neurology 2006;66:193–7.
45. Kavuk I, Yavuz A, Cetindere U, et al. Epidemiology of chronic daily headaches. Eur J Med Res 2003;8:236–40.
46. Hershey AD, Powers SW, Bentti AL, et al. Effectiveness of amitriptyline in the prophylactic management of childhood headaches. Headache 2000;40:539–49.
47. Saper JR, Silberstain SD, Lake AE III, et al. Double-blind trial of fluoxetine: chronic daily headache and migraine. Headache 1994;34:497–502.
48. Galli F, Patron L, Russo PM, et al. Chronic daily headache in childhood and adolescence: clinical aspects and a 4-year follow-up. Cephalalgia 2004;24:850–8.
49. Fischer PR, Brands CK, Porter CJ, et al. High prevalence of orthostatic intolerance in adolescents in a general pediatric referral clinic. Clin Auton Res 2005; 15:340.
50. Stewart JM. Chronic orthostatic intolerance and the postural tachycardia syndrome. J Pediatr 2004;145:725–30.
51. Johnson JN, Mack KJ, Kuntz NL, et al. Postural orthostatic tachycardia syndrome: a clinical review. Pediatr Neurol 2010;42:77–85.
52. Gazit Y, Nahir AM, Grahame R, et al. Dysautonomia in the joint hypermobility syndrome. Am J Med 2003;115:33–40.
53. Rowe PC, Barron DR, Calkins H, et al. Orthostatic intolerance and chronic fatigue syndrome associated with Ehlers-Danlos syndrome. J Pediatr 1999;135:494–9.
54. Shannon JR, Flatten NL, Jordan J, et al. Orthostatic intolerance and tachycardia associated with norepinephrine-transporter deficiency. N Engl J Med 2000;342: 541–9.
55. Chia JK, Chia AY. Chronic fatigue syndrome is associated with chronic enterovirus infection of the stomach. J Clin Pathol 2008;61:43–8.
56. Thieben MR, Sandroni P, Sletten DM, et al. Postural orthostatic tachycardia syndrome: the Mayo clinic experience. Mayo Clin Proc 2007;82:308–13.

57. Kanjwal MY, Kosinksi DJ, Grubb BP. Treatment of postural orthostatic tachycardia syndromes and inappropriate sinus tachycardia. Curr Cardiol Rep 2003;5:402–6.

58. Medow MS, Stewart JM. The Postural Tachycardia Syndrome. Cardiol Rev 2007; 15:67–75.

59. El-Sayed H, Hainsworth R. Salt supplement increases plasma volume and orthostatic intolerance in patients with unexplained syncope. Hear 1996;75:134–40.

60. Lai CC, Fischer PR, Brands CK, et al. Outcomes in adolescents with postural tachycardia syndrome treated with midodrine and beta-blockers. Pacing Clin Electrophysiol 2009;32:234–8.

61. Jacob G, Shannon JR, Black B, et al. Effects of volume loading and pressor agents in idiopathic orthostatic tachycardia. Circulation 1997;96:575–80.

62. Neimensivu R, Pyykko I, Valanne L, et al. Value of imaging studies in vertiginous children. Int J Pediatr Otorhinolaryngol 2006;70(9):1639–44.

63. Davies RA, Luxon LM. Dizziness following head injury: a neuro-otological study. J Neurol 1995;242:222–30.

Head Injury and Blast Exposure: Vestibular Consequences

Faith W. Akin, PhD[a,b,*], Owen D. Murnane, PhD[a,b]

KEYWORDS

- Dizziness • Traumatic brain injury • Blast injuries
- Vestibular function tests • Saccule and utricle
- Postural balance • Vestibular labyrinth

It is well established that head injury can result in symptoms of vertigo, dizziness, and imbalance, and the symptoms are often related to vestibular dysfunction. Robert Bárány[1] observed vestibular symptoms from head injuries in soldiers in a Russian prisoner-of-war camp during the World War I. Caveness and Nielson[2] evaluated 407 Korean conflict veterans with head injury and found that 56% complained of giddiness (dizziness) and vertigo. In recent wars, many soldiers have been exposed to blasts from improvised explosive devices (IEDs) or roadside bombs, and traumatic brain injury (TBI) has been called the signature condition of combat veterans returning from Iraq and Afghanistan. Postconcussive symptoms related to vestibular dysfunction include vertigo, dizziness, and imbalance, and reports indicate that the incidence of dizziness or imbalance secondary to mild TBI (mTBI) ranges from 24% to 83%.[3–5] Numerous studies have demonstrated that vestibular symptoms often last for 6 months or longer after the head trauma.[6,7] In fact, the presence of dizziness 6 months

This work was supported by the Merit Review grants and by the Auditory and Vestibular Dysfunction Research Enhancement Award Program. All funding was sponsored by the Rehabilitation Research and Development Service, Department of Veterans Affairs, Washington, DC.

The contents of this publication do not represent the views of the Department of Veterans Affairs or the United States Government.

[a] Vestibular/Balance Laboratory, Audiology Service, Veterans Affairs Medical Center, Mountain Home, TN 37684, USA

[b] Department of Audiology and Speech Pathology, East Tennessee State University, TN 37614, USA

* Corresponding author. Department of Audiology and Speech Pathology, East Tennessee State University, TN 37614.

E-mail address: faith.akin@va.gov

Otolaryngol Clin N Am 44 (2011) 323–334
doi:10.1016/j.otc.2011.01.005
0030-6665/11/$ – see front matter. Published by Elsevier Inc.

after injury is an adverse prognostic indicator and may be the most persistent symptom of mTBI that adversely affects clinical outcome as well as disease course.[8,9]

The definition of TBI has not been consistent and tends to vary according to medical specialties and circumstances. The terms *brain injury* and *head injury* have been used synonymously, although not all injuries to the head result in TBI, and previously the term *concussion* has been used synonymously with mTBI. In an effort to develop a common definition of TBI, the Department of Defense/Veterans Affairs (DoD/VA) Definition and Symptomatic Taxonomy Working Group[10] and other joint consensus panels recently defined TBI as "a traumatically induced structural injury and/or physiologic disruption of brain function as a result of an external force that is indicated by new onset or worsening of at least one of the following clinical signs immediately following the event:

1. Any period of loss of or a decreased level of consciousness
2. Any loss of memory for events immediately before or after the injury
3. Any alteration in mental state at the time of the injury (confusion, disorientation, slowed thinking, etc.)
4. Neurologic deficits (weakness, loss of balance, change in vision, praxis, paresis/plegia, sensory loss, aphasia, etc.) that may or may not be transient
5. Intracranial lesion."

The DoD/VA definition of mTBI is

1. Normal structural imaging
2. Loss of consciousness for 0 to 30 minutes
3. Alteration of consciousness/mental state for a moment to 24 hours
4. Posttraumatic amnesia for 0 to 1 day
5. Glasgow Coma scale, 13 to 15.

mTBI in combat veterans is often related to blast exposure; thus, the same insult that produces TBI can cause trauma to the inner ear. A blast is caused by the detonation of an explosive (eg, IED) that causes a peak positive pressurization (shock wave) followed in time by a negative pressurization. In a typical blast, the positive pressure phase is initially faster than the speed of sound (5 m/s and very brief) with pressure ranging from hundreds to thousands of lb/in^2. The negative pressure phase occurs immediately after the peak pressure wave and is longer in duration and slower in velocity (30 m/s).[11] Primary blast injuries resulting from the impact of the shock wave affect air- and fluid-filled organs such as the lungs and sensory structures of the middle and inner portions of the ears. Secondary blast injuries can result from flying debris and bomb fragments, and tertiary blast injuries can result from the impact with another object when thrown by a blast wind. In general, the severity of blast injury is reduced the farther away the victim is from the blast.

Otologic injuries caused by blast exposure include tympanic membrane perforations, hearing loss, tinnitus, and otalgia. Dizziness and imbalance also can occur after blast exposure,[12,13] and damage to the vestibular sensory organs has been described in blast survivors.[14] With the exception of benign paroxysmal positional vertigo (BPPV), which is attributed directly to the effects of the blast, some investigators have presumed that dizziness and balance disorders following blast exposure are related to central nervous system (CNS) damage caused by the TBI rather than peripheral vestibular system damage from the blast pressure wave.[11,15] Consequently, most studies have focused on the effect of head trauma or TBI, and there has been little investigation on the effect of blast exposure on peripheral vestibular function.

HORIZONTAL SEMICIRCULAR CANAL FUNCTION

The vestibular system is composed of 2 types of sensory organs (the semicircular canals and the otolith organs) that contribute to gaze and postural stability. Three semicircular canals (superior, posterior, and horizontal) are positioned orthogonally to each other to sense rotational head movement or angular acceleration in the yaw, pitch, and roll planes. For example, the purpose of the horizontal semicircular canals is to provide sensory input to the vestibuloocular reflex (VOR) regarding head rotation in the yaw (horizontal) plane. The primary goal of the semicircular canals is to provide input via the VOR for gaze stability when the head is in motion. The horizontal VOR, therefore, contributes to gaze stability when the head is rotated laterally. Clinical tests of horizontal semicircular canal function have been widely available for many years and include the bithermal binaural caloric test and rotational tests. These tests have been the predominant measure of vestibular function in studies examining the effects of head injury on the vestibular system.

It is well established that head injury can result in peripheral vestibular hypofunction (or unilateral weakness on the caloric test),[16] and it is reasonable to presume that peripheral vestibular system abnormalities associated with TBI are likely due to the head injury rather than the resulting brain injury. Reports reveal that the incidence of horizontal semicircular canal (VOR) dysfunction ranges from 32% to 71% in patients with dizziness after head injury. Davies and Luxon[17] performed electronystagmography testing on 100 consecutive patients who experienced dizziness after head injury and reported that 71% had positive vestibular test findings that included abnormal calorics, the presence of spontaneous nystagmus, or both. Similarly, Toglia and colleagues[18] reported a high incidence of abnormal calorics (63%) and spontaneous nystagmus in patients with head injury. In contrast, Gannon and colleagues[19] reported abnormal vestibular findings in 32% of patients with head injury.

A few studies have examined the effect of blast exposure on horizontal semicircular canal function, and the findings have been inconclusive. Shupak and colleagues[12] examined 5 patrol boat crew members who were injured by close-range explosion of a trinitrotoluene device. The investigators reported that 2 crew members had vestibular abnormalities on tests of horizontal canal function (caloric weakness and/or phase lead on rotary chair) and 1 crew member had BPPV and spontaneous nystagmus. In contrast, Cohen and colleagues[6] reported no caloric abnormalities in 7 survivors who complained of dizziness after a suicide terrorist attack on a municipal bus in Israel. Van Campen and colleagues[13] measured vestibular function using the caloric test in 30 survivors of the Oklahoma City Federal Building bombing who had complaints of dizziness or imbalance. Only 2 survivors demonstrated abnormal caloric findings, and 8 had positional/spontaneous nystagmus.

OTOLITH ORGAN FUNCTION

Two otolith organs sense linear acceleration, head tilt, and gravity, with the primary function to provide input for postural stability via the vestibulospinal tract. The otolith organs are composed of the saccule and the utricle that contribute to postural stability by providing sensory input regarding linear acceleration and changes in gravity. In an upright position, the saccule is positioned vertically and senses linear acceleration in the vertical plane. In contrast, the utricle is positioned horizontally (3.5–4 cm from midline) and senses linear acceleration in the lateral plane. Both the utricle and the saccule respond to acceleration in the anterior-posterior plane.

Until recently, tests to measure otolith function have been used experimentally rather than clinically. Experimental methods include the measurement of the otolith-ocular response during stimulation of the otolith organs with linear acceleration using parallel sleds and swings. However, these methods of otolith stimulation are cumbersome and not sensitive to unilateral otolith hypofunction; therefore, their use has been limited to experimental purposes. More recently, research has focused on the development of clinical tests of otolith function. The cervical vestibular evoked myogenic potential (cVEMP) has been established as a clinical test of saccular and/or inferior vestibular nerve function.[20] cVEMPs are short latency electrical potentials evoked by high-level acoustic stimuli recorded from surface electrodes over the tonically contracted sterno-cleidomastoid (SCM) muscle. The cVEMP waveform consists of an early positive-negative component that depends on the integrity of vestibular afferents because it is abolished after vestibular nerve section but preserved in subjects with severe to profound sensorineural hearing loss.[21] The neurophysiological and clinical data indicate that cVEMPs are mediated by an ipsilateral pathway that includes the saccular macula, inferior vestibular nerve, vestibular nucleus, medial vestibulospinal tract, and motoneurons of the SCM muscle.[22]

The subjective visual vertical (SVV) test has been used as a clinical test of utricular function. The SVV angle is the angle between the gravitational axis (true earth vertical) and the position of a visual linear marker adjusted vertically by a subject. The otolith organs contribute to the estimation of the physical vertical orientation, and normal subjects align the SVV angle within 2° of true vertical (0°). Impaired SVV test results have been documented in patients with unilateral vestibular disorders and in patients with central vestibular disorders, such as brainstem and thalamic infarctions.[23] The SVV angle can also be measured during off-axis yaw rotation to the right or left (unilateral centrifugation) to measure ear-specific utricular function and determine chronic (compensated) vestibular dysfunction.[24,25] In individuals with normal vestibular function, the SVV angle tilts symmetrically during unilateral centrifugation. That is, when the subject is positioned to the right side of the axis of rotation, the SVV is tilted toward the left, and when the subject is positioned to the left side of the axis of rotation, the SVV is tilted in a similar magnitude to the right. Patients with chronic unilateral vestibular loss exhibit an SVV asymmetry when measured during off-axis (eccentric) yaw rotation.[25,26] Specifically, when the lesioned ear is centrifuged, the SVV angle does not shift because the utricle does not respond to the gravitoinertial force vector (linear acceleration).[24]

Both circumstantial and direct evidence suggest that otolith function may be compromised by head trauma.

First, Schuknecht and Davison[27] reported damage to the membranous walls of the utricle and saccule and degenerative changes in the saccular macula in a cat after multiple blows to an unrestrained head. The investigators theorized that the linear acceleration and deceleration of the head blow damaged the otolith organs that sense linear acceleration. Similarly, a histologic study of 10 human victims of a bomb blast demonstrated rupture of the saccule and utricle.[11]

Second, numerous studies have determined that BPPV occurs in 10% to 25% of head trauma patients,[17,28,29] and it is presumed that a blow to the head dislodges otoconia from the utricular otolithic membrane, resulting in free-floating particles (otoconia) that produce endolymphatic fluid flow in the semicircular canals (canalithiasis). Davies and Luxon[17] performed audiovestibular testing on 100 consecutive patients with a history of head injury and determined that audiovestibular organs are interdependently vulnerable to trauma, but the otolith organs are the most vulnerable because of the high incidence of BPPV.

Third, some patients with head injury experience dizziness and imbalance yet have normal horizontal semicircular canal test findings.[7]

Finally, postural instability or imbalance is a common symptom in patients with head trauma, and the otolith organs contribute to postural stability by serving as gravity sensors to the vestibulospinal pathways.

Ernst and colleagues[30] provided the most direct and compelling evidence that otolithic involvement is a common sequela of head trauma by demonstrating a high incidence of cVEMP and SVV abnormalities, in patients with head injury. Furthermore, Basta and colleagues[31] determined that postural stability was correlated with otolith disturbances in patients with mild blunt head injury. Because the vestibulospinal reflex (VSR) uses otolith input to a greater extent than the VOR, this finding is not surprising and suggests that otolith disorders are a likely source of posttraumatic imbalance.

CENTRAL VESTIBULAR SYSTEM/CNS FUNCTION

Sensory input to the vestibular sensory organs and nerves is processed by the central vestibular system, and the origin for dizziness can occur anywhere along these pathways. The central vestibular system includes the brainstem and cerebellum, but pathways also project to higher centers in the midbrain and cerebral cortex. Ocular motor testing can be used as a screening measure for determining CNS function independent from peripheral vestibular system function. In addition, fixation suppression of vestibular nystagmus requires intact connections between the cerebellum and vestibular nuclei and thus has been used as a clinical test for central vestibular involvement. Many CNS disorders cause gaze-evoked nystagmus that can be observed during clinical assessment.

It has been proposed that unsteadiness or imbalance related to head injury is due to central involvement when tests of horizontal semicircular canal (eg, caloric test) or auditory function are within normal limits.[32–34] There is evidence, however, that suggests central vestibular involvement is less common than peripheral involvement in patients after head injury. Davies and Luxon[17] found that only 8 of 100 patients had central findings that included either abnormal ocular motor tests and/or incomplete vestibular suppression. In contrast, Tuohimaa[35] reported a high incidence of central disturbances in patients shortly after head trauma (60%), although the patients with central findings were older than the patients without central findings and the incidence of central involvement decreased to 12% at 6 months after the head trauma.

To the authors' knowledge, central vestibular pathology has not been investigated in victims of blast exposure. Animal studies have determined enlarged ventricles, minor bleeding, and diffuse axonal injury resulting from primary blast injury,[36,37] although few clinical studies have examined the effects of blast on the human brain.[38] Recent developments in neuroimaging techniques may lead to the development of biomarkers for blast-related TBI.[39–41]

POSTURAL STABILITY

Although postural stability is a multisensory task that depends on reliable input from the vestibular, somatosensory, and visual systems, the vestibular system, particularly the otolith organs, provides important information about gravity. Postural control is modulated via the VSRs, and the lateral vestibulospinal tract receives most of its input from the otolith organs and cerebellum and aids in tonic contractions of the antigravity muscles in the upper and lower extremities. Because the otolith organs play an important role in postural control, a decrease in otolith function affects postural stability. Paloski and colleagues[42] reported changes in postural control related to gravitational input to the otolith organs in astronauts returning from space (microgravity environments). Similarly, reduced postural control has been demonstrated in patients with otolithic disturbances.[31,43]

Postural instability/unsteadiness is a common sequela of head injury. Kaufman and colleagues[44] demonstrated that patients with TBI had poorer performance on subjective and objective measurements of balance than normal controls. Posturography has been used extensively to measure postural stability in head-injured patients and the key findings are the following:

> Patients with mTBI have higher magnitudes of anterior-posterior movement when deprived of accurate visual cues.[45–47]
>
> Postural stability can remain abnormal after other neurologic symptoms are resolved.[48]

Because of the multisensory nature of postural stability, some investigators concluded that abnormal postural stability suggests a multisensory or central cause of imbalance.[45] In contrast, Basta and colleagues[31] demonstrated that otolith disorders may be the cause of postural instability in some patients with head injury.

Few studies have examined the effect of blast exposure on postural stability. Cohen and colleagues[6] measured posturography in blast survivors of a terrorist bombing on a bus in Israel. Of the 7 survivors who complained of imbalance, 6 had abnormal posturography. Similarly, Van Campen and colleagues[13] found that 10 of 25 blast survivors had abnormal posturography shortly after the blast exposure, and 5 had abnormal posturography 1 year after blast.

PRELIMINARY DATA

Table 1 summarizes clinical vestibular test results for 31 consecutive veterans with a history of blast and/or mTBI who were referred to the Mountain Home VAMC Vestibular/Balance Laboratory for complaints of dizziness and/or imbalance. The patients ranged in age from 23 to 76 years (mean, 37 years), and most were veterans of the wars in Iraq and/or Afghanistan (n = 25). Twenty-two veterans (71%) had experienced single or multiple blast exposures (typically from IEDs), 18 (58%) had a diagnosis of mTBI, and 9 (29%) veterans had a history of blast exposure and a diagnosis of mTBI. No radiological evaluations were available because imaging is not a local standard clinical protocol for veterans diagnosed with mTBI.

Vestibular and balance assessment included tests of horizontal semicircular canal function (rotary chair and videonystagmography) and otolith function (cVEMPs and SVV tests during unilateral centrifugation); tests for BPPV (Dix-Hallpike and roll tests), central vestibular function (ocular motor and fixation tests), and postural stability (sensory organization test [SOT]); and self-percieved handicap (the Dizziness Handicap Inventory).

Abnormal vestibular testing findings were defined as: (1) the presence of gaze-evoked nystagmus or saccadic pursuit, a consistent abnormal saccadic accuracy, velocity, or latency, or asymmetrical optokinetic nystagmus on ocular motor tests, (2) failure of fixation suppression >50% for caloric testing, (3) the presence of spontaneous/positional nystagmus, (4) a unilateral weakness of >20% on bithermal caloric testing, (5) phase, gain, and asymmetry data on rotary chair testing outside the normal threshold values at 0.01 through 0.64 Hz, (6) absent or asymmetrical cVEMPs (asymmetry ratio of >40%), (7) off-axis SVV angle – on-axis SVV angle <4°, or (8) consistent abnormal equilibrium score in a given condition and an abnormal composite equilibrium score on the sensory organization test.

Table 1
Summary of vestibular test findings in 31 consecutive veterans with a history of blast exposure and/or TBI

Pt	Hx	Age (y)	OM	Fix	Nyst	Caloric	Rot	cVEMP	SVV[a]	SOT	DHI
1	Blast	37	−	−	−	+	+	−	+	DNT	54
2	Both	60	−	−	−	−	−	+	+	+	74
3	Blast	33	−	−	−	−	−	+	+	−	44
4	Blast	23	−	DNT	−	−	−	−	DNT	−	84
5	Blast	59	−	−	−	−	−	−	DNT	+	56
6	mTBI	76	−	−	−	−	−	+	+	+	52
7	Blast	26	−	−	−	+	−	−	+	+	58
8	Blast	24	−	−	−	−	−	DNT	+	−	20
9	Both	33	−	−	−	−	−	−	+	+	32
10	Both	28	−	−	−	−	+	−	+	+	62
11	Both	24	−	−	+	DNT	−	+	+	+	96
12	Blast	24	−	−	−	DNT	−	+	+	−	56
13	Blast	34	−	−	−	−	−	−	+	−	48
14	mTBI	36	−	−	−	−	−	−	+	+	62
15	Blast	39	−	−	−	+	−	−	+	−	68
16	mTBI	54	−	−	−	−	+	+	+	+	68
17	mTBI	42	−	−	−	−	DNT	−	+	+	30
18	Both	36	−	−	−	−	−	+	+	+	94
19	Both	42	−	−	−	+	−	+	+	−	16
20	Blast	38	−	−	−	−	−	+	+	DNT	34
21	Blast	25	−	−	−	DNT	−	+	+	DNT	24
22	Blast	55	+	−	−	+	−	+	+	+	54
23	Both	39	−	−	−	−	−	+	+	+	32
24	Both	25	−	−	−	−	−	−	+	+	44
25	Both	42	−	−	−	−	−	+	+	+	80
26	mTBI	63	−	−	−	−	−	−	+	−	36
27	mTBI	34	−	−	−	+	+	−	+	DNT	20
28	mTBI	31	−	−	−	−	DNT	+	DNT	+	28
29	mTBI	45	−	−	−	+	+	−	+	DNT	54
30	mTBI	44	−	−	−	−	DNT	+	−	−	26
31	Blast	31	−	−	−	−	−	−	DNT	DNT	54

Negative test findings are indicated by −, and positive test findings are indicated by +. In the Hx column, both indicates a history of blast exposure and mTBI.

Abbreviations: caloric, caloric test; DHI, Dizziness Handicap Inventory; DNT, did not perform test on a patient; Fix, failure of fixation tests; Hx, history; Nyst, spontaneous/positional nystagmus; OM, ocular motor tests; Pt, patient; Rot, rotary chair; SOT, sensory organization test (computerized dynamic posturography).

[a] SVV static and/or dynamic conditions.

The preliminary data are shown in **Table 1** and reveal horizontal semicircular canal dysfunction (caloric weakness and/or abnormal rotational testing) in 9 (29%) patients and otolith dysfunction (abnormal cVEMP and/or SVV in static and/or dynamic conditions) in 26 (84%) patients. These data are consistent with the work of Basta and colleagues[31] who showed a higher incidence of otolith disturbance than horizontal semicircular canal involvement in patients with head injury. The DHI scores ranged from 16 to 96 (mean, 50), suggesting mild to severe self-perceived balance handicap. All patients had negative test results for BPPV with the exception of 1 patient who had anterior and horizontal canalithiasis. The composite equilibrium score on the SOT was abnormal in 16 patients (52%), suggesting postural instability and were consistent with symptoms of imbalance. Of 16 patients, 10 with abnormal SOT findings had abnormal otolith findings (63%) and 4 with abnormal SOT findings had both horizontal canal and otolith involvement (25%). In contrast, none of the patients with horizontal canal findings alone had abnormal SOT results. These results are consistent with the findings of Basta and colleagues[31] who demonstrated that postural instability may be related to otolith disorders, and not necessarily horizontal canal dysfunction, in some patients with head injury. Only 1 patient (3%) had positive central vestibular findings, and these results are consistent with those of Davies and Luxon[17] who observed a low incidence of central vestibular findings in patients after head injury.

Fig. 1 shows vestibular test results from a patient who complained of imbalance after a concussion from an IED blast exposure during deployment in Afghanistan. After the blast exposure, the patient noted unsteadiness and imbalance when standing on a ladder or rooftop at his place of employment. The DHI yielded a score of 32 out of 100, suggesting moderate self-perceived balance handicap. The Dix-Hallpike and roll test results were negative for BPPV. The ocular motor test and the failure of fixation

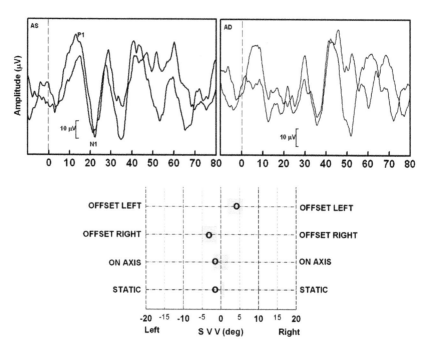

Fig. 1. Otolith test findings from a patient who complained of imbalance after a concussion from an IED blast exposure during deployment in Afghanistan. (*Top*) cVEMPs were recorded from the left side (AS) at 85 dBnHL (P1/N1 = 58 μV); however, cVEMPs were absent from the right side (AD). (*Bottom*) The static SVV was −2°, and SVV (difference angle: offset SVV angle − on-axis SVV angle) during centrifugation to the left was 6° and −2° during centrifugation to the right. The results of the cVEMP and centrifugation SVV tests suggest otolith dysfunction on the right side and normal otolith function on the left side.

test (rotary chair and caloric stimulation) results were negative, suggesting normal central vestibular function. The monothermal warm caloric test revealed normal and symmetric nystagmic responses. Phase, gain, and asymmetry were essentially within normal limits for the sinusoidal harmonic acceleration test on the rotary chair (Micromedical System 2000 rotational chair; Micromedical Technologies, Inc, Chatham, IL, USA). No spontaneous nystagmus or positional nystagmus was present. These results suggest normal horizontal semicircular canal function for this individual.

Otolith function was assessed using cVEMP and SVV during static and dynamic conditions, and the results are shown in **Fig. 1**. cVEMPs were recorded from the left side at 85 dBnHL (amplitude, P1/N1 = 58 μV); however, cVEMPs were absent from the right side. The static SVV was −2°, and SVV during centrifugation to the left and right was 6° and −2°, respectively. The results of the cVEMP and centrifugation SVV tests suggest otolith dysfunction on the right side and normal otolith function on the left side. Computerized dynamic posturography was consistent with a visual/vestibular pattern of dysfunction.

SPECIAL CONSIDERATIONS FOR TESTING BLAST VICTIMS

Posttraumatic stress disorder (PTSD) is an anxiety disorder that develops in reaction to traumatic events. For veterans of recent wars, a history of TBI is often associated with exposure to a traumatic event (eg, blast exposure) that increases the risk of PTSD. According to a Rand Corporation study,[49] nearly 20% of military service members who have returned from Iraq and Afghanistan (approximately 300,000 soldiers) report symptoms of PTSD or major depression. In the authors' preliminary data shown in **Table 1**, 23 of the 31 veterans (74%) who complained of dizziness and/or imbalance also suffered from PTSD. Three veterans were unable to complete testing because of anxiety related to PTSD during the vestibular testing session, and their test results were not included in **Table 1**. Common triggers for anxiety during vestibular and balance assessment included answering questions regarding history of blast exposure, placement in the rotational chair enclosure, restraint of the head for rotational testing, darkening of the test environment, tracking a light bar target during ocular motor testing, and undergoing caloric testing. An awareness of these potential triggers by clinicians working with patients who have experienced blast exposure is important.

Hoge and colleagues[50] suggested that many symptoms associated with TBI, including dizziness and imbalance, were mediated by PTSD or depression. However, some recent studies examining the relationship between blast exposure and/or TBI and vestibular disorders have used subjective measurements such as questionnaires, the presence of symptoms, or screening tests to assess vestibular function.[4,5,7] It seems likely that subjective measurements of dizziness are more influenced by the effects of PTSD than objective measurements of vestibular function. To avoid the potential confounding effects of PTSD, quantitative laboratory tests to determine vestibular involvement are recommended for this patient population.

SUMMARY

Dizziness and imbalance are frequent complaints in patients who have experienced head injury and/or blast exposure. Preliminary results in the authors' laboratory suggest that otolith testing may be an important component of the vestibular test battery in patients with mTBI and/or blast exposure. Vestibular symptoms often last for 6 months or longer after the head trauma, and these findings are inconsistent with vestibular adaptation processes that occur within several months after damage to the semicircular canals and thus suggest a different mechanism causing dizziness in patients with TBI. There is less known about the adaptation process that occurs after damage to the otolith organs; however, Basta and colleagues[51] have shown that traditional vestibular rehabilitation therapy (VRT) is not effective for many patients with otolith disorders. Because there is direct and circumstantial evidence that otolith damage is a common sequela of head trauma, it is important to determine the specific vestibular organ damage associated with blast exposure and/or TBI to optimize treatment outcomes. Further evidence is needed to determine whether or not alternative methods of vestibular rehabilitation would be more effective than traditional VRT in patients with otolith disorders.

REFERENCES

1. Bárány R. Nobel lectures, physiology or medicine 1901–1921. Amsterdam: Elsevier Publishing Company; 1967.
2. Caveness WF, Nielsen KC. Sequelae of cerebral concussion. N Y State J Med 1961;61:871–5.
3. Griffiths MV. The incidence of auditory and vestibular concussion following minor head injury. J Laryngol Otol 1979;93(3):253–65.
4. Jury MA, Flynn MC. Auditory and vestibular sequelae to traumatic brain injury: a pilot study. N Z Med J 2001;114:286–8.
5. Gottshall KR, Gray NL, Drake AI, et al. To investigate the influence of acute vestibular impairment following mild traumatic brain injury on subsequent ability to remain on activity duty 12 months later. Mil Med 2007;172:852–8.
6. Cohen JT, Ziv G, Bloom J, et al. Blast injury of the ear in a confined space explosion: auditory and vestibular evaluation. Isr Med Assoc J 2002;4(7):559–62.
7. Scherer M, Burrows H, Pinto R. Characterizing self-reported dizziness and oto-vestibular impairment among blast-injured traumatic amputees: a pilot study. Mil Med 2007;172(7):731–7.
8. Chamelian L, Feinstein A. Outcome after mild to moderate traumatic brain injury: the role of dizziness. Arch Phys Med Rehabil 2004;85:1662–6.
9. Yang CC, Tu YK, Hua MS, et al. The association between the postconcussion symptoms and clinical outcomes for patients with mild traumatic brain injury. J Trauma 2007;62:657–63.
10. Defense and veterans brain injury center working group on the acute management of mild traumatic brain injury in military operational settings. Washington, DC: Clinical Practice Guidelines & Recommendations; 2006.
11. Kerr AG, Bryne JE. Concussive effects of bomb blast on the ear. J Laryngol Otol 1975;89(2):131–43.
12. Shupak A, Doweck I, Nachtigal D, et al. Vestibular and audiometric consequences of blast injury to the ear. Arch Otolaryngol Head Neck Surg 1993;119:1362–7.
13. Van Campen LE, Dennis JM, King SB, et al. One-year vestibular and balance outcomes of Oklahoma City bombing survivors. J Am Acad Audiol 1999;10(9):467–83.
14. Kerr AG. Trauma and the temporal bone. The effects of blast on the ear. J Laryngol Otol 1980;94(1):107–10.
15. Pahor AL. The ENT problems following the Birmingham bombing. J Laryngol Otol 1981;95:399–406.
16. Lachman J. The importance of vestibular examination in post-concussion vertigo. Acta Med Orient 1955;14(2/3):44–66.
17. Davies RA, Luxon LM. Dizziness following head injury: a neuron-otological study. J Neurol 1995;242:222–30.

18. Toglia JU, Rosenberg PE, Ronis ML. Posttraumatic dizziness: vestibular, audiologic, and medicolegal aspects. Arch Otolaryngol 1970;92(5):485–92.
19. Gannon RP, Willson GN, Roberts ME, et al. Auditory and vestibular damage in head injuries at work. Arch Otolaryngol 1978;104:404–8.
20. Colebatch JG. Vestibular evoked potentials. Curr Opin Neurol 2001;14(1):21–6.
21. Colebatch JG, Halmagyi GM. Vestibular evoked potentials in human neck muscles before and after unilateral vestibular deafferentation. Neurology 1992; 42:1635–6.
22. Halmagyi G, Curthoys I. Otolith function tests. In: Herdman SJ, editor. Vestibular rehabilitation. 3rd edition. Philadelphia: F.A. Davis Co; 2007. p. 144–61.
23. Dieterich M, Brandt T. Ocular torsion and tilt of the subjective visual vertical are sensitive brainstem signs. Ann Neurol 1993;33:292–9.
24. Wetzig J, Reiser M, Martin E, et al. Unilateral centrifugation of the otoliths as a new method to determine bilateral asymmetries of the otolith apparatus in man. Acta Astronaut 1990;21:519–25.
25. Clarke A, Schonfeld U, Hamann C, et al. Measuring unilateral otolith function via the otolith-ocular response and the subjective visual vertical. Acta Otolaryngol Suppl 2001;545:84–7.
26. Bohmer A, Mast F. Chronic unilateral loss of otolith function revealed by the subjective visual vertical during off center yaw rotation. J Vestib Res 1999;9:413–22.
27. Schuknecht HF, Davison RC. Deafness and vertigo from head injury. AMA Arch Otolaryngol 1956;63(5):513–28.
28. Proctor B, Gurdjinan ES, Webster JE. The ear in head trauma. Laryngoscope 1956;66:16–30.
29. Barber HO. Positional head injury, especially after head injury. Laryngoscope 1964;74:891–944.
30. Ernst A, Basta D, Seidl RO, et al. Management of posttraumatic vertigo. Otolaryngol Head Neck Surg 2005;132:554–8.
31. Basta D, Todt I, Scherer H, et al. Postural control in otolith disorders. Hum Mov Sci 2005;24(2):268–79.
32. Ylikoski J, Palva T, Sanna M. Dizziness after head trauma: clinical and morphologic findings. Am J Otol 1982;3(4):343–52.
33. Sanna M, Ylikoski J. Vestibular neurectomy for dizziness after head trauma: a review of 28 patients. ORL J Otorhinolaryngol Relat Spec 1983;45:216–25.
34. Kisilevski V, Podoshin L, Ben-David J, et al. Results of otovestibular tests in mild head injuries. Int Tinnitus J 2001;7(2):118–21.
35. Tuohimaa P. Vestibular disturbance after acute mild head injury. Acta Otolaryngol Suppl 1978;359:7–61.
36. Cernak I, Savic J, Malicevic Z, et al. Involvement of the central nervous system in the general response to pulmonary blast injury. J Trauma 1996;40(Suppl 3):S100–4.
37. Cernak I, Wang Z, Jiang J, et al. Ultrastructural and functional characteristics of blast injury-induced neurotrauma. J Trauma 2001;50(4):695–706.
38. Kocsis JD, Tessler A. Pathology of blast-related brain injury. J Rehabil Res Dev 2009;46(6):667–72.
39. Huang MX, Theilmann RJ, Robb A, et al. Integrated imaging approach with MEG and DTI to detect mild traumatic brain injury in military and civilian patients. J Neurotrauma 2009;26:1213–26.
40. Jantzen KJ. Functional magnetic resonance imaging of mild traumatic brain injury. J Head Trauma Rehabil 2010;25(4):256–66.
41. Niogi SN, Mukherjee P. Diffusion tensor imaging of mild traumatic brain injury. J Head Trauma Rehabil 2010;25(4):241–55.

42. Paloski WH, Black FO, Reschke MF, et al. Vestibular ataxia following shuttle flights: effects of microgravity on otolith-mediated sensorimotor control of posture. Am J Otol 1993;14(1):9–17.

43. de Waele C, Tran Ba Huy P, Diard JP, et al. Saccular dysfunction in Ménière's disease. Am J Otol 1999;20:223–32.

44. Kaufman KR, Brey RH, Chou LS, et al. Comparison of subjective and objective measurements of balance disorders following traumatic brain injury. Med Eng Phys 2006;28:234–9.

45. Rubin AM, Woolley SM, Dailey VM, et al. Postural stability following mild head or whiplash. Am J Otol 1995;16(2):216–21.

46. Guskiewicz KM, Perrin DH, Gansneder BM. Effect of mild head injury on postural stability in athletes. J Athl Train 1996;31(4):300–6.

47. Basford JR, Chou LS, Kaufmann KR. An assessment of gait and balance deficits after traumatic brain injury. Arch Phys Med Rehabil 2003;84:343–9.

48. Geurts AC, Ribbers GM, Knoop JA, et al. Identification of static and dynamic postural instability. Arch Phys Med Rehabil 1996;77(7):639–44.

49. Tanielian T, Jaycox LH. Invisible wounds of war: psychological and cognitive injuries, their consequences, and services to assist recovery. Santa Monica (CA): Rand; 2008.

50. Hoge CW, Castro CA, Messer SC, et al. Combat duty in Iraq and Afghanistan, mental health problems, and barriers to care. N Engl J Med 2004;351:13–22.

51. Basta D, Singbartl F, Todt I, et al. Vestibular rehabilitation by auditory feedback in otolith disorders. Gait Posture 2008;28(3):397–404.

Evaluation of Dizziness in the Litigating Patient

Gerard J. Gianoli, MD[a,b,*], James S. Soileau, MD[a]

KEYWORDS

- Vertigo • Dizziness • Lawsuit • Litigation • Disability
- Worker's compensation • Malingering • Exaggeration

R.G. is a 50-year-old man describing nonspecific dizziness. He states that the dizziness is constant and does not come in spells. He indicates that his symptoms wax and wane in severity with no consistent pattern for time of day or inciting activity. He reports associated symptoms of headache and neck pain, which are also constant, and bilateral tinnitus. He denies hearing loss. He states that his past medical history is negative, and his physical examination is unremarkable. Toward the end of the appointment, he indicates that all his symptoms began after a motor vehicle crash and that his lawyer specifically referred him to you for evaluation, because ...you are the best doctor in town.

DIZZINESS IN LITIGATING PATIENTS

Dizziness is one of the most frequent chief complaints that brings patients to their physician's office.[1] Dizziness is also a frequent complaint among litigants who have suffered accidental or job-related injuries. Worker's compensation, disability claims, and lawsuits are filed for financial compensation because of this complaint. As physicians, we inevitably will become embroiled as either expert witnesses in our patients' lawsuits or as experts sought out by entities being sued by individuals for the alleged injury related to the complaint of dizziness. A competent evaluation of this entity is frequently sought from otolaryngologists in the position as an expert witness. This review puts forth some guidelines in dealing with this type of patient and the legal system. Although this article is entitled "Evaluation of Dizziness in the Litigating Patient," the principles set forth in it are applicable for patients who are seeking disability status, worker's compensation claims, and any other situations in which there is significant potential for secondary gain.

[a] The Ear and Balance Institute, 17050 Medical Center Drive, Suite # 315, Baton Rouge, LA 70816, USA
[b] Departments of Otolaryngology and Pediatrics, Tulane University School of Medicine, 1430 Tulane Avenue, New Orleans, LA 70112, USA
* Corresponding author. The Ear and Balance Institute, 17050 Medical Center Drive, Suite # 315, Baton Rouge, LA 70816.
E-mail address: ggianoli@gmail.com

Otolaryngol Clin N Am 44 (2011) 335–346
doi:10.1016/j.otc.2011.02.001
0030-6665/11/$ – see front matter © 2011 Elsevier Inc. All rights reserved.

oto.theclinics.com

BASIC PRINCIPLES
Physician Role: Patient Advocate Vs Advocate/Agent of Court

As physicians we find ourselves in the role of patient advocate for several different causes and are taught that this is our role as physicians. We advocate for their best interests in relieving their suffering and preventing further harm to their health. We advocate for them to get insurance approval for appropriate health care, and we advocate for their disability application when appropriate. These roles are all ethical and, indeed, laudable positions to find ourselves. However, when we are in the role of expert witness, we are no longer in the role of a patient advocate. When we take on the position of a medical expert, we are, in essence, enjoined as agents of the court, and our role is to provide truthful and objective assessments of an individual's physical condition.[2] To advocate for the patient in this situation would be unethical. This fact is important to keep in mind because the patient's best interests may not be aligned with the best interests of the court and society as a whole.

Extensive Documentation of History and Physical Examination

Extensive documentation of the history and physical examination is an important first step in the evaluation of those who are involved in litigation. Experience has taught the authors to use an extensive pre-visit questionnaire to document the patient's responses in their own handwriting. This questionnaire is filled out in our office waiting room, signed by the patient, dated, and witnessed by one of our staff members. This questionnaire is important to document because so many of our medical opinions and diagnoses are based on information garnered from the history. This procedure may seem elaborate, but there will be times when the patient will later deny statements made in the office. Without documentation to the contrary, the expert will either be forced to change his opinion based on this "new" historical information or will be caught in a "my word against his word" confrontation. Of course, if the above-mentioned documentation occurs, any future changes in the medical history are problematic for the patient and will denigrate his reliability. Any historical information provided by the patient (or the attorney) must be corroborated by medical records, physical findings, test results, and so forth. Memory is often swayed by potential million-dollar settlements. At the same time our intake questionnaire is completed, we have the patient sign a consent form for evaluation and testing, which includes consent for photograph or video documentation. If this is not signed, we do not see the patient.

Extensive Objective Testing to Verify Complaints

Do not be cost-conscious. In this day of escalating health care costs, many physicians have been made ever so aware of ordering unnecessary testing. However, in the context of litigation, the concern of being cost-conscious is misplaced. A complete and thorough evaluation including history, physical examination, audiological testing, vestibular testing, imaging, and any other ancillary tests needed is unlikely to exceed $10,000. Any (non-nuisance) litigation concerning dizziness almost certainly seeks redress exceeding several hundred thousand dollars and frequently exceeds a million dollars. Consequently, the costs of the evaluation by the medical expert in these cases are almost always negligible. If an attorney is reticent to proceed with a full evaluation because of the costs, this is a good clue that he does not have a case and is looking to settle for a nuisance fee.

Corroboration of Objective and Subjective Findings

Because litigation involving the complaint of dizziness often involves the possibility of very large monetary awards, there is considerable incentive for plaintiffs to malinger or to exaggerate their symptoms. Lawyers, judges, and juries are also aware of these factors, sometimes more so than physicians. Consequently, it is imperative that any subjective complaint be verified objectively and quantified as best as possible. This process will often either bolster the plaintiff's case or destroy the case entirely. However, sometimes the result is a mixture of these outcomes, helping some aspects of the case while harming the others. To the expert witness, whatever the result, it should not matter.

Make Sure All Pieces Fit: Do Symptoms and Severity Correlate with Objective Findings?

Among dizzy patients who are undergoing litigation, approximately 25% will have symptoms that are corroborated by objective testing and 25% will have nonphysiologic test results, with no objective findings to corroborate their subjective complaints (**Fig. 1**). These 2 groups would seem to be fairly straightforward—one group that seems to be fairly honest and legitimate and the other group that is highly suspicious for malingering. However, there is another larger group of patients representing approximately 50% of litigating patients complaining of dizziness who have characteristics of both–some verification of subjective findings by objective testing and some nonphysiologic results suggesting malingering or exaggeration. Putting all 3 groups together, one could reasonably say that 75% of all patients complaining of dizziness and involved in litigation are either malingering or exaggerating their problems. Or, one could also reasonably state that 75% of these patients have a legitimate pathologic condition. Both statements would be correct. Separating the true pathologic condition from exaggeration is the main role of the expert witness.[3]

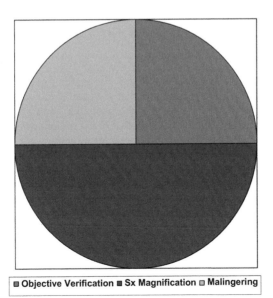

☐ Objective Verification ■ Sx Magnification ☐ Malingering

Fig. 1. Among dizzy patients involved in litigation, objective verification of symptoms is found in approximately 25%, nonphysiologic results suggesting frank malingering in roughly 25%, and exaggeration of symptoms in about 50%.

Assessment of Causation

Once the evaluation of the objective pathologic condition has been performed, causation must be considered. The legal hurdle for most expert witness testimony is the determination of probability. Probability is defined as more than 50% likelihood; consequently, absolute certainty is not required when determining causation, although it is best to be more certain than not. Remember, anything is possible, but the courts want to know what is probable.

Two factors that need to be considered are the timing and mode of injury. Timing refers to the time sequence of events in question relative to the pathologic condition causing the litigant's dizziness. Mode of injury refers to the mechanism, such as blunt head trauma, noise trauma, and explosion. Obviously, in a patient with immediate onset of vertigo after a sledgehammer impacted his occiput, both the timing and mode of injury would seem reasonable to accept as more probable than not, the head trauma is the cause of the vertigo. However, if you later find out that the patient did not have any vertigo or dizziness until 1 year after the sledgehammer incident, you would likely conclude that the vestibular problem was more probable than not to be unrelated to the head trauma. Similarly, for a situation in which a plaintiff complains of dizziness immediately after a tap on the shoulder, one might reasonably conclude that although the timing might be appropriate for causation, the mode of injury is inconsistent with the pathologic condition observed. Consequently, one would accept as more probable than not, that the shoulder tapping did not cause the dizziness. The 2 main questions to be answered are the following:

1. Is the mechanism of trauma appropriate for the injury?
2. Is the timing appropriate to link the pathologic condition to the alleged incident?

A word of caution is that it is inappropriate to take the patient's (or the attorney's) word for the mechanism of injury. You are the expert, and it is your job to make this determination. Both the patient and the attorneys (defense and plaintiff) have a significant stake in the outcome of your determination. Remain objective and verify anything you are told with objective findings, such as the medical record or test results.

Prognosis

After determination of the objective pathology, causation, and probability, the next step is determination of the prognosis. In this regard, you need to consider the average, that is, the best and the worst-case scenarios. You also need to consider sequelae that may be many years in the future. For the patient who has been seriously affected, this litigation may be their only chance for monetary recompense. The basis for the plaintiff's award is entangled in the prognosis. Any future medical and nonmedical needs should be considered. A recent conversation with a plaintiff's attorney was enlightening. I had seen his patient and treated her benign paroxysmal positional vertigo (BPPV). I informed him that he had a good case and that his client was already cured. He took this information as a good news/bad news moment. He had a good case, but because the client was cured, there would be little monetary award for future medical or other needs.

Dealing with Lawyers

Many physicians mistakenly believe that attorneys who hire an expert want that expert merely to support their case, a "hired gun." Although this belief may be true for a small minority of attorneys, our experience has been quite the opposite. Some of the most thankful attorneys were the ones to whom we had to give bad news. Plaintiff attorneys sink a lot of their own money into their cases, and the amount of money invested is often substantial. The last thing a plaintiff attorney wants to do is to get all the way to a trial (read: large outlay of his own money on an expensive court trial) and then finally find out that his client is malingering. Similarly, a defense attorney who finds out that the plaintiff is legitimate and will likely win at trial is much more willing to offer a generous settlement in pretrial negotiations rather than risk losing at trial.

HISTORY AND PHYSICAL EXAMINATION

Our evaluation of litigating patients starts with an extensive questionnaire as mentioned earlier. This questionnaire is reviewed during the case history interview in order to clarify any points that may have caused some confusion. Some important points to identify during the history are the following:

1. Details of the alleged trauma or inciting event
2. Time course for onset of symptoms
3. Important associated events
4. Progression of symptoms
5. Evaluation and therapeutic interventions used
6. Prior history of dizziness, vertigo, tinnitus, hearing loss, or other otologic diseases
7. Extensive medical history including:
   - Surgical history
   - Significant medical illnesses
   - Hospitalizations
   - Medication use
   - Prior trauma
   - Alcohol, tobacco, and drug use
   - Occupational history including military history, criminal convictions, and prison stay
   - Family history.

The physical examination must include a complete head and neck examination as well as an extensive neurotologic examination. Specifically, this examination should include microscopic otoscopy, documentation of facial nerve function, global neurologic examination, and eye examination using infrared videography. The eye examination should include examination of ocular movements and examination for spontaneous nystagmus (with and without visual fixation) in all cardinal positions of gaze. Headshake and head thrust maneuvers should also be performed. Some physicians perform Dix-Hallpike testing during the physical examination, whereas others reserve this component for the formal electronystagmographic (ENG) or videonystagmographic (VNG) examination. The neurologic examination should include tests of the cranial nerves, cerebellar function, Romberg test, Fukuda test, and gait analysis.

Refer to the authors' "Dizziness Questionnaire" from The Ear and Balance Institute in the Appendix in this publication.

TESTING

As mentioned, objective testing is mandatory in cases involving litigation or other situations with potential for a secondary gain, such as worker's compensation or disability claims. Before objective testing is performed, there are 2 requirements: equipment calibration and properly trained ancillary personnel. If either of these is not present, you cannot rely on the test results. Many physicians depend on their audiologists for the laboratory assessment of vestibular function. Whereas many audiologists are quite good at vestibular testing, others have had limited vestibular educational exposure and limited experience with vestibular testing. If this is the case, appropriate continuing education and training are required.

Audiological Testing

Audiometric evaluation should include a comprehensive audiogram, including air conduction and bone conduction testing (regardless of how good the hearing seems to be), speech audiometry, tympanometry, and acoustic reflex testing. Appropriate validation tests (eg, Stenger test) should be performed when there is a significant hearing asymmetry between the ears. One should take note of the pure tone average (PTA) in comparison to the speech reception threshold (SRT) in that there should be less than 6 dB difference between the PTA and SRT. In addition, the sound level of conversation at which the patient is instructed in the audiometric test booth should not be lower than the PTA or SRT. Other factors that should be noted include whether the patient reported hearing unmasked bone stimulation appropriately, whether the patient responded with "half spondees" (eg, the patient is requested to repeat the word "baseball" and replies "base....something"), whether bone conduction responses were present at higher sensation levels than air conduction responses, and whether acoustic reflexes were present in an ear that was reported as having profound hearing loss or conductive hearing loss. The physician should ask the individual performing the audiometric tests for a general impression of patient performance as well as the level of cooperation and reliability. Finally, the pure tone pattern should be assessed for physiologic character suggesting an organic pathologic condition or a non-physiologic pattern. In addition to the above-mentioned audiometric testing, we strongly advise that any abnormality should be corroborated by otoacoustic emissions and auditory evoked potential testing for threshold. We also find that adjunct testing, such as electrocochleography, is helpful in objectively identifying the pathologic condition. However, the decision to include such testing should be larboratory-specific and depends on the reliability of that particular laboratory's experience with the testing.

Vestibular Testing

Vestibular testing should include a comprehensive analysis of all aspects of the vestibular system that can be evaluated objectively. Current technology allows assessment of vestibular responses with a variety of stimuli. Among these, a bare minimum would include ENG/VNG, rotary chair testing, and computerized dynamic posturography. Additional studies that may prove to be helpful would include vestibular evoked myogenic potentials and high-frequency vestibuloocular reflex (VOR) testing. Throughout these tests, the clinician should look for patterns consistent with known pathologic conditions and should be suspicious of poor results, unusual results, or failure to obtain any result at all. Poor cooperation should be noted. The clinician should also keep in mind that all these tests can be separated into 2 categories determined by whether the response is voluntary or involuntary. A common mistake for inexperienced clinicians is to interpret abnormalities on the oculomotor tests as being evidence of central vestibular dysfunction. Although this interpretation may be true, one should keep in mind that these tests require the patient's cooperation and that abnormal results could also be the result of poor cooperation or malingering on the part of the patient. The clinician should be especially suspicious in cases in which the patient gives non-physiologic results in any of the testing protocols. Input from the individual performing the vestibular assessment can be very helpful in cases in which results vary significantly from the norm. It should be considered standard for the examiner to report any erratic behavior of the patient or deviation from the test protocol. These patients should never be left alone in the examination or testing rooms, and ideally, a clinic chaperone should be present as a witness to all events that take place. We have also used video recording in various locations throughout our office. This evidence helps to eliminate contrary claims of patient experiences while in our office.

Imaging

We think that imaging (both high-resolution computed tomographic [CT] scan and magnetic resonance imaging [MRI]) should be performed in all cases involving litigation. Because the history may not be as straightforward as we would like, a detailed analysis of the inner ear and skull base anatomy is often elucidating. Consider the example of a patient who falls in a big-box store claiming hearing loss and balance dysfunction as a result of the fall. She has a CT scan of temporal bones that does not show any abnormality and an audiovestibular testing that demonstrates unilateral hearing loss and unilateral vestibular loss. The patient claims that the hearing loss and balance dysfunction occurred immediately after the fall. It would be easy to concur that the fall caused this patient's problem had you not ordered the MRI scan that shows a 3-cm acoustic neuroma in the affected ear. Yes, the hearing loss could have occurred when she fell, although this seems unlikely. Even so, the fact that she has a 3-cm acoustic neuroma in the affected ear certainly changes the complexion of the entire case.

REVIEW OF MEDICAL RECORDS

Medical records should be reviewed whenever possible. We find that the most helpful information is anything having to do with testing that gives objective results and almost any information before the event that is being litigated. Review of the police accident report, emergency medical technician report, emergency room report, and initial hospitalization can provide information that many patients may not remember. These reports can also be used to corroborate the patient's history as well as to corroborate any information that is provided by the attorneys. It is wise to exhaustively review the pertinent medical records before any courtroom testimony.

MALINGERING

Malingering is the false and fraudulent simulation or exaggeration of disease, performed to obtain money, drugs, evade duty or criminal responsibility or other reasons readily understood from the individual's circumstances, rather than learning the individual's psychology.[4]

Although a patient may be suspected of malingering, malingering is only part of the differential diagnosis in such cases. Remember that non-physiologic test results can also be otherwise explained. Alternative explanations include technical malfunction of equipment, poor understanding of the requirements of the test (as would be seen in young children and those with a mental illness), and panic disorder. In your capacity as an expert witness, it is better practice to avoid the formal diagnosis of malingering and instead expound upon whether or not the patient meets the *Diagnostic and Statistical Manual of Mental Disorders (Fourth Edition)* (DSM-IV) criteria for malingering. After that, the judge and jury will decide whether malingering is an appropriate explanation of the litigant's behavior.

Malingering is suspected if any combination of the following DSM-IV criteria for malingering[5] is observed:

1. Medical/legal context of presentation
2. Marked discrepancy between the person's claimed stress of disability and objective findings
3. Lack of cooperation during the diagnostic evaluation and in complying with the prescribed treatment regimen
4. The presence of antisocial personality disorder.

Malingering by Imputation

Many think that the most difficult form of malingering to encounter is malingering by imputation. In this case, the litigant has a legitimate pathologic condition and is very consistent, cooperative, and honest in dealing with the clinicians, that is, with the exception of 1 or 2 details leading to the causation of the pathologic condition. In general, the only way to identify this type of malingering is by a thorough review of the existing medical records. Even so, litigants, being aware that this review is a liability to them, may have worked hard to conceal any prior records identifying the pathologic condition as a premorbid condition. When the individual is not forthcoming with regard to a condition that is eventually identified, it is likely to be a case of malingering by imputation. On the other hand, a patient who is forthright about a prior condition and claims worsening of this condition by the event that is being litigated presents a situation that is not so straightforward. The question then becomes whether the alleged incident did indeed worsen the pathologic condition, which becomes a judgment call by the clinician dictated by the specifics of the case. Of course, admission of the premorbid condition will likely reduce monetary rewards on behalf of the plaintiff.

Red Flags

Certain findings should be red flags for the clinician to raise suspicions of malingering or symptom exaggeration regarding plaintiffs complaining of dizziness. Obviously, this includes the finding of nonphysiologic test results, but there are also more subtle issues to consider. The patient who either refuses testing or is unable to complete testing should raise suspicions. In our experience, we rarely encounter a non-litigating patient who cannot complete testing, and, in general, the more severely affected the patient the more motivated is he or she to complete testing. When the symptoms seem too severe for the disorder identified, one must consider whether exaggeration of symptoms is occurring. Frequent falls should raise suspicion of malingering or exaggeration. Although falls are the concern for patients with dizziness, vertigo, and poor balance, frequent falls are not commonly found in patients complaining of dizziness with no potential for a secondary gain. Patients may have 1 or 2 falls and then generally recognize this tendency. Subsequently, adaptations are made by either avoiding situations likely to cause falls or by taking other measures, such as the use of a cane or walker, to aid balance. Similarly, patients with episodic vertigo are typically mindful of their safety and use fall-avoidance behaviors at the first signs of vertigo. Difficulty in categorizing the plaintiff's complaints with a diagnosis should also cause some unease among clinicians. Patients who malinger or exaggerate tend to defy diagnostic categorization. And of course, behavioral inconsistencies such as lies, obvious exaggerations, and poor cooperation should certainly raise the specter of malingering in the mind of the clinician. Remember that those who will lie to you over small things will certainly lie to you over big things. There could be legitimate explanations for all the abovementioned findings, but if any of these are present, a good explanation for their presence is warranted.

What not to miss
Obvious nonphysiologic test results
Patient who refuses testing or is unable to complete testing
Frequent falls with no attempt to report them or take measures to avoid them
Behavioral inconsistencies from the patient.

THE "NORMAL EVALUATION" PATIENT

Another vexing situation is the normal patient, a cooperative, reliable patient with a plausible history but normal findings on all of the objective tests performed. Because there are no objective findings on testing or physical examination, the entire case rests on the credibility of the patient. In our experience, patients in this category are more likely to represent the true pathologic condition. We must remember that all currently available vestibular tests only evaluate a small portion of the vestibular system. Consequently, it is not unreasonable to envision a patient who has pathologic condition outside the bounds of conventional testing. Vestibular function and symptoms can also fluctuate. Keep in mind that the test findings are a snapshot in time of that patient's vestibular status, allowing for the possibility of a normal evaluation in a patient with a vestibulopathy. If one doubts this, consider the case of BPPV. One of the major characteristics of BPPV is fatigability, the phenomenon in which repeated testing of a positive result becomes negative. When patients have an abnormal result during the Dix-Hallpike maneuver, there is no doubt that they have BPPV; however, it cannot be determined with certainty that a patient with normal results during the Dix-Hallpike testing does not have BPPV. In the latter scenario, the patient may have BPPV that has already "fatigued." For someone suspicious for BPPV with normal Dix-Hallpike results, repeat testing is recommended. Our recommendation for the patient in litigation is similar, repeat testing.

ASSUMPTIONS/PEARLS
Your Work and Your Credentials Will be Scrutinized

As an expert witness, you must be prepared to explain your findings and conclusions, knowing that the opposing attorney has hired an expert who will be reviewing your work. Alternative explanations of your findings will be brought forth, and you will need to expound upon whether these theories are more or less likely than your conclusions. Many physicians find it unsettling for their diagnoses and conclusions to be questioned. However, such questioning is the rule rather than the exception when litigation is involved. Many experts will have scientific publications within the area being litigated. You can rest assured that a good opposing legal team will have reviewed your publications and any deviation from your prior opinions will make your testimony seem suspect. You may be required to explain excerpts from your prior papers that are placed out of context. In addition, your qualifications as an expert will be routinely examined and scrutinized by the attorney who hired you (usually before you are hired) and by the opposing counsel (at your deposition). Again, while this examination and scrutiny is unsettling for some, it is routine for expert witness work.

Never Assume Any Prior Diagnosis is Correct

Frequently, a prior diagnosis is assumed to be correctly made and is used as a shortcut to treat the patient. Whereas this is not good practice in general, it is a big mistake in the face of litigation. Physicians who examined and diagnosed the patient previously may not have been aware of any potential for secondary gain and accepted the patient at their word rather than objectively documenting any pathologic condition. Consequently, their prior diagnosis may have been made based on faulty information.

Cannot Assume a Normal Premorbid State

As mentioned earlier, you cannot assume that the patient had a normal premorbid state. A review of existing medical records is important in this regard, in search of past history of ear-related problems, dizziness, and associated testing. Only if there is no prior documentation can one infer that no prior pathologic condition existed. Even in this scenario, however, many patients will have pathologic condition of which they may not have been aware. We find that the most common example of this is noise-induced hearing loss. Easily identified by the 4 kHz notch on the audiogram, this pathologic condition creeps up on patients slowly and in its early phases may not present with symptoms. If noise-induced hearing loss has no reasonable association with the alleged injury, it is likely a premorbid state.

Appropriate Referrals

Pathologic condition outside our areas of expertise should be evaluated by the appropriate professional. Extreme reservation should be used in giving expert opinions in areas outside of one's specific field. For example, a common complaint among patients with closed head injury is cognitive dysfunction. A neuropsychology referral is warranted to quantify this issue objectively and to separate organic pathologic condition from nonorganic causes. Similarly, anxiety and panic disorder should be referred for appropriate treatment.

Financial Incentives Obscure the Picture

It is helpful to understand the financial motivation of all parties involved in litigation. The easiest to understand is that of the plaintiff, which is monetary recompense for the alleged injury. The expert witness must always keep in mind this bias and how it may result in exaggeration or malingering. The defense obviously wants to avoid any payout to the plaintiff and is in direct conflict with the plaintiff. The defense attorneys, while wanting to make a good defense, are usually paid on an hourly basis and have an incentive to drag out the proceedings as long as possible regardless of the outcome. The plaintiff attorneys are more interested in shorter proceedings because they typically invest their own money into the case and do not have unlimited resources for a protracted litigation. In fact, unless a case can win a certain sum of money, regardless of the case's merits, a plaintiff attorney may either decline a case or become very passive in its prosecution. In any event, many more cases settle out of court rather than proceeding to trial.

Litigation May Become Protracted

If you are acting as an expert witness, you need to prepare yourself for the possibility that your services may be required for one case many years after the fact. Both authors have been involved in cases that have taken beyond 10 years to resolve. It is not unusual for litigation to spawn additional litigation or repeat lawsuits. It seems that some litigants become "frequent flyers" in the court system.

Be Prepared to Change Your Opinion as New Evidence Arises

Sometimes when you are evaluating a patient in the context of litigation, you are not privy to all the information concerning the plaintiff. Because of an inevitable bias of either side in the litigation, your opinion may be swayed by information informally relayed to you that you eventually find out is not correct. Consequently, a change in your opinion during the course of evaluation may be warranted. There is no reason that an expert witness cannot change his opinion as new evidence surfaces. In fact, the merits of the case should be re-evaluated and a new opinion produced when any new pertinent evidence arises. This situation is more common than many realize.

Payment

Although many physicians are uncomfortable discussing fees, it is important to be upfront about your fees when dealing with any case involving litigation. If at all possible, you should have a signed contract with the attorney who has hired you before seeing the patient. This contract should detail all your fees, including office visits, testing, reports, phone conferences, depositions, and trial appearances. Because the time, effort, and intellectual energy expended in these cases are considerably more than those with routine patients, one should not accept discounted Medicare or insurance rates for the clinical components in the evaluation of these patients. It is advisable to require payment in advance for your services and to decline cases with contingency fees. Accepting a contingency fee for a case compromises your impartiality and credibility and is unethical. While depositions can be scheduled at your convenience, trial appearances cannot. Providing courtroom testimony will typically absorb most, if not all, of your working day and more than a day if there is any significant travel involved. More trial appearances will be scheduled than actually occur because many cases settle at the last minute. Because it is difficult to reschedule a clinical day at the last minute, payment in advance and a cancellation fee are reasonable approaches for such occurrences.

CONCLUSIONS ON EVALUATION OF THE DIZZY PATIENT IN LITIGATION

Evaluation of the dizzy patient who is involved in ongoing litigation is a challenging endeavor. However, recognizing the challenges and appropriate management of these patients, in addition to the legal entanglements associated with them, can lead to a fruitful endeavor. The role of the physician in this situation is not that of a patient advocate but rather of an agent of the court in pursuit of a truthful unbiased analysis of disability, causation, and prognosis.

What not to miss

- Physician as agent of the court
- Extensive documentation of history and physical examination
- Extensive objective verification of complaints
- Extensive objective testing to exclude other pathologies
- Corroboration of objective and subjective findings
- Assessment of disability, causation, prognosis, and future needs
- Evaluation of possible malingering or exaggeration.

REFERENCES

1. McLemore T, Delozier J. 1985 Summary: National ambulatory medical care survey. In: National Center for Health Statistics (Hyattsville, MD) Advance data from vital statistics. No 128. Washington, DC: Government Printing Office; 1987. US Dept of Health and Human Services Publication No. (PHS) 87–1250.
2. Patient Safety and Professional Liability Committee, American College of Surgeons. Statement on the physician acting as an expert witness. Bull Am Coll Surg 2007;92(12):24–5.
3. Gianoli G, McWilliams S, Soileau J, et al. Posturographic performance in patients with the potential for secondary gain. Otolaryngol Head Neck Surg 2000;122:11–8.
4. Gorman WF. Defining malingering. J Forensic Sci 1982;27:401–7.
5. American Psychiatric Association, 2000 Malingering and illness deception. In: Halligan PW, Bass C, Oakley DA, editors. DSM-IV-TR. Washington, DC: Oxford University Press; 2003. UK.

Positional Vertigo: As Occurs Across All Age Groups

Edward I. Cho, MD, Judith A. White, MD, PhD*

KEYWORDS

- Posterior semicircular canal • Lateral semicircular canal
- Vertigo • Nystagmus • BPPV • Dix-hallpike
- Canalith repositioning

J.W. is a pleasant, articulate 71-year-old man describing motion-provoked, position-dependent vertigo. He states that his symptoms began suddenly 3 weeks ago after spending 2 days supervising landscapers pruning the trees in his yard looking up for hours. He reports that on rolling over in bed to turn off the alarm clock, he became vertiginous and noted that everything in the room was swirling around. He states that he tried to sit up and call to his wife for help, but fell backward onto the bed feeling very dizzy and disoriented. He indicates that he lay still for a few minutes and the symptoms subsided, only to return when he attempted to sit up again. He indicates that his wife did come to his aid and she noticed that his eyes would "jump around" every time she tried to help him sit up. Later that morning, the symptoms improved and he was able to go about his day, but only if he moved very slowly. He notes that since this time he experiences 15 to 30 seconds of true vertigo when he transitions from sitting to supine positions, rolls onto his right side in bed, or bends over. He denies associated auditory symptoms. He states that his medical history is significant for hypertension, cardiac bypass surgery 8 years ago, high cholesterol, arthritis in his knees and hands, frequent heartburn, and seasonal sinus problems.

POSITIONAL VERTIGO

Benign paroxysmal positional vertigo (BPPV) is one of the most common vestibular disorders with an estimated lifetime prevalence of 2.4% in the general adult population.[1] Of the 5.6 million clinic visits per year in the United States for dizziness, it is estimated that between 17% and 42% of patients with vertigo are diagnosed with BPPV.[2–4] Although this disorder affects people across their lifespan, it tends to

The authors have nothing to disclose.
Section of Vestibular and Balance Disorders, The Cleveland Clinic Head and Neck Institute, A71, 9500 Euclid Avenue, Cleveland, OH 44195, USA
* Corresponding author.
E-mail address: whitej3@ccf.org

Otolaryngol Clin N Am 44 (2011) 347–360
doi:10.1016/j.otc.2011.01.006
0030-6665/11/$ – see front matter © 2011 Elsevier Inc. All rights reserved.

affect individuals aged 50 to 70 years and therefore has some noteworthy societal burdens.[5] For example, it is estimated that $2000 is spent on average to diagnose BPPV and that 86% of patients have interruption in their daily activities and lost work days because of the vertigo symptoms.[1,6–8] Furthermore, older patients with BPPV have a greater incidence of falls and impairments to their daily activities. These falls can cause secondary injuries, including hip fractures, and can lead to additional costs from hospital and nursing home admissions.[9] (See article by Barin and Dodson in this publication). Therefore, this disorder affects not only an individual's quality of life but also the society.

The true incidence and prevalence of BPPV is difficult to accurately estimate. For example, a study in Japan estimated the incidence to be 0.01%,[10] whereas one done in Minnesota estimated it to be 0.06% with an increase of 38% with each decade of life.[11] However, it is likely that these early epidemiologic studies were underestimates because they included only those patients who presented to physicians with their acute vestibular problem and did not include those who never reported to physicians. A recent study in Germany looked at the estimated prevalence and incidence of BPPV in the general adult population. The investigators used a cross-sectional nationally representative survey of the general adult population in Germany and found a prevalence of 2.4% overall with a prevalence of 3.2% in females and 1.6% in males. The 1-year incidence was calculated at 0.6%, which is approximately 10 times higher than earlier estimates.[1] In this study, the 1-year prevalence was also broken down by age. In patients aged 18 to 39 years, the estimated prevalence was 0.5%. From 40 to 59 years of age, the prevalence was 1.7%. Finally, for patients older than 60 years, the estimated prevalence was 3.4%.[1]

BPPV ACROSS THE LIFESPAN

There are very few published reports of BPPV in patients younger than 18 years. However, one series of case reports by Giacomini and colleagues[12] described 9 patients who developed BPPV after intense physical activity. Of these 9 patients, 7 were younger than 36 years. One 16-year-old girl developed BPPV after an intense dolphin stroke–style swimming activity. She was diagnosed with posterior semicircular canal (PSC) BPPV on the left. Personal communication with Giacinto Asprella-Libonati, MD, in 2010, showed that, in his experience, approximately 1% of BPPV seen per year affects the pediatric population aged 3 to 14 years. He reports that it is important to examine these children within 24 to 48 hours because BPPV was diagnosed in only 25% of those referred by pediatricians. There was a higher spontaneous resolution of BPPV in children, possibly because of their continuous head movements when playing games. PSC-BPPV was the most common form (about 80% of cases), followed by BPPV of lateral semicircular canal (LSC) (20% of cases). The BPPV cases were generally related to recent minor head trauma in the previous 24 to 48 hours (domestic injuries, sports injuries, school injuries, dental care). However, recurrent cases of BPPV usually occurred in children with a family history of migraine. These patients had more episodes of typical BPPV not preceded by head injury with involvement of multiple channels (LSC and PSC) in subsequent episodes. (Giacinto Asprella-Libonati, MD, Italy, personal communication, August 2010).

In the authors' experience with adults aged 18 to 39 years, risk factors for BPPV include certain activities such as yoga, pounding activities such as running on pavement, working underneath objects such as cars, and repetitively reaching high up, as would be common for ceiling painters. Giacomini and colleagues[12] also found that activities such as intense aerobic exercise, jogging, running on the treadmill, and swimming caused BPPV in this age group.

Finally, common causes of BPPV in people older than 40 years include head trauma or association with other ear disorders such as vestibular neuritis or labyrinthitis.[13–15] As with the 18- to 39-year-olds, certain positions are most likely to provoke vertigo, including lying back in bed, arising quickly, looking up, or reclining for dental or hairdressing procedures.

Recent work has suggested a correlation of recurrent episodes of positional vertigo with migraine, and because migraine is more prevalent in females, it may be a factor in the higher prevalence of BPPV in females.[1] Migraine-associated vertigo may cause episodic positional nystagmus that is difficult to differentiate from BPPV. The short duration of episodes (1 to 2 days) and frequent recurrence in otherwise healthy young patients with a history of migraine meeting the International Headache Society criteria often aid in making this diagnosis. Repositioning maneuvers are usually not effective in migraine-associated vertigo. Positional vertigo nystagmus during migraine-associated vertigo attacks may also appear atypical or have central features.

PATHOPHYSIOLOGY OF BPPV

Regardless of age, the pathophysiology of BPPV does not change. It is likely caused by otoconia that fall into the PSC or LSC after detaching from the utricle. The reasons for detachment are many but include increasing age, trauma, and infection. Schuknecht[16] was the first to suggest that these basophilic deposits on the cupula of the posterior canal caused BPPV. However, further work and intraoperative observations suggest that these canaliths are likely to be floating in the PSC or LSC where they render the canal gravitationally sensitive by acting as a plunger.[17,18]

Approximately 94% of BPPV cases involve the PSC-BPPV.[19] Dix and Hallpike[20] first observed this occurrence in 1952 when they developed the head maneuver that produces the characteristic ipsidirectional torsional nystagmus used to identify BPPV. During this maneuver, the patient's head is turned 45° to one side while he is seated. The patient is then moved quickly to a supine position with the neck slightly extended and the head remaining turned. The characteristic ipsidirectional torsional nystagmus is seen when the undermost ear is affected. The patient is then brought back up to a sitting position, and the nystagmus is noted to reverse direction as the canaliths fall back into the canal by gravity. The characteristics of the nystagmus include onset after several seconds, a decline after 10 to 30 seconds, and diminished effect with repeated positional testing in the same sitting (**Fig. 1**).[20,21] Although the maneuver needs no special equipment, visualization of the nystagmus can be aided by the use of infrared video or optical Frenzel lenses, which eliminate visual fixation.

Lateral (horizontal) canal involvement is the next most common variant of BPPV, constituting between 5% to 15% of BPPV cases.[22,23] LSC-BPPV was first described by Cipparrone and colleagues[24] and McClure[25] in 1985 and is characterized by nystagmus provoked by supine bilateral head turns with beating toward the undermost ear. The two distinct subtypes of LSC-BPPV based on the direction of horizontal nystagmus during supine head turns are geotropic and apogeotropic. Geotropic LSC-BPPV beats toward the undermost ear on supine positional testing. The horizontal nystagmus has a short latency and prolonged duration with poor fatigability. It is thought to be caused by canaliths moving under the influence of gravity within the long arm of the LSC. This, in turn, causes stimulation of utriculopetal endolymph flow in the supine position with the affected ear down (**Fig. 2**). Apogeotropic LSC-BPPV is characterized by a similar short latency and prolonged duration horizontal

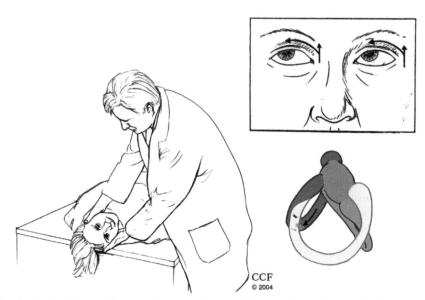

Fig. 1. Dix-Hallpike positioning. Lying position (head turned 45° to the right). Characteristic upbeat and right torsional nystagmus is illustrated (inset); canalith material has traveled down the long arm of the PSC, causing ampullofugal endolymph flow and stimulation of the cupula. (*From* White J. Benign paroxysmal positional vertigo: how to diagnose and quickly treat it. Cleve Clin J Med 2004;71(9):724. Copyright © 2004. The Cleveland Clinic Foundation. All rights reserved; with permission.)

nystagmus, but the direction of beating is away from the undermost ear on supine positional testing. Apogeotropic LSC-BPPV was not reported until later by Pagnini and colleagues[26] and Baloh and colleagues in 1995.[27] Different factors are likely responsible for apogeotropic LSC-BPPV, which includes otoconial debris that adhere to the cupula of the lateral canal causing the cupula to become gravity sensitive (cupulolithiasis) or otoconia trapped in the proximal segment of the lateral canal near the cupula (**Fig. 3**).[25–29]

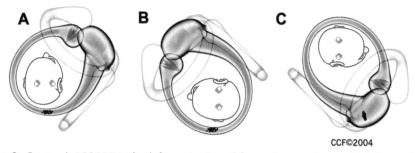

Fig. 2. Geotropic LSC-BPPV. The left ear is viewed from above as the patient lies supine. Head position is indicated. (*A*) The patient is supine and canalith material is in the distal LSC. (*B*) The patient has rolled onto the left ear and the canalith material moves toward the left LSC cupula, causing an ampullopetal endolymph current that is excitatory. (*C*) The patient has rolled onto the right ear and the canalith material moves away from the cupula, causing an ampullofugal endolymph flow that is inhibitory. Nystagmus beats toward the undermost ear. (*Courtesy of* Cleveland Clinic Foundation, copyright, 2004; with permission.)

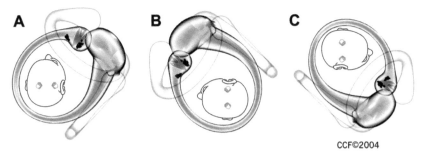

CCF©2004

Fig. 3. Apogeotropic LSC-BPPV. The left ear is viewed from above as the patient lies supine. Head position is indicated. (*A*) The patient is supine and canalith material is in the proximal LSC, possibly adherent to the cupula. (*B*) The patient has rolled onto the left ear, causing an ampullofugal endolymph current that is inhibitory. (*C*) The patient has rolled onto the right ear, causing an ampullopetal endolymph flow that is excitatory. Nystagmus beats away from the undermost ear. (*Courtesy of* Cleveland Clinic Foundation, copyright, 2004; with permission.)

DIAGNOSIS AND TREATMENT

Initially, BPPV treatments were exercise based and emphasized compensation and habituation.[30] However, specific canalith repositioning maneuvers based on an improved understanding of the pathophysiology of BPPV have been developed in the last 20 years and are now the standard of treatment, including the maneuvers described by Semont and colleagues,[31] and Epley[32] and the particle repositioning maneuvers for PSC-BPPV, which is a modified Epley maneuver without mastoid vibration (**Fig 4**).[18] Vestibular suppressant medication is not as effective as repositioning maneuvers and vestibular therapy.[33,34]

Although Dix-Hallpike positioning is highly effective for diagnosing PSC-BPPV, it lacks sensitivity in LSC-BPPV. For this reason, positional testing should include Dix-Hallpike positioning to head hanging right and left positions and also supine positional testing in the head centered supine, right ear down, and left ear down positions. Dix-Hallpike positional testing was entirely negative in case reports of 2 patients whose horizontal nystagmus with lateral supine head turns reached 12 degrees/second and 16 degrees/second.[35] In 4 other patients, the horizontal nystagmus observed in Dix-Hallpike positions appeared to beat in the contralateral direction to that observed during supine positional testing (1 geotropic and 3 apogeotropic). Furthermore, in most of the other patients, the Dix-Hallpike positioning nystagmus had a lesser velocity than that seen on supine positional testing.[35]

The identification of the involved ear in LSC-BPPV can be especially difficult because the canals are coplanar and nystagmus is seen in both lateral supine positions. Order effect and head tilt may also affect the direction of nystagmus.[36] In geotropic LSC-BPPV, the nystagmus is worse with the affected ear down. Treatment of geotropic LSC-BPV consists of 360° roll maneuvers toward the unaffected ear at 90° increments every 30 to 60 seconds, beginning with the patient in the supine position with the head flexed 0° to 30° and laterally rotated toward the affected ear.[37] The Gufoni maneuver is also highly effective and is performed with the patient beginning in the sitting position, lying quickly to the unaffected side, and then rotating the head 45° downwards, maintaining the position for 2 to 3 minutes, as described by Casani and colleagues.[29]

Treatment of apogeotropic LSC-BPPV consists of a variety of maneuvers because none are universally effective. Identification of the affected ear can be more

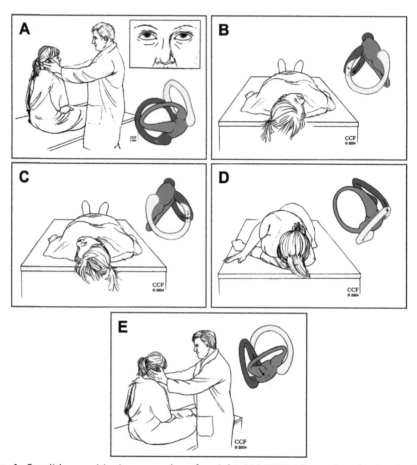

Fig. 4. Canalith repositioning procedure for right PSC-BPPV. The patient begins in the seated position with the head turned 45° toward the examiner (*A*). The patient is placed in the right Dix-Hallpike position and the characteristic nystagmus may be observed (*B*). The patient remains supine and the head is slowly rotated toward the opposite ear (*C*). The patient rolls onto the opposite shoulder and directs the head into a nose-down position (*D*). After any nystagmus subsides, the patient is assisted in returning to the original position (*E*). (*From* White J. Benign paroxysmal positional vertigo: how to diagnose and quickly treat it. Cleve Clin J Med 2004;71(9):725. Copyright © 2004. The Cleveland Clinic Foundation. All rights reserved; with permission.)

challenging in apogeotropic LSC-BPPV. Nystagmus is usually worse with the affected ear uppermost, and spontaneous nystagmus is occasionally seen in the supine position, which usually beats toward the involved side. The Lempert 360° roll maneuver toward the unaffected ear may be used first. The modified Gufoni maneuver can also be performed with the patient beginning in the sitting position and lying quickly to the affected side and then rotating the head 45° upwards, maintaining the position for 2 to 3 minutes, as described by Appiani and colleagues.[38] The Vannucchi-Asprella maneuvers are performed with the patient rapidly moving from the sitting to the supine position, then turning the head rapidly to the unaffected side, and returning to sitting position in which the head is then returned to midline. This maneuver is repeated 5 to 8 times in rapid succession.[39]

Finally, anterior semicircular canal BPPV is a controversial entity. Some investigators suggest that the paroxysmal nystagmus has a pure or torsional downbeat component in contrast to that seen with posterior canal involvement, which has a vertical upbeat component. Because the same maneuvers used to treat posterior canal BPPV seem effective for possible anterior canal involvement (although they may be performed on the contralateral side in some reports), the question may have more theoretical than clinical relevance.

EFFICACY OF TREATMENT

Multiple studies have looked at the efficacy of treatment by comparing a subjective assessment of a patient's self-reported vertigo frequency and severity and an objective assessment using repeated Dix-Hallpike testing. These studies have noted a poor correlation between self-report and Dix-Hallpike testing results. Studies by Pollak and colleagues,[40] Dornhoffer and Colvin,[41] and Ruckenstein[42] found that 22% to 38% of patients continue to report symptoms despite negative results of Dix-Hallpike testing, whereas Sargent and colleagues[43] noted reports of subjective improvement despite persistent positive results of Dix-Hallpike testing in their study sample. Lynn and colleagues[44] suggested that objective Dix-Hallpike testing should be considered the gold standard of outcome measures in BPPV. Controlled trials performed without Dix-Hallpike testing at outcome are generally excluded from evidence-based reviews.[45]

The effect of canalith repositioning on the quality of life in patients with benign positional vertigo has been demonstrated using the Medical Outcomes Study 36-Item Short Form Health Survey (SF-36)[46] and the Dizziness Handicap Inventory Short Form, (DHI-S).[47] In one study, patients with active benign positional vertigo scored worse than population norms on both measures, which improved 1 month after canalith repositioning maneuvers were performed (DHI-S mean decrease 8.1, $P<.001$, N = 40).[48] In addition, the SF-36 subscales normalized ($P<.05$).[49]

Recurrence is common after successful canalith repositioning for BPPV. One or two treatments are commonly effective in eliminating the current episode in more than 90% of cases, but will not prevent additional episodes.[50] Although the average recurrence rate is approximately 15% per year,[32,50,51] reported rates have ranged from 5% per year[52] to 45% at 30 weeks.[53]

Conversion between the posterior and horizontal canals can occasionally occur when patients are retested with Dix-Hallpike positioning after canalith repositioning has been performed. When conversion occurs, patients develop a brisk horizontal nystagmus that responds well to a 360° supine roll maneuver toward the unaffected side. In a study by the authors' group, it was found that of 241 cases there was LSC conversion in 15 cases, a rate of 6.2%. Repeat Dix-Hallpike testing after repositioning increases the diagnostic sensitivity for lateral canal conversions, which allows for rapid identification and quick management when they occur (**Fig. 5**).[54]

The use of postural restrictions after repositioning has declined in recent years. Patients were initially advised to keep their head elevated for 24 to 48 hours after the positioning procedure and avoid lying on the affected side for 5 days, all of which theoretically allowed the free-floating canalith debris to settle back into the utricle rather than returning to the semicircular canal. But, several studies have suggested that these instructions do not increase treatment efficacy.[55–57] Massoud and Ireland[56] studied the outcomes for the particle repositioning maneuver (N = 46) in patients who were randomized to post-procedure restrictions or control, with follow-up at 1 week.[56] The BPPV resolved in 96% of the 23 patients in the control group compared with 88%

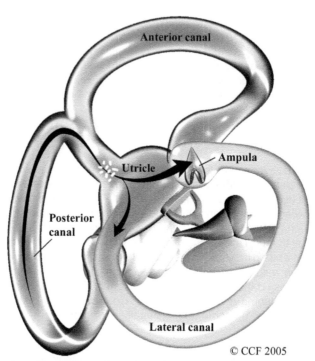

© CCF 2005

Fig. 5. Conversion of posterior to lateral canal BPPV. Canalith material leaves the PSC and can move onto the cupula of the LSC or into its long arm. In the first instance, the nystagmus on supine positioning is apogeotropic horizontal; in the latter instance, it is geotropic horizontal. (*Courtesy of* Cleveland Clinic Foundation, copyright, 2004; with permission.)

of the patients who received post-procedure restrictions. The difference did not reach statistical significance, possibly because of the small sample size. However, some centers continue to observe post-procedure restrictions based on anecdotal experience.

Other complications from repositioning include an isolated report of fainting, sweating, pallor, and hypotension during maneuvers accompanied by severe vertigo, possibly reflecting a vasovagal response.[58]

In an evidence-based review published in 2005, White and colleagues[59] found that the efficacy for a single treatment session for PSC-BPPV was 78% (range, 53% to 99% including 22 studies). The treatment efficacy increased with repeated sessions and usually reached at least 90%. Overall, 9 placebo-controlled trials consisting of 505 patients were evaluated in this meta-analysis. The risk of persistent BPPV without treatment was 69% compared with the 28% risk of persistent BPPV after a single canalith repositioning treatment, with a statistically significant difference (z, 9.09; $P<.001$). Therefore, the relative risk (risk of BPPV in the treatment group compared with the control group) was 39% (95% confidence interval, 0.32–0.48), representing a relative risk reduction of 61% (1−relative risk). The absolute risk reduction was 41% (used to estimate the treatment effect considering the actual frequency of the disorder in both groups). The number needed to treat was 2 (whole number rounded from 2.38). This number indicates that 2 patients would need to be treated to achieve a favorable outcome compared with no treatment. A number needed to treat within the range of 2 to 3 indicates that a treatment is very effective.[60]

The efficacy of canalith repositioning for LSC-BPPV depends on whether the nystagmus is geotropic or apogeotropic. For geotropic nystagmus, which beats toward the undermost ear on supine positional testing, repositioning treatments can alleviate symptoms in 75% to 100% of patients.[29,35,39] These same maneuvers are also used to treat the apogeotropic variant, which is characterized by nystagmus beating away from the undermost ear on supine positional testing. The apogeotropic variant is more difficult to treat, however, because the treatment depends on the mobilization of the otoconial debris. When the otoconial debris can be mobilized by repositioning maneuvers from near the cupula into the posterior portion of the LSC, the apogeotropic nystagmus can be converted to geotropic nystagmus, which is predictive of an excellent treatment response.[39] Casani and colleagues[29] used the Gufoni procedure in 9 patients with apogeotropic LSC-BPPV with a 44% success rate.[29] Asprella Libonati and colleagues[39] have described related techniques of rapid supine head turns in the Vannucchi-Asprella technique with somewhat better results, and White and colleagues[35] reported a 50% success rate. Therefore, cupulolithiasis of the horizontal semicircular canal explains many of the features of apogeotropic LSC-BPPV, including its persistence and resistance to treatments shown successful with canalithiasis, such as roll maneuvers.

In addition, it is possible that some apogeotropic LSC-BPPV cases represent a subtype of vestibular neuritis, which is a more central lesion. The superior vestibular nerve innervates the LSC crista, superior canal crista, macula utriculi, and dorsum of the macula sacculi. Nadol[61] showed that superior division vestibular neuritis caused degeneration of the lateral canal crista. The neuritis could also affect the utricular nerve, thus removing otolith inhibition from the LSC efferents at the level of the vestibular nuclei. Animal experiments have demonstrated that apogeotropic horizontal nystagmus develops in cats after unilateral utricular nerve inactivation.[62] Gacek[63] theorizes that a loss of inhibitory otolith input is responsible for some cases of PSC-BPPV, a model that can also be considered in apogeotropic LSC-BPPV. Otolith-canal mismatch or neural degeneration may also explain the persistence of apogeotropic LSC-BPPV despite aggressive therapy aimed at particle repositioning or liberation.

In the authors' published series, treatment resolved the geotropic LSC-BPPV in all 10 patients.[35] The affected ear was identified as the side provoking the worst nystagmus in the supine head turn, and roll maneuvers were performed toward the unaffected ear in each patient during the initial office visit. Symptoms resolved immediately in 7 of 10 patients. The symptoms resolved in 2 more patients with roll maneuvers in physical therapy. Also, 1 patient required additional physical therapy to resolve nystagmus and vertigo including repeated roll procedures and modified Brandt-Daroff habituation exercises.

Only 5 of the 10 patients in the apogeotropic group experienced complete resolution of vertigo and nystagmus. Of these 5 patients, 1 responded to treatment in the first session, which consisted of vigorous 120° head shaking for 1 minute. This treatment was used because the patient was unable to roll or engage in a physical therapy program after a traumatic fall with orthopedic injuries. Subsequent follow-up with supine head turn testing demonstrated complete resolution of nystagmus. In the 4 additional successfully treated apogeotropic patients, roll maneuvers were effective. The remaining 5 patients with apogeotropic LSC-BPPV continued to experience persistent nystagmus. One patient reported substantial symptomatic improvement but continued to show apogeotropic positional nystagmus and was treated with roll maneuvers and modified Brandt-Daroff habituation exercises in physical therapy before declining further treatment. The other 4 patients continued physical therapy with mildly persisting symptoms. Treatment included roll maneuvers, modified Brandt-Daroff habituation exercises, Gufoni maneuvers, Vannucchi-Asprella maneuvers, and vestibular rehabilitation. Chi-square testing revealed that the outcome was statistically significantly poorer in the apogeotropic group than in the geotropic group (χ^2, 7.3; df, 1; $P<.007$).[35]

Finally, there is an association between BPPV and postural control because patients experience postural instability with BPPV. Increased anterior-posterior sway has been documented on computerized dynamic posturography (CDP).[64–67] Some residual postural instability has been observed even after successful treatment of BPPV.[65,66] Theories regarding this persistent postural instability include receptor sensitivity alteration, residual scant debris in the semicircular canal of the inner ear, otolith dysfunction, or dysfunctional central adaptation.[66]

The elderly may be more affected by residual postural instability after successful BPPV treatment. Blatt and colleagues[65] suggested that younger subjects were more likely to show recovery of postural stability after successful BPPV treatment. Their study sample size was small (33 patients aged 38–91 years) and did not specifically report data on the number and outcome of the elderly patients. Conditions more common in the elderly, including orthopedic problems, deconditioning, and medical conditions, such as diabetes, neuropathy, and neurologic disorders, may complicate the assessment of postural control in this age group. To examine the recovery of the elderly from BPPV, follow-up is necessary to compare postural stability before and after successful BPPV treatment.

The authors' experience has revealed significant improvement in postural control after canalith repositioning for PSC-BPPV in elderly patients (J. White, MD, PhD, Cleveland, OH, unpublished observations, July 2005.) It was found that the most sensitive measure was the Dynamic Gait Index (DGI) ($P = .011$), particularly the horizontal head turn condition ($P = .02$). The improvement in baseline to posttreatment scores of 3.4 points exceeds the 3-point criteria for clinically significant improvement suggested in other published studies using the DGI to assess fall risk reduction.[68] This improvement suggests that canalith repositioning for BPPV reduces fall risk in elderly patients with BPPV.

CDP results were consistent with DGI findings and with previously published reports noting impaired postural stability in patients with active PSC-BPPV.[64–67] Total CDP score and vestibular subscale scores showed a trend toward improvement after treatment, although significance may have been limited by the small sample size. Improvement after canalith repositioning was also reflected in a highly significant change in self-reported Dizziness Handicap Inventory ($P = .027$).

SURGICAL TREATMENT

Plugging of the involved semicircular canal may be a consideration in cases of BPPV with unquestionable localization to the semicircular canal involved and persistent symptoms. This procedure has been used successfully in cases of resistant PSC-BPPV.[69] Difficulties in definitively identifying the affected side make the procedure less appealing in LSC-BPPV than in PSC-BPPV. Horii and colleagues[70] reported a case of LSC-BPPV that did not improve when treated with plugging of the LSC and required additional treatment on the unoperated side.

SUMMARY

BPPV is one of the most common causes of vertigo. As the world population continues to age, it is expected that the societal burdens from BPPV will increase. This increase is a result of the higher risk of falls with injury in the elderly that occur because of vertigo and postural instability. BPPV does occur across the lifespan, but there are very few published reports on its occurrence in children. However, when it does occur in children aged 3 to 14 years, it is typically associated with minor traumatic activities or migraine headache. Regardless of age, the pathophysiology of BPPV does not change. BPPV is thought to be caused by otoconia that fall into the PSC or LSC after they detach from the utricle. This detaching and falling of otoconia can be secondary to trauma, infection, aging, or other factors. Approximately 94% of these cases occur when the otoconia fall into the PSC and can be diagnosed with the Dix-Hallpike maneuver. Approximately 5% to 15% of these cases occur when the otoconia fall into the LSC. These cases can be diagnosed with supine bilateral head turns. The geotropic form, which is characterized by canaliths moving under the influence of gravity within the long arm of the LSC, can be effectively treated with a 360° log roll or the Gufoni maneuver. The apogeotropic form, on the other hand, is more difficult to treat because it is either caused by adherence of the otoconia to the cupula or a more central cause such as a subtype of vestibular neuritis.

Strong evidence exists for the efficacy of canalith repositioning. Efficacy for treatment of PSC-BPPV is estimated to be up to 90% after 1 to 2 sessions. The efficacy for LSC-BPPV depends on whether the nystagmus is geotropic or apogeotropic. For geotropic forms, the efficacy of canalith repositioning is approximately 75% to 100%. The efficacy of canalith repositioning for apogeotropic LSC-BPPV, on the other hand, is approximately 44% to 50%, because some forms may represent cupulolithiasis, other vestibular dysfunctions, or central disorder.

If positioning therapy is not successful, surgery is an option for PSC-BPPV. Plugging of the involved semicircular canal has been used in cases of resistant PSC-BPPV. However, this treatment has been more difficult for LSC-BPPV because of the difficulty in locating the correct side.

Continuing education of otolaryngologists and primary care providers in BPPV will help to decrease the incidence of falls and fractures secondary to vertigo and will ultimately decrease the potential societal burden as the population continues to age.

REFERENCES

1. von Brevern M, Radtke A, Lezius F, et al. Epidemiology of benign paroxysmal positional vertigo: a population based study. J Neurol Neurosurg Psychiatry 2007;78(7):710–5.
2. Schappert SM. National ambulatory medical care survey: 1989 summary. Vital Health Stat 13 1992;110:1–80.
3. Katsarkas A. Benign paroxysmal positional vertigo (BPPV): idiopathic versus post-traumatic. Acta Otolaryngol 1999;119(7):745–9.
4. Hanley K, O'Dowd T, Considine N. A systematic review of vertigo in primary care. Br J Gen Pract 2001;51(469):666–71.
5. Baloh RW, Honrubia V, Jacobson K. Benign positional vertigo: clinical and oculographic features in 240 cases. Neurology 1987;37(3):371–8.
6. Nedzelski JM, Barber HO, McIlmoyl L. Diagnoses in a dizziness unit. J Otolaryngol 1986;15(2):101–4.
7. Neuhauser HK. Epidemiology of vertigo. Curr Opin Neurol 2007;20(1):40–6.
8. Li JC, Li CJ, Epley J, et al. Cost-effective management of benign positional vertigo using canalith repositioning. Otolaryngol Head Neck Surg 2000;122(3): 334–9.

9. Oghalai JS, Manolidis S, Barth JL, et al. Unrecognized benign paroxysmal positional vertigo in elderly patients. Otolaryngol Head Neck Surg 2000;122(5):630–4.

10. Mizukoshi K, Watanabe Y, Shojaku H, et al. Epidemiological studies on benign paroxysmal positional vertigo in Japan. Acta Otolaryngol Suppl 1988;447: 67–72.

11. Froehling DA, Silverstein MD, Mohr DN, et al. Benign positional vertigo: incidence and prognosis in a population-based study in Olmsted County, Minnesota. Mayo Clin Proc 1991;66(6):596–601.

12. Giacomini PG, Ferraro S, Di Girolamo S, et al. Benign paroxysmal positional vertigo after intense physical activity: a report of nine cases. Eur Arch Otorhinolaryngol 2009;266(11):1831–5.

13. Schuknecht HF. Mechanism of inner ear injury from blows to the head. Ann Otol Rhinol Laryngol 1969;78(2):253–62.

14. Barber HO. Positional nystagmus, especially after head injury. Laryngoscope 1964;74:891–944.

15. Barber HO. Head injury audiological and vestibular findings. Ann Otol Rhinol Laryngol 1969;78(2):239–52.

16. Schuknecht HF. Cupulolithiasis. Arch Otolaryngol 1969;90(6):765–78.

17. Hall SF, Ruby RR, McClure JA. The mechanics of benign paroxysmal vertigo. J Otolaryngol 1979;8(2):151–8.

18. Parnes LS, Price-Jones RG. Particle repositioning maneuver for benign paroxysmal positional vertigo. Ann Otol Rhinol Laryngol 1993;102(5):325–31.

19. Honrubia V, Baloh RW, Harris MR, et al. Paroxysmal positional vertigo syndrome. Am J Otol 1999;20(4):465–70.

20. Dix MR, Hallpike CS. The pathology symptomatology and diagnosis of certain common disorders of the vestibular system. Proc R Soc Med 1952;45(6): 341–54.

21. Baloh RW, Sakala S, Honrubia V. The mechanism of benign paroxysmal positional nystagmus. Adv Otorhinolaryngol 1979;25:161–6.

22. Cakir BO, Ercan I, Cakir ZA, et al. What is the true incidence of horizontal semicircular canal benign paroxysmal positional vertigo? Otolaryngol Head Neck Surg 2006;134(3):451–4.

23. Parnes LS, Agrawal SK, Atlas J. Diagnosis and management of benign paroxysmal positional vertigo (BPPV). CMAJ 2003;169(7):681–93.

24. Cipparrone L, Corridi G, Pagnini P. Cupulolitiasi. In: V Giornata Italiana di Nistagmografia Clinica. Nistagmografia e patologia vestibolare periferica. Milano Italia; 1985. p. 36–53.

25. McClure JA. Horizontal canal BPV. J Otolaryngol 1985;14(1):30–5.

26. Pagnini P, Vannucchi P, Nuti D. Le nystagmus apogeotrpique dans le vertige paroxystique positionelle benin du canal semicirculaire horizontal. La revue d'Otoneurologie Francaise 1994;12:304–7.

27. Baloh RW, Yue Q, Jacobson KM, et al. Persistent direction-changing positional nystagmus: another variant of benign positional nystagmus? Neurology 1995; 45(7):1297–301.

28. Fife TD. Recognition and management of horizontal canal benign positional vertigo. Am J Otol 1998;19(3):345–51.

29. Casani AP, Vannucci G, Fattori B, et al. The treatment of horizontal canal positional vertigo: our experience in 66 cases. Laryngoscope 2002;112(1):172–8.

30. Brandt T, Daroff RB. Physical therapy for benign paroxysmal positional vertigo. Arch Otolaryngol 1980;106(8):484–5.

31. Semont A, Freyss G, Vitte E. Curing the BPPV with a liberatory maneuver. Adv Otorhinolaryngol 1988;42:290–3.
32. Epley JM. The canalith repositioning procedure: for treatment of benign paroxysmal positional vertigo. Otolaryngol Head Neck Surg 1992;107(3):399–404.
33. McClure JA, Willett JM. Lorazepam and diazepam in the treatment of benign paroxysmal vertigo. J Otolaryngol 1980;9(6):472–7.
34. Fujino A, Tokumasu K, Yosio S, et al. Vestibular training for benign paroxysmal positional vertigo. Its efficacy in comparison with antivertigo drugs. Arch Otolaryngol Head Neck Surg 1994;120(5):497–504.
35. White JA, Coale KD, Catalano PJ, et al. Diagnosis and management of lateral semicircular canal benign paroxysmal positional vertigo. Otolaryngol Head Neck Surg 2005;133(2):278–84.
36. Bisdorff AR, Debatisse D. Localizing signs in positional vertigo due to lateral canal cupulolithiasis. Neurology 2001;57(6):1085–8.
37. Lempert T, Tiel-Wilck K. A positional maneuver for treatment of horizontal-canal benign positional vertigo. Laryngoscope 1996;106(4):476–8.
38. Appiani GC, Catania G, Gagliardi M, et al. Repositioning maneuver for the treatment of the apogeotropic variant of horizontal canal benign paroxysmal positional vertigo. Otol Neurotol 2005;26(2):257–60.
39. Asprella Libonati G, Gagliardi G, Cifarelli D, et al. "Step by step" treatment of lateral semicircular canal canalolithiasis under videonystagmoscopic examination. Acta Otorhinolaryngol Ital 2003;23(1):10–5.
40. Pollak L, Davies RA, Luxon LL. Effectiveness of the particle repositioning maneuver in benign paroxysmal positional vertigo with and without additional vestibular pathology. Otol Neurotol 2002;23(1):79–83.
41. Dornhoffer JL, Colvin GB. Benign paroxysmal positional vertigo and canalith repositioning: clinical correlations. Am J Otol 2000;21(2):230–3.
42. Ruckenstein MJ. Therapeutic efficacy of the Epley canalith repositioning maneuver. Laryngoscope 2001;111(6):940–5.
43. Sargent EW, Bankaitis AE, Hollenbeak CS, et al. Mastoid oscillation in canalith repositioning for paroxysmal positional vertigo. Otol Neurotol 2001;22(2):205–9.
44. Lynn S, Pool A, Rose D, et al. Randomized trial of the canalith repositioning procedure. Otolaryngol Head Neck Surg 1995;113(6):712–20.
45. Blakley BW. A randomized, controlled assessment of the canalith repositioning maneuver. Otolaryngol Head Neck Surg 1994;110(4):391–6.
46. Ware JE Jr, Sherbourne CD. The MOS 36-item short-form health survey (SF-36). I. Conceptual framework and item selection. Med Care 1992;30(6):473–83.
47. Jacobson GP, Newman CW. The development of the dizziness handicap inventory. Arch Otolaryngol Head Neck Surg 1990;116(4):424–7.
48. Lopez-Escamez JA, Gamiz MJ, Fernandez-Perez A, et al. Impact of treatment on health-related quality of life in patients with posterior canal benign paroxysmal positional vertigo. Otol Neurotol 2003;24(4):637–41.
49. Gamiz MJ, Lopez-Escamez JA. Health-related quality of life in patients over sixty years old with benign paroxysmal positional vertigo. Gerontology 2004;50(2):82–6.
50. Nunez RA, Cass SP, Furman JM. Short- and long-term outcomes of canalith repositioning for benign paroxysmal positional vertigo. Otolaryngol Head Neck Surg 2000;122(5):647–52.
51. Furman JM, Cass SP. Benign paroxysmal positional vertigo. N Engl J Med 1999;341(21):1590–6.

52. Sakaida M, Takeuchi K, Ishinaga H, et al. Long-term outcome of benign paroxysmal positional vertigo. Neurology 2003;60(9):1532–4.

53. Beynon GJ, Baguley DM, da Cruz MJ. Recurrence of symptoms following treatment of posterior semicircular canal benign positional paroxysmal vertigo with a particle repositioning manoeuvre. J Otolaryngol 2000;29(1):2–6.

54. White JA, Oas JG. Diagnosis and management of lateral semicircular canal conversions during particle repositioning therapy. Laryngoscope 2005;115(10): 1895–7.

55. Marciano E, Marcelli V. Postural restrictions in labyrintholithiasis. Eur Arch Otorhinolaryngol 2002;259(5):262–5.

56. Massoud EA, Ireland DJ. Post-treatment instructions in the nonsurgical management of benign paroxysmal positional vertigo. J Otolaryngol 1996;25(2):121–5.

57. Nuti D, Nati C, Passali D. Treatment of benign paroxysmal positional vertigo: no need for postmaneuver restrictions. Otolaryngol Head Neck Surg 2000;122(3): 440–4.

58. Yimtae K, Srirompotong S, Sae-Seaw P. A randomized trial of the canalith repositioning procedure. Laryngoscope 2003;113(5):828–32.

59. White J, Savvides P, Cherian N, et al. Canalith repositioning for benign paroxysmal positional vertigo. Otol Neurotol 2005;26(4):704–10.

60. Smeeth L, Haines A, Ebrahim S. Numbers needed to treat derived from meta-analyses–sometimes informative, usually misleading. BMJ 1999;318(7197): 1548–51.

61. Nadol JB Jr. Vestibular neuritis. Otolaryngol Head Neck Surg 1995;112(1): 162–72.

62. Fluur E. Positional and positioning nystagmus as a result of utriculocupular integration. Acta Otolaryngol 1974;78(1–2):19–27.

63. Gacek RR. Pathology of benign paroxysmal positional vertigo revisited. Ann Otol Rhinol Laryngol 2003;112(7):574–82.

64. Black FO, Nashner LM. Postural disturbance in patients with benign paroxysmal positional nystagmus. Ann Otol Rhinol Laryngol 1984;93(6 Pt 1):595–9.

65. Blatt PJ, Georgakakis GA, Herdman SJ, et al. The effect of the canalith repositioning maneuver on resolving postural instability in patients with benign paroxysmal positional vertigo. Am J Otol 2000;21(3):356–63.

66. Di Girolamo S, Paludetti G, Briglia G, et al. Postural control in benign paroxysmal positional vertigo before and after recovery. Acta Otolaryngol 1998;118(3): 289–93.

67. Voorhees RL. The role of dynamic posturography in neurotologic diagnosis. Laryngoscope 1989;99(10 Pt 1):995–1001.

68. Hall CD, Schubert MC, Herdman SJ. Prediction of fall risk reduction as measured by dynamic gait index in individuals with unilateral vestibular hypofunction. Otol Neurotol 2004;25(5):746–51.

69. Parnes LS. Update on posterior canal occlusion for benign paroxysmal positional vertigo. Otolaryngol Clin North Am 1996;29(2):333–42.

70. Horii A, Imai T, Mishiro Y, et al. Horizontal canal type BPPV: bilaterally affected case treated with canal plugging and Lempert's maneuver. ORL J Otorhinolaryngol Relat Spec 2003;65(6):366–9.

Vestibular Neuritis

John C. Goddard, MD[a], Jose N. Fayad, MD[a,b],*

KEYWORDS

- Vestibular neuritis • Vestibular neuronitis
- Labyrinthitis • Vertigo • Dizziness

L.R. is a 40-year-old woman referred by her primary care physician with a chief complaint of acute, severe, room-spinning vertigo. She stated that she awoke at 4 AM when the sensation of vertigo came on very suddenly, was quite violent, and was accompanied by nausea and vomiting. She recalled having to crawl on the floor to make it to the bathroom and felt that the room continued to spin any time she opened her eyes. She eventually made it back to her bed and had to lie still, without moving her head, to minimize the waves of nausea and episodes of vomiting. She felt a "heavy" sensation in her head for several days afterward. Although it was difficult to remember the details, she did not recall a loss of hearing or any associated ringing in her ears with the episode. The patient felt a bit nauseated the day before the vertigo began, but otherwise had been in good health. The patient was ultimately taken to the emergency room by her spouse, where she was hydrated intravenously and given vestibular suppressants and antiemetics. Several days after the onset of the vertigo, the patient described feeling quite unsteady, especially with any rapid movement of her head or body.

INTRODUCTION

Vestibular neuritis is characterized by the acute onset of vertigo with associated nausea, vomiting, and generalized imbalance. The acute phase is often severe and can last from a few hours to several days, while a more subtle sense of imbalance and unsteadiness may linger for weeks. Auditory symptoms are uncommon, although patients may occasionally report fullness and tinnitus. Patients with accompanying hearing loss are believed to have a slightly different pathophysiological entity termed acute labyrinthitis.

The precise etiology of vestibular neuritis remains elusive. Several theories have been postulated and supported, at least partially, within the literature. Dix and Hallpike[1] in the 1950s suggested that an infectious process affecting "Scarpa's" ganglion or the vestibular nerve might be responsible. Lindsay and Hemenway[2] felt that an ischemic process might be responsible, although they found no direct

The authors have nothing to disclose.
[a] House Clinic, 2100 West Third Street, Los Angeles, CA 90057, USA
[b] University of Southern California, 1200 North State Street, Los Angeles, CA 90031, USA
* Corresponding author.
E-mail address: jfayad@hei.org

Otolaryngol Clin N Am 44 (2011) 361–365
doi:10.1016/j.otc.2011.01.007
0030-6665/11/$ – see front matter © 2011 Elsevier Inc. All rights reserved.

evidence of vascular occlusion. More recent efforts have suggested that a viral agent may be the underlying cause.[3–7] While individual studies have demonstrated the presence of herpes simplex virus DNA within vestibular nerve fibers and "Scarpa's" ganglion, others have demonstrated histologic changes within the vestibular nerve suggestive of viral-induced atrophy and inflammation.[6–8] Anatomic studies have also demonstrated that the superior vestibular nerve, which supplies the utricle, superior, and horizontal semicircular canals, is more likely to be involved in cases of vestibular neuritis.[2,9] Goebel and colleagues[10] have shown an anatomic basis for this observation related to the increased length, reduced diameter, and increased bony trabeculae of the bony canal housing the superior vestibular nerve (and its divisions) as compared with the inferior vestibular nerve.

Despite an inability to clearly identify the cause of vestibular neuritis, a thorough understanding of its clinical course and management has been established. The typical onset is one of intense vertigo, oftentimes described upon awakening. Patients may have a tendency to fall toward the involved side and will frequently demonstrate spontaneous nystagmus whose direction is similar in various positions of gaze. Head or body movements exacerbate the symptoms, and patients will often try to minimize any such movements by lying completely still. While the initial vertigo symptoms do subside over a period of days, patients will often have a longer period of continued imbalance. This imbalance may manifest as difficulty making quick movements or turns, slight swaying during walking, or a generalized feeling of unsteadiness. Patients also often complain of a heavy feeling in their head or simply feeling "off" for days to weeks after the initial episode. Benign paroxysmal positional vertigo (BPPV) is more common in patients who have suffered from vestibular neuritis, but it can occur at varying intervals after the acute attack. Why BPPV seems to occur more frequently in these patients is not known, Schucknecht suggested that utricular otoconia might be loosened with the initial neuritis.[11] Repeated bouts of vestibular neuritis have also been described, which many contend lends evidence toward a possible viral reactivation process as seen in herpes zoster oticus.[5]

As with most vestibular disorders of peripheral origin, a diagnosis of vestibular neuritis is primarily reached through a complete and thorough history and physical examination. A history of chronic ear disease should be elicited, as complications of chronic otitis media are quite common and may present with vertigo (ie, labyrinthine fistula or cerebellar abscess). The duration of the vertigo attack is a critical component in the history of any patient with a complaint of dizziness and is particularly helpful in diagnosing vestibular neuritis. However, variability in the duration of the initial attack of vertigo is possible (ie, hours to days), while recurrent episodes of intense vertigo may occur with years of time between individual events. Equally important as the duration of the vertigo attack is whether any neurologic symptoms are present. As there are several potentially dangerous causes of dizziness, one must always maintain a high degree of suspicion (**Box 1**). Directed questioning regarding associated symptoms is of paramount importance in ruling out vertigo of central etiology. In particular, one should ask about any weakness or change in sensation (pain, temperature, or numbness) of the limbs or face, slurred speech, vision changes, memory loss, or ataxia. These symptoms are indicative of a central insult and require a distinctly different management paradigm than that used in patients with vestibular neuritis. Brainstem/cerebellar infarct or hemorrhage may present with some form of dizziness but will invariably be accompanied by other neurologic symptoms. These patients will oftentimes be unable to stand or walk. In such cases, imaging is diagnostic, with magnetic resonance imaging (MRI) being the preferred modality. Although rare, compromise of the posterior cerebral circulation may manifest with neck pain (from

Box 1
Differential diagnosis of acute vertigo

Cerebellar hemorrhage or ischemia	Multiple sclerosis
Brainstem hemorrhage or ischemia	Labyrinthitis
Vertebral artery dissection	Traumatic disruption of otic capsule
	Ménière's disease

trauma or vertebral artery dissection) and associated dizziness and requires prompt neurosurgical consultation.

Physical examination should be performed to confirm the absence or presence of neurologic involvement. In addition to a complete head and neck examination with an otoscopic examination and testing of all cranial nerves, tuning fork testing, cerebellar testing, gait assessment, and a full neurologic examination should be performed. Chronic ear disease and any associated complications are usually discernible from a combination of history and physical examination including a careful microscopic otoscopic examination. High-resolution computed tomography (CT) imaging of the temporal bones should be obtained if intracranial pathology of otologic origin is suspected, and the appropriate treatment should be instituted accordingly. Any neurologic abnormalities on physical examination should prompt further investigation into a central cause with dedicated imaging of the brain, preferably in the form of MRI. Patients with vestibular neuritis may sway toward the side of the involved ear while standing, but an inability to stand without assistance is also indicative of a central lesion and demands dedicated imaging. Cases of vestibular neuritis present with characteristic spontaneous nystagmus that is both horizontal and rotary, has a fast phase directed toward the uninvolved ear, and improves with fixation. Head thrust testing toward the affected ear will often demonstrate catch-up saccades indicating a peripheral vestibular insult.[12] Formal vestibular testing, though not performed in practice in the acute setting, has been performed in research settings and typically demonstrates reduced caloric responses.[1] Imaging studies are not required in classic cases of vestibular neuritis, but as outlined previously, the presence of any additional or unusual symptoms demands an assessment for the presence of a central lesion.

In clinics specializing in vestibular disorders, vestibular neuritis accounts for between 3% and 10% of diagnoses.[13] An annual incidence of vestibular neuritis approximating 3.5 cases per 100,000 persons was reported by Sekitani and colleagues,[14] but further literature on the subject is lacking. In this same report, which was based on a large Japanese population, the peak age distribution for vestibular neuritis was between 30 and 50 years, with a range of 3 to 88 years. Furthermore, approximately 12% of patients in this study were over age 65.[14] Dix and Hallpike,[1] in their review of 100 cases of vestibular neuritis, found that 94% of cases occurred among patients between the ages of 20 and 59. While middle-aged individuals do seem to be more commonly affected, the authors' experience would suggest that vestibular neuritis likely accounts for a larger percentage of vestibular diagnoses than outlined in these reports. This may be a consequence of differences in geographic referral patterns, variations in health care access, and a general lack of follow-up in patients achieving rapid resolution of symptoms. Additionally, it is possible that some practitioners may confuse vestibular neuritis with other diagnoses, including migraine-associated vertigo (MAV). MAV is most often seen in patients having some prior history of headaches or a family history of migraines[15] (see article by Cherchi and Hain in this publication). In patients with MAV, the headache itself may occur before or after the onset of dizziness, while the sensation of dizziness may represent true vertigo or merely a sense of disequilibrium. The variability of symptom duration in patients with MAV, with dizziness lasting from several hours to even a whole day, may explain why there might be some difficulty in properly distinguishing between this entity and cases of vestibular neuritis. MAV occurs in both adults and children, although in pediatric cases it is commonly referred to as benign paroxysmal vertigo of childhood[15] (see articles by McCaslin and colleagues, and O'Reilly and colleagues in this publication). Cases of pediatric vestibular neuritis have been reported, yet such a diagnosis among children is fairly uncommon.[16,17] Reasons for this apparent predilection for middle-aged individuals is not known, and further investigation into the etiology of vestibular neuritis, viral or otherwise, is likely to aid in understanding this disease process.

Management of patients with vestibular neuritis is primarily supportive. The acute phase is best managed with vestibular suppressants, antiemetics, and in some cases, intravenous hydration. Common medications employed in this acute phase have been extensively reviewed elsewhere.[12] Patients who are more susceptible to dehydration, including children, the elderly, and individuals with underlying systemic disorders, may require hospitalization for a brief period of time. It has been suggested that the early administration of steroids may improve the rate and extent of recovery of vestibular function, although controversy remains as to the best method of assessing vestibular recovery and whether there is truly an improvement in clinical symptomatology.[18–21] The use of antiviral medications has also been proposed as an adjunctive treatment, yet evidence supporting their effectiveness is lacking.[19]

Once the acute phase of vestibular neuritis has passed, treatment efforts are aimed at improving central compensation through vestibular rehabilitation. In addition to minimizing the use of vestibular suppressants, early exercise is encouraged, and patients are instructed on various vestibular exercises designed to enhance ocular stability and improve the tolerance of various head and body movements. The degree of compensation is somewhat variable and likely depends on a number of factors, including patient age and underlying functional status, degree of initial vestibular injury (and any subsequent end-organ recovery), as well as patient motivation. While many patients may be able to compensate with the help of home vestibular exercise programs, others may require formal vestibular rehabilitation under the supervision of a dedicated vestibular therapist (see article by Alrwaily and Whitney in this publication). Elderly individuals and patients with prolonged recovery would likely be excellent candidates for such a course of treatment. In rare instances, when prolonged vestibular therapy is not effective and patients are debilitated by their symptoms, surgical intervention may be warranted. In such patients, the authors feel that an MRI of the brain as well as videonystagmography should be performed preoperatively to document the absence of an eighth nerve or central lesion and to determine the degree of peripheral vestibular dysfunction. Surgical options in the setting of chronic vestibular neuritis include vestibular nerve section if hearing is present, or labyrinthectomy in cases of a dead or unserviceable ear. Although surgical intervention is considered a solution of last resort, it can be quite effective in improving patient symptoms.[22,23]

CONCLUSION

In summary, vestibular neuritis is characterized by the acute onset of severe vertigo, nausea, and imbalance; an absence of neurologic deficits; and the presence of normal hearing. History and physical examination alone are usually adequate for diagnosis, although one must ensure that a central insult is not at fault. Imaging is generally not required if the history and physical examination support a diagnosis of vestibular neuritis. However, CT imaging should be considered in the setting of chronic ear disease with MRI reserved for cases that are suggestive of a central (ie, brainstem or cerebellar) cause. Management of the acute phase of vestibular neuritis is primarily medical, while long-term treatment is designed to improve vestibular compensation.

REFERENCES

1. Dix M, Hallpike C. The pathology, symptomatology, and diagnosis of certain common disorders of the vestibular system. Proc R Soc Med 1952;45(6):341–54.
2. Lindsay JR, Hemenway WG. Postural vertigo due to unilateral partial vestibular loss. Ann Otol Rhinol Laryngol 1956;65:692–708.
3. Furata Y, Takasu T, Fukuda S, et al. Latent herpes simplex virus type 1 in human vestibular ganglia. Acta Otolaryngol Suppl 1993;503:85–9.
4. Hirata Y, Gyo K, Yanagihara N. Herpetic vestibular neuritis: an experimental study. Acta Otolaryngol Suppl 1995;519(Suppl):93–6.
5. Gacek R, Gacek M. The three faces of vestibular ganglionitis. Ann Otol Rhinol Laryngol 2002;111(2):103–14.
6. Theil D, Arbusow V, Deurfuss T, et al. Prevalence of HSV-1 LAT in human trigeminal, geniculate, and vestibular ganglia and its implication for cranial nerve syndromes. Brain Pathol 2001;11(4):408–13.
7. Baloh RW, Ishiyama A, Wackym P, et al. Vestibular neuritis: clinical–pathological correlation. Otolaryngol Head Neck Surg 1996;114:586–92.
8. Schuknecht HF, Kitamura K. Vestibular neuronitis. Ann Otol Rhinol Laryngol 1981; 78:1–19.
9. Nadol JB. Vestibular neuritis. Otolaryngol Head Neck Surg 1995;112:162–72.
10. Goebel J, O'Mara W, Gianoli G. Anatomic considerations in vestibular neuritis. Otol Neurotol 2001;22:512–8.
11. Schuknecht HF. Positional vertigo: clinical and experimental observations. Trans Am Acad Ophthalmol Otolaryngol 1962;66:319–31.
12. Baloh R. Vestibular neuritis. N Engl J Med 2003;348:1027–32.
13. Neuhauser H. Epidemiology of vertigo. Curr Opin Neurol 2007;20:40–6.
14. Sekitani T, Imate Y, Noguchi T, et al. Vestibular neuronitis: epidemiological survey by questionnaire in Japan. Acta Otolaryngol Suppl 1993;503:9–12.
15. Reploeg MD, Goebel JA. Migraine-associated dizziness: patient characteristics and management options. Otol Neurotol 2002;23(3):364–71.
16. Wiener-Vacher SR. Vestibular disorders in children. Int J Audiol 2008;47:578–83.
17. Bower CM, Cotton RT. The spectrum of vertigo in children. Arch Otolaryngol Head Neck Surg 1995;121:911–5.
18. Kitahara T, Kondoh K, Morihana T, et al. Steroid effects on vestibular compensation in humans. Neurol Res 2003;25:287–91.
19. Strupp M, Zingler V, Arbusow V, et al. Methylprednisolone, valacyclovir, or the combination for vestibular neuritis. N Engl J Med 2004;351(4):354–61.
20. Shupak A, Issa A, Golz A, et al. Prednisone treatment for vestibular neuritis. Otol Neurotol 2008;29:368–74.
21. Goudakos J, Markou K, Franco-Vidal V, et al. Corticosteroids in the treatment of vestibular neuritis: a systematic review and meta-analysis. Otol Neurotol 2010;31: 183–9.
22. Benecke JE. Surgery for non-Meniere's vertigo. Acta Otolaryngol Suppl 1994; 513:37–9.
23. Pappas D, Pappas D. Vestibular nerve section: long-term follow up. Laryngoscope 1997;107:1203–9.

Migraine-Associated Vertigo

Marcello Cherchi, MD, PhD[a,b],*, Timothy C. Hain, MD[a,b,c,d]

KEYWORDS

• Migraine • Vertigo • Headache • Aura • Vestibular • Otologic

DG is a 31-year-old woman who presents with a 6-week history of episodic dizziness that she describes, "As if I am standing on a boat." The dizziness can last the entire day and may occur 2 to 3 times per week. The dizziness is worse with movement but can even be present when she remains still while looking at a computer screen. Although she has had some of her usual headaches, they do not coincide with the episodes of dizziness. She was easily susceptible to carsickness during childhood. Since her teenage years she has had unilateral throbbing headaches associated with photophobia and nausea, but they are infrequent now and usually respond to over-the-counter analgesics. She delivered her first child 6 months ago and recently finished nursing. She has already seen her obstetrician, who ordered an MRI of the brain that came back as normal.

MIGRAINE-ASSOCIATED VERTIGO

Migraine-associated vertigo (MAV) is defined as vertigo or dizziness caused by migraine. Approximately 10% of the population has migraine headaches,[1] and one-third of persons with migraine experience dizziness,[2] so the prevalence of MAV can be estimated as approximately 3% of the population. Using stricter criteria (outlined on the following page), the prevalence has been estimated at nearly 1% of the population.[3] By way of comparison, the prevalence of Ménière's disease has been estimated to be 2 per 1000, or 0.2%.[4] Thus, MAV is approximately 5 to 10 times more common than Ménière's disease.

Disclosures: The authors have no financial disclosures or conflicts of interest to report.
[a] Department of Neurology, Northwestern University Feinberg School of Medicine, 303 East Chicago Avenue, Ward 10-185, Chicago, IL 60611, USA
[b] Chicago Dizziness and Hearing, 645 North Michigan Avenue, Suite 410, Chicago, IL 60611-5800, USA
[c] Department of Otolaryngology - Head and Neck Surgery, Northwestern University Feinberg School of Medicine, 676 North St Clair Street, Suite 1325, Chicago, IL 60611, USA
[d] Department of Physical Therapy and Human Movement Sciences, Northwestern University Feinberg School of Medicine, 645 North Michigan Avenue, Suite 1100, Chicago, IL 60611, USA
* Corresponding author. Chicago Dizziness and Hearing, 645 North Michigan Avenue, Suite 410, Chicago, IL 60611-5800.
E-mail address: m-cherchi2@md.northwestern.edu

The literature concerning migraines in general is immense, and an exhaustive review is impractical. The literature specifically about MAV is also large, and there are several excellent recent reviews of this topic.[3,5,6] This article focuses on the salient features of dizziness as a manifestation of migraine, concentrating on the points of diagnosis and management of interest to the otolaryngologist.

DEFINITION OF MIGRAINE-ASSOCIATED VERTIGO

Although there is no universally recognized definition for MAV, several recent studies have employed criteria originally proposed by Neuhauser and Lempert.[3] These criteria are extensions of the definition of migraine as proposed in the *International Classification of Headache Disorders* (2nd Edition) (*ICHD-II*)[7] and are as follows:

Definite vestibular migraine
1. Episodic vestibular symptoms of at least moderate severity.
2. One of the following:
   - Current or previous history of migraine according to the *ICHD-II*.
   - Migrainous symptoms during two or more attacks of vertigo (Migrainous headache, photophobia, phonophobia, visual aura, or other aura).
3. Other causes ruled out by appropriate investigations.

Probable vestibular migraine
1. Episodic vestibular symptoms of at least moderate severity.
2. One of the following:
   - Current or previous history of migraine according to the *ICHD-II*.
   - Migrainous symptoms during vestibular symptoms.
   - Migraine precipitants of vertigo in more than 50% of attacks (food triggers, sleep irregularities, or hormonal change)
   - Response to migraine medications in more than 50% of attacks.
3. Other causes ruled out by appropriate investigations.

PATHOPHYSIOLOGY OF MIGRAINE-ASSOCIATED VERTIGO

Migraine has been recognized for centuries and has been studied intensively, yet its pathophysiology remains poorly understood. The mechanistic framework used throughout this review combines the ideas that migraine sufferers are more sensitive to many types of unpleasant sensory input and that when there is an overload of adverse sensory input, a threshold is triggered resulting in a cortical event followed by brainstem events, causing even more sensory input to be perceived as noxious, generally resulting in severe headache and temporary shutdown of the individual.

There is good evidence that the brain of persons with migraine is hyperexcitable.[8] Persons with migraine are more likely to experience discomfort from bright light, loud sound, smells, and motion as well as many other sensory inputs that are not disturbing to non-migraineurs. Some studies report thickening of sensory cortex.[9] Migraine sufferers are almost always extraordinarily sensitive during their headaches[10] but also are often more sensitive at baseline, even outside of their migraine headaches. As an example, patients with migraines often give a history of susceptibility to motion sickness. Studies have found that 45% of children with migraines[11] and 50% of adults with migraines[12] report a history of being highly susceptible to motion sickness. In other words, migraines are hard-wired.

The vascular theory of headache proposes that migraine aura represents vasoconstriction and cortical hypoxia. It is now believed that vascular dysregulation is only part of the pathophysiology. Migraine aura is now thought to represent a cortical neuronal process.[13] Research on migraine aura, such as the cortical spreading depression of Leão[14,15] and the changes in blood flow in the occipital cortex demonstrated in migraineurs with certain visual auras,[16] implicates both vascular dysregulation and abnormal electrical activity.

Research regarding the pain associated with migraines as well as the response to serotonin agonists, such as triptans, implicates dysfunction of trigeminal brainstem circuits.[17] The vasodilator peptide, calcitonin gene–related peptide (CGRP), is found in the cell bodies of trigeminal neurons. CGRP probably modulates vascular nociception and has been heavily implicated in the headache of migraine. There may be a positive feedback loop in which sensory overload triggers cortical circuitry that causes release of CGRP, which increases painful input.[18] Triptans, acting as 5-hydroxytryptamine1B/D agonists, block these responses.

In MAV, the same general mechanisms have been proposed. Patients with MAV commonly report unusual discomfort from motion as well as visual input. Motion sickness symptoms, punctuated by dizziness attacks, may occur with or without headache.

COMMON HISTORICAL FEATURES OF MIGRAINE-ASSOCIATED VERTIGO

Although this article uses the term *vertigo*, patients may use a variety of descriptions for the disequilibrium that they experience. One recent study of MAV found that the most common vestibular symptom was rotational vertigo (70%), followed by intolerance of head motion (48%) and positional vertigo (42%).[19] Intolerance of visual motion is another common complaint. Less common symptoms include a sensation of motion sickness, floating, rocking, tilting, walking on an uneven surface, and lightheadedness. The chronology is similarly variable, with onset ranging from gradual to abrupt. Neuhauser and colleagues[19] found the most common duration to be 5 to 60 minutes (33%), followed by 1 to 24 hours (21%), seconds to 5 minutes (18%), and more than 24 hours (2%). Cutrer and Baloh[20] proposed that the mechanism of short vertigo attacks was aura whereas longer attacks were due to processes resembling central sensitization.

MAV and migraine headaches need not be simultaneous. Neuhauser and colleagues[19] reported that during symptoms of MAV, 45% of patients consistently have migraine headache, 48% of patients sometimes have migraine headache, and 6% of patients never have migraine headache. During MAV, 70% of patients have photophobia, 64% have phonophobia, and 36% have auras other than vertigo.[19]

A minority of patients are able to identify triggers for MAV, and these usually are similar to triggers for other migraines. Putative triggers documented in clinical practice can be numerous, but some recur far more frequently than others. Common weather-related triggers include storm fronts (ie, rapid changes in barometric pressure) and changes of season. Common activity triggers include physical exertion, dehydration, sleep deprivation, menses, and exposure to bright light. Common dietary triggers include caffeine (or change in the pattern of caffeine intake), chocolate, alcohol, aged cheeses, monosodium glutamate, and nitrites. Although the time lapse between trigger exposure and symptom manifestation is usually on the order of minutes to hours, occasionally the trigger is delayed. For this reason, it is worthwhile for patients to spend several weeks maintaining a symptom and dietary log.

Patients with migraines also have aural complaints. Of patients with both migraines and dizziness, 66% report phonophobia, 63% report tinnitus, 32% report hearing loss, and 11% report fluctuating hearing loss and aural fullness.[21]

DEMOGRAPHICS AND RISK FACTORS OF MIGRAINE-ASSOCIATED VERTIGO

The prevalence of MAV using the criteria discussed previously has been estimated at 0.98%.[3] Similar to migraine in general,[22] it affects women approximately 3 times more frequently than men.

Migraine in general occurs with greater than chance frequency in association with several important otologic disorders. Approximately 10% of the general population has migraine. Approximately one-third of patients with BPPV have migraines,[23] with a higher percentage in female (43%) than male patients (21%).[24] Radke and coworkers[25] reported that 56% of patients with Ménière's disease also have symptoms meeting criteria for migraines. The mechanism for the association between otologic entities and MAV remains unclear.

PHYSICAL EXAMINATION IN MIGRAINE-ASSOCIATED VERTIGO

A patient who has MAV and no other illnesses typically has a normal examination. One exception to this is that patients with migraine (including MAV) may have nystagmus[12,26] that, although usually not observable on direct inspection, may be discernible with video Frenzel goggle examination.[27]

TESTING FOR MIGRAINE-ASSOCIATED VERTIGO

MAV is a diagnosis of exclusion. Usually the most significant overlap is with otologic disorders, and, for this reason, a screening otologic and vestibular work-up is advisable. In clinical practice, the most useful tests include audiometry (to exclude Ménière's disease or labyrinthitis) and vestibular evoked myogenic potentials or videonystagmography (to exclude peripheral vestibular hypofunction). In cases where doubt remains, brain imaging is warranted.

Myriad studies have been published suggesting that there might be diagnostic tests to rule in a diagnosis of migraine, such as otoacoustic emissions,[28] brain auditory evoked responses,[21,29] vestibular evoked myogenic potentials,[30] rotary chair testing,[31–33] posturography,[31,34,35] and caloric testing.[34,35] Although these tests can exclude other disorders, the authors' experience has been that there are no tests that can be relied on to confirm a diagnosis of MAV. This is hardly surprising because persons with MAV function normally during most of their lives.

Oculomotor testing, especially at the bedside, can be helpful to exclude other conditions. von Brevern and colleagues[26] reported that there are minor oculomotor abnormalities in 70% of patients with acute MAV. There may be weak nystagmus with horizontal, vertical, or torsional components. The nystagmus can be positional.

Brain imaging is usually normal in patients with MAV. A recent meta-analysis concluded, however, that approximately 23% of migraine patients accumulate white matter abnormalities not attributable to other disorders, and that migraine patients are at approximately a fourfold higher risk for developing white matter abnormalities than patients without migraine, even after controlling for vascular risk factors.[36] The imaging findings typically involve scattered punctate foci of T2 and fluid-attenuated inversion recovery signal hyperintensity in the deep cerebral white matter.

There are rare cases of hearing loss in patients with MAV.[37–39] Such hearing loss is usually episodic,[40] creating challenges for differentiating MAV from Ménière's disease. Cases involving permanent unilateral hearing loss are attributed to presumed migrainous infarction. There are no data on hearing loss specifically in patients with MAV. The authors' clinical experience suggests that almost all patients with MAV have normal hearing, except when MAV is combined with Ménière's disease.

DIFFERENTIAL DIAGNOSIS OF MIGRAINE-ASSOCIATED VERTIGO

When headache and dizziness coincide, MAV is by far the most likely diagnosis. MAV is more challenging to diagnose in persons who have headaches and dizziness at different times or in persons who have no headaches at all. An additional complication to the differential diagnosis is that migraines may be triggered by dizziness, as reported in a recent study.[41]

The main difficulty in Ménière's disease patients with headache is allocating impairment between Ménière's disease per se and the commonly accompanying migraine. Approximately 50% of patients diagnosed with Ménière's disease also meet the criteria for migraine.[25] This can be particularly problematic when a destructive treatment of Ménière's disease, such as low-dose gentamicin, is considered, because, to the authors' knowledge, MAV does not respond to either gentamicin or vestibular nerve section. Practically, the authors think it best simply to make a reasonable attempt to treat MAV (**Fig. 1**) before embarking on a destructive procedure.

Vertebrobasilar insufficiency can usually be distinguished from MAV based on history and lack of headache. Typical vertebrobasilar patients are older and have multiple vascular risk factors. Vertebrobasilar insufficiency typically causes multiple cranial nerve symptoms (eg, visual abnormalities, diplopia or oscillopsia, dizziness, or dysphagia) and may culminate in frank syncope. (See article by Ishiyama and Ishiyama in this publication.)

Episodic ataxias (EA) can sometimes be difficult to distinguish from MAV. EA type 2 is a dominantly inherited condition, so there is usually a family history of similar symptoms. Half of patients with EA type 2 also have migraines. EA type 2 typically manifests in the second decade of life with episodes of truncal ataxia, sometimes associated with vertigo, nausea, and vomiting. Physical examination during an episode reveals truncal ataxia and spontaneous nystagmus. Between episodes, EA2 patients may have gaze-evoked nystagmus, rebound nystagmus, suppression of the vestibuloocular reflex, and downbeat nystagmus.[42] As the disease progresses, patients may begin to exhibit subtle cerebellar signs even between attacks, resulting in mild, chronic ataxia. Although genetic testing is available, sometimes a good response to acetazolamide or carbamazepine provides adequate support for the diagnosis. (See article by Cherchi in this publication.)

Cyclic vomiting syndrome manifests as recurrent episodes of nausea and vomiting. It is often coincident with migraine,[43] which has led to speculation that it is a variant of migraine. The age of onset is 2 to 49 years.[44] The duration of the episodes is 2 to 4 days. An evaluation (sometimes involving endoscopy or imaging) should be undertaken to exclude primary gastrointestinal disorders. The authors have observed that cyclic vomiting often responds to migraine prophylaxis, especially to verapamil.

Benign paroxysmal vertigo of childhood (not to be confused with benign paroxysmal positional vertigo) is a vertiginous disorder of childhood. One study estimated that between the ages of 6 and 12 years, vertigo attributable to migraine has a prevalence of 2.8%,[45] and such cases could be reasonably viewed as MAV. (See articles by McCaslin and colleagues, O'Reilly and colleagues, and Taylor and Goodkin in this publication.)

TREATMENT OF MIGRAINE-ASSOCIATED VERTIGO

Patients should be encouraged to keep a log or diary of symptoms, with the goal of discerning triggers of their migraines. Even if a trigger cannot be altered (eg, weather changes), its recognition can at least provide some predictability to symptoms.

If no triggers are found or if trigger avoidance is not possible, then MAV can be treated pharmacologically. There are only a few published randomized trials of

Migraine and MAV prevention Flowchart

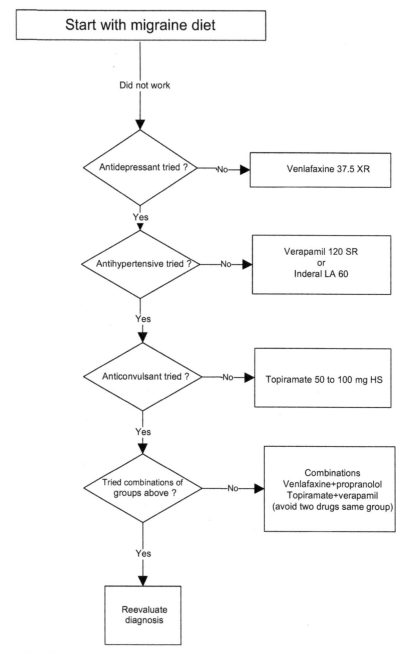

Fig. 1. Sample algorithm for migraine prophylaxis medications.

Table 1
Common prophylactic medications for MAV

Group	Medication	Initial Dose	Target Dose
Antidepressant	Venlafaxine	One-third of one capsule of 37.5 qam, increased by another one-third every week	37.5 to 75
Anticonvulstant	Topiramate	25 mg hs, increase by 25 mg every week	50 to 100 mg hs
β-Blocker	Propranolol	60 mg qhs	120 mg qhs
Calcium channel blocker	Verapamil	120 mg hs	2 mg/kg

medications specifically for MAV,[46] so in clinical practice it is managed similarly to other migraines. Prophylactic strategies are favored when attacks are frequent (ie, more than once per week) or severe (eg, making driving dangerous). Prophylactic strategies are also necessary for long-duration symptoms.

There are three main groups of prophylactic medications that can be employed: anticonvulsants, antihypertensives, and antidepressants (see **Fig. 1**). Agents from each group can be combined in refractory situations. It is critical to start with very low doses of any chosen medication, because the sensory hypersensitivity of migraine often extends to medications. Medication trials usually are performed over 2 to 4 weeks and are terminated by either significant side effects or attainment of the dose indicated in **Table 1** for a month.

In the authors' practice, treatment most commonly starts with the antidepressant, venlafaxine, followed by the anticonvulsant, topiramate, and then β-blockers (eg, propranolol). Many detailed reviews of migraine prophylactic strategies[47–49] and abortive strategies[50] are available. A practical algorithm is provided in **Fig. 1** and relevant dosing in **Table 1**.

Migraine abortives that the authors use for headaches include the triptans (eg, sumatriptan and rizatriptan), Midrin (isometheptene, dichloralphenazone, and acetaminophen), Fioricet (butalbital, acetaminophen, and caffeine), and Fiorinal (butalbital, aspirin, and caffeine).

PROGNOSIS OF MIGRAINE-ASSOCIATED VERTIGO

The prognosis of MAV is probably similar to that of migraines in general, although no study has specifically explored this. In the general population, women can expect migraines to persist during their childbearing years but decrease in frequency and severity after menopause.

With respect to medical management, most patients with MAV are able to bring symptoms under a reasonable degree of control, meaning that the frequency is significantly reduced and breakthrough symptoms can be curtailed or ameliorated with migraine abortive therapies.

REFERENCES

1. Stewart W, Shechter A, Rasmussen B. Migraine prevalence. A review of population based studies. Neurology 1994;44(Suppl 4):S17–23.
2. Selby G, Lance JW. Observations on 500 cases of migraine and allied vascular headache. J Neurol Neurosurg Psychiatry 1960;23:23–32.

3. Neuhauser H, Lempert T. Vestibular migraine. Neurol Clin 2009;27(2):379–91.

4. Wladislavosky-Waserman P, Facer GW, Mokri B, et al. Meniere's disease: a 30-year epidemiologic and clinical study in Rochester, Mn, 1951–1980. Laryngoscope 1984;94(8):1098–102.

5. Cha YH, Baloh RW. Migraine associated vertigo. J Clin Neurol 2007;3(3):121–6.

6. Eggers SD. Migraine-related vertigo: diagnosis and treatment. Curr Neurol Neurosci Rep 2006;6(2):106–15.

7. Headache Classification Subcommittee of the International Headache Society. The international classification of headache disorders: 2nd edition. Cephalalgia 2004;24(Suppl 1):9–160.

8. Aurora SK, Wilkinson F. The brain is hyperexcitable in migraine. Cephalalgia 2007;27(12):1442–53.

9. DaSilva AF, Granziera C, Snyder J, et al. Thickening in the somatosensory cortex of patients with migraine. Neurology 2007;69(21):1990–5.

10. Burstein R, Yarnitsky D, Goor-Aryeh I, et al. An association between migraine and cutaneous allodynia. Ann Neurol 2000;47(5):614–24.

11. Barabas G, Matthews WS, Ferrari M. Childhood migraine and motion sickness. Pediatrics 1983;72(2):188–90.

12. Kayan A, Hood JD. Neuro-otological manifestations of migraine. Brain 1984; 107(Pt 4):1123–42.

13. Schreiber CP. The pathophysiology of migraine. Dis Mon 2006;52(10):385–401.

14. Leão AAP. Spreading depression of activity in the cerebral cortex. J Neurophysiol 1944;7:359–90.

15. Leão AAP, Morison RS. Propagation of spreading cortical depression. J Neurophysiol 1945;8:33–46.

16. Olesen J, Friberg L, Olsen TS, et al. Timing and topography of cerebral blood flow, aura, and headache during migraine attacks. Ann Neurol 1990;28(6): 791–8.

17. Welch KM. Concepts of migraine headache pathogenesis: insights into mechanisms of chronicity and new drug targets. Neurol Sci 2003;24(Suppl 2):S149–53.

18. Ramadan NM. Targeting therapy for migraine: what to treat? Neurology 2005; 64(10 Suppl 2):S4–8.

19. Neuhauser H, Leopold M, von Brevern M, et al. The interrelations of migraine, vertigo, and migrainous vertigo. Neurology 2001;56(4):436–41.

20. Cutrer FM, Baloh RW. Migraine-associated dizziness. Headache 1992;32(6): 300–4.

21. Dash AK, Panda N, Khandelwal G, et al. Migraine and audiovestibular dysfunction: is there a correlation? Am J Otolaryngol 2008;29(5):295–9.

22. Lipton RB, Bigal ME, Diamond M, et al. Migraine prevalence, disease burden, and the need for preventive therapy. Neurology 2007;68(5):343–9.

23. Uneri A. Migraine and benign paroxysmal positional vertigo: an outcome study of 476 patients. Ear Nose Throat J 2004;83(12):814–5.

24. von Brevern M, Radtke A, Lezius F, et al. Epidemiology of benign paroxysmal positional vertigo: a population based study. J Neurol Neurosurg Psychiatry 2007;78(7):710–5.

25. Radtke A, Lempert T, Gresty MA, et al. Migraine and Meniere's disease: is there a link? Neurology 2002;59(11):1700–4.

26. von Brevern M, Zeise D, Neuhauser H, et al. Acute migrainous vertigo: clinical and oculographic findings. Brain 2005;128(Pt 2):365–74.

27. Polensek SH, Tusa RJ. Nystagmus during attacks of vestibular migraine: an aid in diagnosis. Audiol Neurootol 2010;15(4):241–6.

28. Bolay H, Bayazit YA, Gunduz B, et al. Subclinical dysfunction of cochlea and cochlear efferents in migraine: an otoacoustic emission study. Cephalalgia 2008;28(4):309–17.

29. Bayazit Y, Yilmaz M, Mumbuc S, et al. Assessment of migraine-related cochleo-vestibular symptoms. Rev Laryngol Otol Rhinol (Bord) 2001;122(2):85–8.

30. Baier B, Stieber N, Dieterich M. Vestibular-evoked myogenic potentials in vestibular migraine. J Neurol 2009;256(9):1447–54.

31. Furman JM, Sparto PJ, Soso M, et al. Vestibular function in migraine-related dizziness: a pilot study. J Vestib Res 2005;15(5/6):327–32.

32. Arriaga MA, Chen DA, Hillman TA, et al. Visually enhanced vestibulo-ocular reflex: a diagnostic tool for migraine vestibulopathy. Laryngoscope 2006;116(9):1577–9.

33. Cass SP, Furman JM, Ankerstjerne K, et al. Migraine-related vestibulopathy. Ann Otol Rhinol Laryngol 1997;106(3):182–9.

34. Celebisoy N, Gokcay F, Sirin H, et al. Migrainous vertigo: clinical, oculographic and posturographic findings. Cephalalgia 2008;28(1):72–7.

35. Teggi R, Colombo B, Bernasconi L, et al. Migrainous vertigo: results of caloric testing and stabilometric findings. Headache 2009;49(3):435–44.

36. Swartz RH, Kern RZ. Migraine is associated with magnetic resonance imaging white matter abnormalities: a meta-analysis. Arch Neurol 2004;61(9):1366–8.

37. Lee H, Lopez I, Ishiyama A, et al. Can migraine damage the inner ear? Arch Neurol 2000;57(11):1631–4.

38. Lee H, Whitman GT, Lim JG, et al. Hearing symptoms in migrainous infarction. Arch Neurol 2003;60(1):113–6.

39. Viirre ES, Baloh RW. Migraine as a cause of sudden hearing loss. Headache 1996;36(1):24–8.

40. Lipkin AF, Jenkins HA, Coker NJ. Migraine and sudden sensorineural hearing loss. Arch Otolaryngol Head Neck Surg 1987;113(3):325–6.

41. Murdin L, Davies RA, Bronstein AM. Vertigo as a migraine trigger. Neurology 2009;73(8):638–42.

42. Baloh RW. Episodic vertigo: central nervous system causes. Curr Opin Neurol 2002;15(1):17–21.

43. Fleisher DR, Matar M. The cyclic vomiting syndrome: a report of 71 cases and literature review. J Pediatr Gastroenterol Nutr 1993;17(4):361–9.

44. Fleisher DR, Gornowicz B, Adams K, et al. Cyclic Vomiting Syndrome in 41 adults: the illness, the patients, and problems of management. BMC Med 2005;3:20.

45. Abu-Arafeh I, Russell G. Paroxysmal vertigo as a migraine equivalent in children: a population-based study. Cephalalgia 1995;15(1):22–5 [discussion: 24].

46. Fotuhi M, Glaun B, Quan SY, et al. Vestibular migraine: a critical review of treatment trials. J Neurol 2009;256(5):711–6.

47. Buchanan TM, Ramadan NM. Prophylactic pharmacotherapy for migraine headaches. Semin Neurol 2006;26(2):188–98.

48. Ramadan NM. Prophylactic migraine therapy: mechanisms and evidence. Curr Pain Headache Rep 2004;8(2):91–5.

49. Ramadan NM, Silberstein SD, Freitag FG, et al. Evidence-based guidelines for migraine headache in the primary care setting: pharmacological management for prevention of migraine. U.S. Headache Consortium; 2000. Available at: http://www.aan.com/professionals/practice/pdfs/gl0090.pdf. Accessed January 31, 2011.

50. Silberstein SD. Practice parameter: evidence-based guidelines for migraine headache (an evidence-based review): report of the Quality Standards Subcommittee of the American Academy of Neurology. Neurology 2000;55(6):754–62.

Is Superior Canal Dehiscence Congenital or Acquired? A Case Report and Review of the Literature

Stefan C.A. Hegemann, MD[a],*, John P. Carey, MD[b]

KEYWORDS

- Vestibular disorder • Phobic vertigo • Autophony
- Hennebert sign • Tullio phenomenon

Superior canal dehiscence syndrome was first described by Minor and colleagues in 1998.[1] Typical symptoms include hyperacusis for bone-conducted sounds with autophony, and vertigo induced by loud sounds (Tullio phenomenon) or increased pressure in the middle ear (Hennebert sign) or intracranial space (eg, during strenuous activities).

The pathophysiology of the dehiscent bone over the superior semicircular canal is still debated. Symptoms and signs of semicircular canal dehiscence syndrome (SCDS) typically occur in adulthood.[2] Nevertheless, a developmental or congenital anomaly is suspected because thinning of the bone overlying the superior canal often occurs bilaterally, as shown in CT and temporal bone dissection studies.[3,4] This thin bone could then presumably be disrupted by trauma or erosion caused by pressure of the overlying temporal lobe.[3] A genetic defect has not yet been identified (Gürtler N, personal communication, 2009). Thin bone overlying the superior semicircular canal on the side contralateral to a dehiscence has been reported both on CT scans[4] and in temporal bones.[3] However, a long-term study with follow-up CT or vestibular evoked myogenic potentials (VEMPs) to assess the development of SCD on the intact side has not been reported. One case report of a 7-year-old girl with SCD on the right[5] and one recent report of a 4-year-old child with a partial dehiscence of the right posterior semicircular canal have been published.[6] Otherwise, SCDS in children seems to be rare, underdiagnosed, or not published.

[a] Department of Otorhinolaryngology, Head & Neck Surgery, Zürich University Hospital, Frauenklinikstrasse 24, 8091 Zürich, Switzerland
[b] Department of Otolaryngology-Head & Neck Surgery, The Johns Hopkins University School of Medicine, 601 North Caroline Street, 6th Floor, Baltimore, MD 21287-0910, USA
* Corresponding author.
E-mail address: stefan.hegemann@usz.ch

Otolaryngol Clin N Am 44 (2011) 377–382
doi:10.1016/j.otc.2011.01.009
0030-6665/11/$ – see front matter © 2011 Elsevier Inc. All rights reserved.

A defect in the bone overlying the superior semicircular canal can also be caused by trauma (although the force needed to create a defect is unknown, and whether a thinning of the bone must exist before the trauma occurs is also unclear), cholesteatoma,[7] vestibular schwannoma,[3] meningioma,[8] or even glioblastoma,[9] but these are rarely found with SCDS, so one or more other causes seem more likely in most cases. No evidence currently supports the theory of osteoporosis as a potential cause of semicircular canal dehiscence. The authors still believe that a developmental defect is the most likely cause for SCDS, especially because the bone overlying the SC is the last part of the temporal bone to form in development.[3] Nevertheless, why the diagnosis is usually first made in adulthood remains an enigma.

This article presents a case report of patient who was diagnosed with SCDS at 37 years of age, whose typical symptoms had begun in the classical form approximately 3 years earlier. However, a detailed and specific history revealed that some symptoms had already begun at approximately 10 years of age.

CASE REPORT

A 37-year-old man was seen in the authors' interdisciplinary center for vertigo and balance disorders in 2005. He complained of periods of dizziness that were usually provoked by loud sounds, especially when he had to speak loudly in conferences or in restaurants with a noisy background. He never experienced true rotatory vertigo. These spells of dizziness increased at 34 years of age, after which his sensitivity to noise also increased, to the point where he could even hear his own eye movements in his right ear and other sounds produced by his own body, such as footsteps and his own voice. Dizziness increased with exertion in sport activities until he could not even jog after 35 years of age.

Physical examination showed normal outer ear canals and eardrums with normal Eustachian tube function, but during Valsalva maneuver he felt a slight shift of the visual scene and dizziness. The Weber tuning fork test lateralized to the right ear, and the Rinne test was positive bilaterally. Hennebert's sign was positive, so that both positive and negative pressure in the right outer ear canal provoked a shifting of the visual scene. When repeating these signs under Frenzel goggles, the authors noted small torsional movements of the eyes toward the left side while positive pressure was applied, which reversed when negative pressure was applied. Vertical and horizontal components could not be seen. This simple investigation alone was sufficient for SCDS to be suspected.

Audiometry supported the clinically suspected air–bone gap at least at 500 Hz, and cervical VEMPs in response to acoustic clicks confirmed a reduced threshold of approximately 46 dB nHL on the right and a normal threshold (82 dB nHL) on the left (**Fig. 1**A). CT of the temporal bones showed dehiscence of the right superior semicircular canal (**Fig. 2**A).

In a more detailed history, the authors found that even beginning at approximately 10 years of age, the patient experienced periodic vague dizziness, especially in train stations, shopping centers, and other noisy public places. His symptoms increased with exertion in sporting activities, especially when riding his bicycle uphill. He felt best in quiet environments and when lying in bed. He avoided common social activities with friends, and later also with colleagues, because he found them too noisy; he preferred quiet. He often told his parents that something must be wrong, and was evaluated by several physicians who considered diagnoses such as vitamin deficiencies and even psychogenic causes. Before presenting to the authors' clinics, the conclusion was simply that he had to live with these symptoms.

The authors saw no indications of panic disorder, depression, or any other psychogenic disturbances. The patient had a good sense of humor, was intelligent and insightful, and was running his own company successfully in a very competitive field. No indication was seen that he was somatizing or overestimating his symptoms. After he learned the diagnosis and the operative treatment option, he chose to wait 3 more years, during which time the symptoms became even stronger and, ultimately, intolerable, at which point he decided to pursue surgical treatment.

The dehiscent canal was plugged using the middle cranial fossa approach without complications. In the immediate postoperative period, air conduction thresholds were almost identical to the preoperative audiogram. Bone conduction thresholds were still slightly better than air-conduction thresholds. In absolute silence he was still able to hear his eyes moving with his right ear, but markedly less so than preoperatively, and it was not bothersome. Vestibular function was reduced only for the plugged superior canal, because he showed evidence of a deficient vestibuloocular reflex for rapid head thrusts exciting the plugged canal but none of the other canals on the ipsilateral side.

Within 48 hours of surgery the patient noted profound changes, even commenting on what seemed like a "new life." First, he noted that he no longer heard his voice, eye movements, or other body sounds in the affected ear. Second, he noted that ambulation, particularly outdoors, felt more stable. Finally, he found that ambient noise no longer seemed to disturb his equilibrium or sense of well-being. Reflecting on this, he commented that only after surgery did he realize how often since childhood he had altered his routine or environment to avoid noisy situations and the associated disequilibrium. He now enjoys going to social events and restaurants, and has been able to resume sporting activities without feeling dizzy. Loud sounds no longer disturb him, and he has no fear of crowds or busy places.

DISCUSSION

The symptoms this patient presented with as an adult seemed typical for SCDS. Nevertheless, the patient's recollections suggest that the right superior canal was dehiscent from at least 10 years of age, because the major symptom of dizziness had already appeared by then. Delays in diagnosing this condition are common,[10] partly because SCDS is still a new diagnosis that is not familiar to clinicians outside of subspecialties dealing commonly with vertigo. Another reason for the delay may be patient reluctance to complain openly of seemingly bizarre symptoms, such as hearing one's eyes move. This case, however, shows that diagnosis may be delayed from childhood into adulthood.

As a child, this patient experienced vague symptoms that he found difficult to communicate to his parents and that seemed to be absent in his peers. Unable to understand these symptoms or relate them to others, the patient simply adjusted his activities to avoid the noisy environments or straining that provoked them. Over time, much of this avoidance became unconscious habit incorporated into his otherwise successful lifestyle.

However, for some reason his symptoms worsened as an adult and led him to seek an explanation and treatment. Whether this worsening of symptoms happened because of an increase in the size of the dehiscence is unknown. However, the patient had no history of head trauma, tumor, or other lesion that might affect the dehiscence. Another possibility is that the dehiscence began to transmit more pressure between

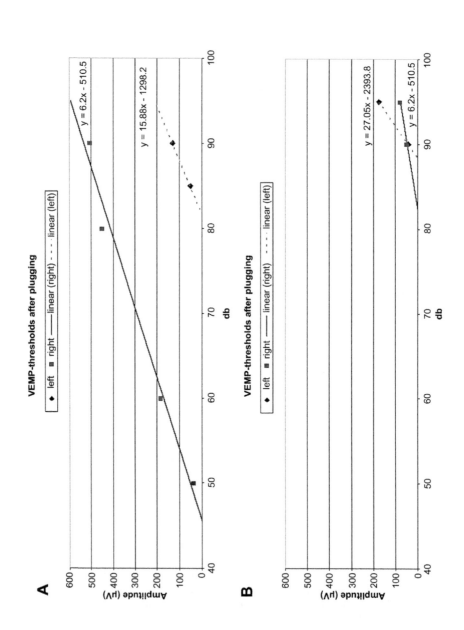

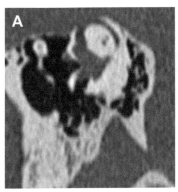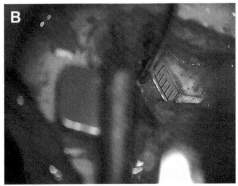

Fig. 2. (A) CT reconstruction in the plane of the right superior semicircular canal. A large dehiscence in the upper part of the semicircular canal can be seen. (B) The dehiscence intra-operatively. Scale ticks are 1 mm.

the inner ear and intracranial space as the patient aged. This effect might occur if the elasticity of the dura changed with age, or if the pressure gradients between the inner ear and intracranial space changed. Another possibility is that the patient experienced the loss of some central compensatory mechanism that had minimized the symptoms in childhood. However, the immediate recovery from all symptoms shortly after the operation argues against a central process that might have slowly deteriorated, because a slow readaptation to the new (plugged) state would then be expected. Instead, the instant resolution of symptoms with the correction of the peripheral defect suggests strongly that some change in the physiology of the dehiscence explained the worsening of symptoms in adulthood. The nature of this change has not been determined.

This case raises the possibility that SCDS symptoms may be present in childhood and go unrecognized. Increased awareness of this diagnosis may help identify more cases of children experiencing symptoms of SCDS. Clinicians evaluating young patients experiencing dizziness should maintain a high degree of suspicion of SCDS. Symptoms such as autophony and hearing one's own body sounds may seem so unusual to children that they may not spontaneously share these complaints with their parents or clinicians. A careful history is essential to diagnosing SCDS, and clinicians may have to inquire about apparent agoraphobia to determine if it is really

Fig. 1. Cervical vestibular evoked myogenic potential thresholds before (A) and after (B) plugging of the superior canal. The threshold is determined by a linear regression through the amplitudes of the potentials at different stimulus intensities. This technique is a very rough way to determine the threshold, but because the change in amplitude with stimulus intensity is usually linear, the authors often use only two stimulus intensities if the threshold has normal values. As can be seen, even with four intensities used in (A) for the threshold of the right sacculus, the amplitudes are close to the linear regression and the threshold is at approximately 46 decibels above normal adult hearing level (dB nHL), which is considerably below normal (75 dB nHL in the authors' laboratory). After plugging, the vestibular evoked myogenic potential threshold is normal on both sides, between 80 and 90 dB nHL. The amplitude at 90 dB nHL is almost identical on both sides. The value of 176 μV at 95 dB nHL may be a little high, but even taking the value of the first measurement (131 μV) would result in a normal threshold.

a manifestation of situational dizziness provoked by noisy, crowded places. Furthermore, the physical examination (looking for characteristic nystagmus in response to loud sounds, Valsalva maneuvers, or pressure changes in the external auditory canal) and appropriate interpretation of audiometric findings (conductive hearing loss or bone conduction hyperacusis with normal stapedial reflexes) provide further clues. Suggestive findings from the history or physical examination should prompt further testing, including high-resolution CT scanning of the temporal bones, with appropriate reconstructions of the superior semicircular canal,[11] and VEMP testing.

REFERENCES

1. Minor LB, Solomon D, Zinreich JS, et al. Sound- and/or pressure-induced vertigo due to bone dehiscence of the superior semicircular canal. Arch Otolaryngol Head Neck Surg 1998;124(3):249–58.
2. Minor LB, Carey JP, Cremer PD, et al. Dehiscence of bone overlying the superior canal as a cause of apparent conductive hearing loss. Otol Neurotol 2003;24(2): 270–8.
3. Carey JP, Minor LB, Nager GT. Dehiscence or thinning of bone overlying the superior semicircular canal in a temporal bone survey. Arch Otolaryngol Head Neck Surg 2000;126(2):137–47.
4. Hirvonen TP, Weg N, Zinreich SJ, et al. High-resolution CT findings suggest a developmental abnormality underlying superior canal dehiscence syndrome. Acta Otolaryngol 2003;123(4):477–81.
5. Zhou G, Ohlms L, Liberman J, et al. Superior semicircular canal dehiscence in a young child: implication of developmental defect. Int J Pediatr Otorhinolaryngol 2007;71(12):1925–8.
6. Paladin AM, Phillips GS, Raske ME, et al. Labyrinthine dehiscence in a child. Pediatr Radiol 2008;38(3):348–50.
7. Brantberg K, Bagger-Sjoback D, Mathiesen T, et al. Posterior canal dehiscence syndrome caused by an apex cholesteatoma. Otol Neurotol 2006;27(4):531–4.
8. Crane BT, Carey JP, McMenomey S, et al. Meningioma causing superior canal dehiscence syndrome. Otol Neurotol 2010;31(6):1009–10.
9. Licht AK, Schulmeyer F, Allert M, et al. Vertigo and hearing disturbance as the first sign of a glioblastoma (World Health Organization grade IV). Otol Neurotol 2004; 25(2):174–7.
10. Minor LB. Clinical manifestations of superior semicircular canal dehiscence. Laryngoscope 2005;115(10):1717–27.
11. Belden CJ, Weg N, Minor LB, et al. CT evaluation of bone dehiscence of the superior semicircular canal as a cause of sound- and/or pressure-induced vertigo. Radiology 2003;226(2):337–43.

Ménière's Disease: A Challenging and Relentless Disorder

Maroun T. Semaan, MD[a],*, Cliff A. Megerian, MD[b]

KEYWORDS

- Ménière's disease • Cochlear hydrops
- Endolymphatic hydrops • Labyrinthectomy
- Vestibular nerve section • Electrocochleography
- Vestibular evoked myogenic potentials

Ménière's disease (MD) is characterized by episodic vertigo, fluctuating hearing loss, aural pressure, and tinnitus. Since its description by Prosper Ménière's[1] in the Gazette Médicale de Paris in 1861, the pathophysiology and management of MD has been a controversial topic. Depending on the geographic location, the incidence of MD varies between 4.3 and 15.3 per 100,000.[2,3] Affected individuals are usually between the fourth and sixth decades of life, with a female/male ratio of 1.3:1.

The Committee on Hearing and Equilibrium of the American Academy of Otolaryngology-Head and Neck Surgery published the defining guidelines of Ménière's disease (**Table 1**).[4] Based on the residual hearing and residual vertigo after treatment, staging systems and classification schemes have been proposed (**Tables 2** and **3**).[4]

The diagnosis of MD, an idiopathic condition, is made after excluding other causes that may mimic the disorder. Several pathologic conditions can masquerade as MD and are best referred to as Ménière's syndrome. These conditions can be infectious (otosyphilis),[5] autoimmune (Cogan syndrome, autoimmune inner ear disease),[6] and neoplastic (eg, intralabyrinthine or vestibular schwannomas, endolymphatic sac tumors).[7]

This article presents a clinical vignette of a patient with MD who ultimately displays the full spectrum of the disease, and discusses the clinical presentation, the diagnostic evaluation, and the different therapeutic modalities. The article provides the essential points that can help guide the assessment and management of this condition.

---

[a] Division of Otology and Neurotology, Department of Otolaryngology and Head & Neck Surgery, University Hospitals Case Medical Center, Louis Stokes Veteran's Affair Medical Center, Case Western Reserve University School of Medicine, 11100 Euclid Avenue, Lakeside 4528, Cleveland, OH 44106, USA
[b] Division of Otology and Neurotology, Department of Otolaryngology and Head & Neck Surgery, University Hospitals Case Medical Center, Case Western Reserve School of Medicine, Lakeside 4528, Cleveland, OH 44106, USA
* Corresponding author.
E-mail address: maroun.semaan@UHHospitals.org

Otolaryngol Clin N Am 44 (2011) 383–403
doi:10.1016/j.otc.2011.01.010
0030-6665/11/$ – see front matter. Published by Elsevier Inc.

oto.theclinics.com

Table 1
Classification of Ménière's disease according to the 1995 guidelines of the Committee on Hearing and Equilibrium of the American Academy of Otolaryngology and Head & Neck Surgery

Definition	Symptoms
Certain Ménière's disease	Definite Ménière's disease plus histopathologic confirmation
Definite Ménière's disease	≥2 definitive spontaneous episodes of vertigo 20 min or longer Audiometrically documented hearing loss on at least 1 occasion Tinnitus or aural fullness in the treated ear Other causes excluded
Probable Ménière's disease	One definitive episode of vertigo Audiometrically documented hearing loss on at least 1 occasion Tinnitus or aural fullness in the treated ear Other causes excluded
Possible Ménière's disease	Episodic vertigo without documented hearing loss, or Sensorineural hearing loss fluctuating or fixed, with dysequilibrium but nonepisodic Other causes excluded

*A.S. is a 34-year-old woman, healthy without any significant past medical history, who presented to the otology clinic 10 years ago for evaluation of a 3-day complaint of a right- sided muffled hearing, sensation of ipsilateral aural fullness and a low-pitched oceanlike sound. She denied vertigo or significant disequilibrium. She denied any recent viral illnesses. The otoscopic examination was normal. She had a similar episode 8 months earlier, which spontaneously resolved. An audiogram performed at that time is shown in **Fig. 1**, which reveals a right-sided, low-frequency rising to normal sensorineural hearing loss with excellent word discrimination score (WDS). Her tympanogram and stapedial reflexes (not shown) were normal. A follow-up audiogram, performed 3 weeks following the initial presentation (**Fig. 2**), showed normal hearing thresholds.*

*A repeat audiogram was performed during the current visit (**Fig. 3**) and revealed a moderate rising to mild, low-frequency sensorineural hearing loss. The WDS was 84%. The Stenger test was negative.*

*A gadolinium-enhanced magnetic resonance imaging (gado-MRI) study, centered on the internal auditory canals, was normal. An electrocochleography showed an increased summating potential (SP)/action potential (AP) ratio at 0.64:0.74 microvolts on the right side (**Fig. 4**), with the contralateral ear showing a normal ratio less than 0.4 (not shown). The presumed diagnosis was cochlear hydrops (CH). She completed a 10-day course of prednisone, and instructions were given for a low-salt diet. Her hearing returned to normal.*

Table 2
Staging of Ménière's disease according to the 1995 guidelines of the Committee on Hearing and Equilibrium of the American Academy of Otolaryngology and Head & Neck Surgery

Stage	Four-tone Average (dB)
1	≤25
2	26–40
3	41–70
4	>70

Table 3
Reporting guidelines according to the 1995 guidelines of the Committee on Hearing and Equilibrium of the American Academy of Otolaryngology and Head & Neck Surgery. Numerical value = (X/Y)×100. X is the average number of definitive spells per month for the 18 to 24 months after therapy, and Y is the average number of definitive spells per month for the 6 months before therapy

Numerical Value	Class
0	A
1–40	B
41–80	C
81–120	D
>120	E
Secondary treatment initiated because of disability from vertigo	F

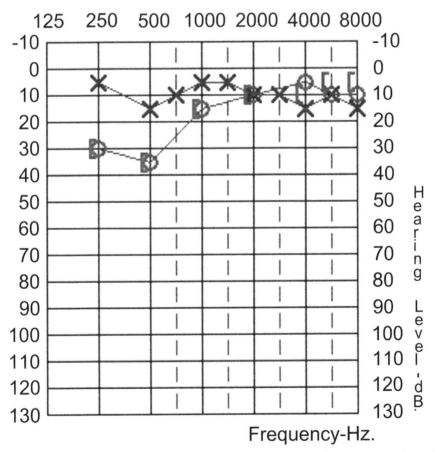

Fig. 1. Audiogram showing normal left-sided hearing and mild low-frequency sensorineural hearing loss on the right side. The word discrimination score (WDS; not shown) is 100%.

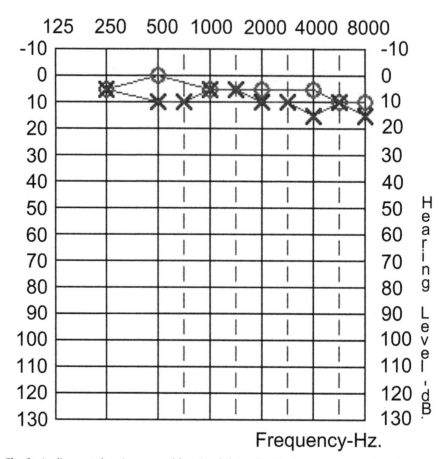

Fig. 2. Audiogram showing normal hearing bilaterally. The WDS (not shown) is 100%.

Six months later the patient developed recurrence of her right-sided hearing loss, aural fullness, roaring right-sided tinnitus, and a vertigo spell that lasted approximately 3 hours and was associated with nausea and vomiting. She also described a subjective sensation of falling backward. On examination, she had a right-beating horizonatal nystagmus, which increased in amplitude on right lateral gaze. A vestibular evoked myogenic potential (VEMP) showed an increased threshold on the left side (**Fig. 5**). The audiogram showed a moderate rising to mild sensorineural hearing loss (**Fig. 6**). The WDS was 76%. She was treated with a course of steroids and started on hydrochlorothiazide and triamterene. The patient's symptoms were consistent with the diagnosis of right-sided probable MD.

WHAT IS CH? WHAT IS ITS SIGNIFICANCE?

The term CH has been used to describe fluctuating hearing loss without associated vertigo, which may represent an earlier phase of a continuum, ranging from mild cochlear involvement to full cochleovestibular dysfunction as seen in MD.

House and colleagues[8] studied the relationship between CH and MD. In their retrospective review of 950 hydropic ears, 71% were diagnosed with unilateral MD and

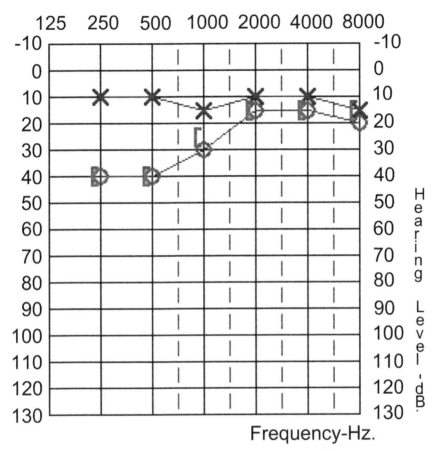

Fig. 3. Audiogram showing normal left-sided hearing and mild low-frequency sensorineural hearing loss on the right side. The WDS (not shown) is 84%.

29% were labeled as unilateral CH. Bilateral MD at presentation was seen in 11%, with another 14% of unilateral MD becoming bilateral MD. Of patients initially diagnosed as having unilateral CH, 33% developed MD during an average of 7.6 years of follow-up.

WHAT IS THE PATHOPHYSIOLOGY OF CH AND MÉNIÈRE'S DISEASE?

Although endolymphatic hydrops (ELH) is felt to be the underlying histopathologic correlate in MD, to date no histopathologic study has confirmed the presence of ELH in patients with CH. Despite the lack of direct evidence of this association, electrophysiologic studies showing increased SP/AP ratios suggest the presence of ELH.[9]

   The pathophysiology of hydrops remains unknown. Several intrinsic (genetic, anatomic, autoimmune, or vascular)[10–14] or extrinsic (allergic, viral, or trauma)[15–17] factors can cause disturbance in the mechanisms involved in the regulation of endolymphatic fluid homeostasis. Whether this disturbance causes a predominant alteration in the longitudinal versus radial flow of endolymph has long been debated.[18,19] However, it remains unclear whether the produced hydrops is the result of cytochemical abnormality or anatomic anomaly.

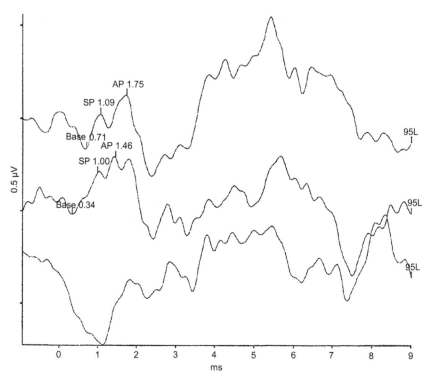

Fig. 4. Electrocochleography results in the affected ear. The SP/AP ratio was increased (0.64/0.74).

The sine qua non relationship of ELH to the symptoms of MD has also been questioned as to whether the observed ELH is the direct pathologic initiator of cochleovestibular dysfunction or is an epiphenomenon of a subtler biochemical perturbation. In a review of their temporal bone registry, Merchant and colleagues[20] found that all 28 patients with Ménière's syndrome had evidence of ELH. However, of the 79 patients with ELH, only 51 had Ménière's symptoms. Classic symptoms were absent in 9 of 35 patients with idiopathic hydrops and in 42 of 44 patients with secondary hydrops.

WHAT IS THE ROLE OF ADJUNCTIVE TESTS IN THE DIAGNOSIS OF MD?

A national survey showed that, depending on the region (west, midwest, northeast, New England, and Atlantic coast), 26.9% to 46.7% of treating otolaryngologists relied on history, physical examination, and audiometry alone to establish the diagnosis of MD.[21] Others obtained adjunctive tests to support their diagnosis.

Electrophysiologic Studies

In recent years, several diagnostic tests have been proposed to study the presence of ELH and complement the diagnosis of CH or MD. Two electrophysiologic tests merit discussion: electrocochleography (ECoG) and VEMPs.

Electrocochleography is an evoked potential in response to condensation and rarefaction click or tone burst stimuli recorded by an intratympanic or extratympanic electrode. The SP and AP of the eighth nerve are recorded. An increased SP/AP ratio (greater than 0.4) and/or a widened AP width (greater than 3 milliseconds) are

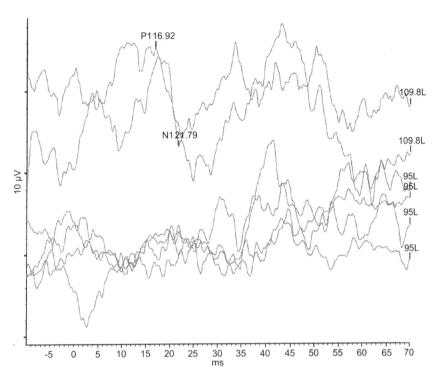

Fig. 5. Increased vestibular evoked myogenic potential (VEMP) threshold on the right side (109.8 dB) compared with the left side.

considered to be significant for ELH. Alteration of the SP and AP in the hydropic ear is believed to result from a mechanical asymmetry in the basilar membrane.[22] Ge and Shea[23] reviewed 1549 patients with MD and found an increased SP/AP ratio in 71.6%. They also showed that the sensitivity of the ECoG increased with duration and severity of disease. The sensitivity increased from 71% in stage 1 disease to 90% in stage 4 disease, and from 43% in MD of less than 1 year duration to 100% when MD had been present for more than 30 years.

The cervical VEMP (cVEMP) is a short latency inhibitory potential of the ipsilateral sternocleidomastoid muscle evoked by a brief and loud (>85 dB) monaural click or tone burst stimuli. The cVEMP is believed to be a recording of the vestibulocollic reflex generated in the saccule, carried via the inferior vestibular nerve. Patients with MD were shown to have increased cVEMP thresholds or absent VEMPs compared with controls.[24] These findings were more common in MD with Tumarkin crisis[25] and were seen in 27% of the contralateral asymptomatic ears of affected individuals.[25] We believe that both VEMP and ECoG should be used to complement the clinical picture and should not be the sole basis for diagnosis.

Caloric Testing and Head-thrust Testing

The role of electronystagmography (ENG) or videonystagmography (VNG) in the diagnosis of MD is limited. Significant caloric weakness is present in 42% to 73% of patients with MD.[26] Complete loss of function is seen in 6% to 11%. Approximately 23% to 29% of patients have abnormal angular vestibulo-ocular reflex (aVOR) on

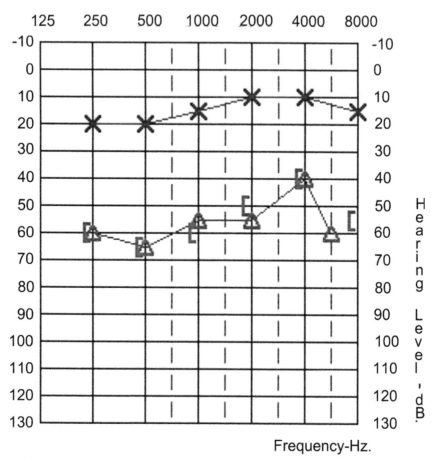

Fig. 6. Normal hearing thresholds on the left and moderate sensorineural hearing loss on the right side. The WDS (not shown) was 76%.

the head-thrust testing (HTT), with gain asymmetry and phase lead being the most common findings.[26,27]

We believe that caloric testing is useful in: (1) assessment of contralateral function before an ablative procedure, (2) assessment of residual function after an ablative procedure, and (3) assessment of ipsilateral function; if residual function is good, we favor a non-destructive procedure.

Retrocochlear Studies

When surveyed for workup of retrocochlear disorders, 57.7% to 93.3% of otologists obtained retrocochlear studies.[21] We believe that Ménière's syndrome becomes MD only after excluding other causes; therefore, we obtain MRI on all of our patients.

*During the following year, our patient had a total of 5 episodes of severe vertigo associated with aural fullness, hearing loss, and tinnitus. During the course of that year, she developed progression of her hearing loss. The audiogram showed moderate low-frequency hearing loss with a WDS of 72% (**Fig. 7**). Three of the spells responded to a steroid taper and a regimen of antiemetics. Two episodes were treated with injections of intratympanic dexamethazone (IT Dex) that gave*

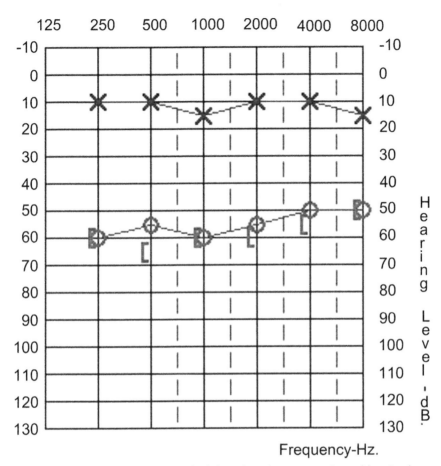

Fig. 7. Normal hearing thresholds on the left and moderate sensorineural hearing loss on the right. The WDS (not shown) is 72%.

temporary relief of vertigo. Her hearing remained unchanged, and she acquired a hearing aid.

Nine months later, she developed recurrence of vertigo spells occurring on a weekly basis. These spells responded less to a combination of oral and intratympanic steroids. A Meniett Device (Medtronic Inc, Minneapolis, MN, USA) was used without success. Her audiogram was unchanged, and she continued to use her hearing aid.

At that time, destructive and nondestructive options were discussed as management options for the weekly vertigo spells. She underwent endolymphatic sac decompression with placement of a shunt (endolymphatic sac surgery [ESS]). The sigmoid was noted to be far forward, requiring decompression. The sac was hypoplastic and inferiorly displaced. The surgery resulted in complete resolution of her vertigo spells. Her hearing remained stable. Nevertheless, she continued to complain of moderate to severe roaring tinnitus and constant sensation of aural fullness.

WHAT IS THE ROLE OF MEDICAL MANAGEMENT?

The medical management of MD includes a low-salt diet, avoidance of caffeine derivatives and alcohol, diuretics, vasodilators, and steroids.

Diuretics and low-sodium diet are effective in controlling the symptoms of MD in 71% to 79% of patients.[28,29]Although intratympanic gentamicin (IT-Gent) injection is a medical form of therapy, it is a destructive treatment that results in chemical labyrinthectomy.

A Cochrane database review of all prospective randomized controlled trials (RCT), between 1966 and 2005 comparing diuretics with placebo failed to show a single trial of sufficient quality to meet standard criteria set for review.[30] Another Cochrane database review of all RCT comparing betahistine (a vasodilator) with placebo between 1966 and 1999 (6 trials with 162 patients) failed to show any benefit.[31]

Steroids, whether administered orally or topically, have been used to treat acute exacerbations of MD. In a series of 129 patients with unilateral MD, Boleas-Aguirre and colleagues[32] showed that dexamethasone (12 mg/mL) administered intratympanically resulted in vertigo control in 91% of patients. Although more than half of the patients responded to 1 or 2 injections, 21% required more than 4 injections.

WHAT IS THE ROLE OF VESTIBULAR REHABILITATION IN THE ACUTE PHASE?

The role of vestibular rehabilitation in the acute phase of the disease has been questioned. Because of the fluctuating and dynamic nature of the vestibular symptoms seen in MD, most physicians believe that vestibular rehabilitation has limited benefit. Although the acute vertiginous spells are usually self-limited, chronic unsteadiness between the episodes of vertigo is a common complaint in patients with MD. Gottshall and colleagues[33] showed that vestibular rehabilitation, even outside the acute care of patients with surgically ablated vestibular function, seems to improve the overall balance function in both reported and objective measures (see article by Alrwaily and Whitney in this publication).

WHAT IS THE INITIAL TREATMENT IF MEDICAL THERAPY FAILS?

In a survey by Kim and colleagues,[21] 50% of otologists proceed with ESS, whereas 39% perform an IT-Gent injection. A minority offer a Meniett Device (9%) or vestibular nerve section (2%).

Controversies with ESS

A detailed review of this topic is beyond the scope of this article. However, some pathophysiologic aspects of ESS and some of the pertinent clinical studies are highlighted.

Whether limited to sac decompression and/or placement of a shunt, the efficacy of sac surgery has been, and continues to be, debated. Decompression of a tight endolymphatic sac (ELS), alteration of neovascularization in the perisaccular region, passive diffusion of endolymph, creation of an osmotic gradient, and decreased production of endolymph have all been proposed as potential mechanisms of action.[18]

Is ESS Better Than Natural History?

Many investigators have questioned the efficacy of this procedure compared with natural history. Others have questioned its long-term efficacy.

Quaranta and colleagues[34] retrospectively evaluated 38 patients with intractable Ménière's disease with a minimum of 7 years' follow-up. Twenty underwent ESS and 18 were offered surgery but declined (natural history group). Eighty-five percent of patients in the ESS group and 74% of natural history patients had complete or substantial control of vertigo. The difference between the 2 groups was not significant at 1 year. However, it was significant at 2 and 4 years' follow-up. At 2 years, patients having ESS had complete or substantial control of vertigo in 65% of the cases, and

85% of patients having ESS had complete or substantial control of vertigo at 4 and 6 years. Only 32% of the natural history patients had complete or substantial control of vertigo at 2 years, but this increased to 50% at 4 years and to 74% at 6 years. Hearing results in the 2 groups were not significantly different.

Silverstein and colleagues[29] performed a retrospective comparison of patients who were offered surgery but declined (natural history group, N = 50) with those who underwent ESS (N = 83). Of the non-operated group, 57% had complete control of vertigo at 2 years; 71% had complete control after an average of 8.3 years. In the ESS group, 40% had complete control of vertigo after 2 years; 70% had complete control after an average of 8.7 years. These results suggest that ESS does not alter the long-term natural course of vertigo control in Ménière's disease.

However, Telischi and Luxford[35] reviewed the long-term vertigo control in 234 patients who underwent ESS and were followed for at least 10 years (mean = 13.5 years). Sixty-three percent did not undergo any further surgery to control vertigo, and an additional 17% had only revisions of the endolymphatic sac shunt. Thus, 80% never required a destructive procedure. Of the 147 patients with only the original ESS, 93% reported no dizziness or mild to no disability. Of the group who underwent only revisions of the original shunt, 96% stated that they had no more dizziness or mild to no disability.

Kato and colleagues,[36] using a disease-specific quality-of-life (QOL) questionnaire, found that the QOL was improved in 87% of 159 patients with MD who underwent an ESS.

Is Sac Decompression Only Without Shunt Placement Effective?

In a recent review of 94 patients with definite MD who underwent an endolymphatic sac-mastoid shunt (54 patients) and endolymphatic sac decompression (40 patients), Brinson and colleagues[37] showed a class A or B vertigo control (see **Table 1**) in 67% of the endolymphatic mastoid shunt group, and in 66% of the endolymphatic sac decompression at 18 to 24 months' follow-up.

Regardless of the nuances in analyzing the outcomes of ELS surgery, it remains a commonly performed, nondestructive procedure.

After 2 years, A.S. had recurrence of her vertigo spells frequently associated with disequilibrium. She described her disequilibrium as a sensation of being off balance and unsteadiness exacerbated by fast or repetitive movement. This sensation was associated with a constant "foggy" feeling in her head.

*She felt disabled by her recurrent symptoms and decided to quit her job and stop driving. A repeat audiogram was unchanged (see **Fig. 7**). Videonystagmography (VNG) showed right-sided reduced vestibular response to caloric stimulation of 81%, and findings consistent with right-sided peripheral vestibular hypofunction (**Fig. 8**). She was counseled regarding chemical and surgical labyrinthectomy versus vestibular nerve section. Because she felt that her hearing was serviceable, she elected to have a retrosigmoid selective vestibular nerve section. Her hearing was preserved, and she was able to continue using her hearing aid. Despite a reduction in the overall frequency of vertigo spells, she continued having attacks 12 months after surgery, describing what seems like an impending sensation of falling backward, and has suffered 2 episodes of Tumarkin crisis. Repeat VNG showed an absent vestibular response to standard caloric stimulation on the right side. Ice caloric testing showed a small response on the right side (**Fig. 9**). Her hearing on that side deteriorated to a severe sensorineural hearing loss (**Fig. 10**), and her WDS decreased to 24%. cVEMPs were absent (**Fig. 11**). She then elected to have IT-Gent injections, using the titration method. This treatment failed to control her vertigo completely, and she then had a transmastoid labyrinthectomy (TML) that resulted in elimination of her vertigo spells. She completed 4 months of vestibular rehabilitation.*

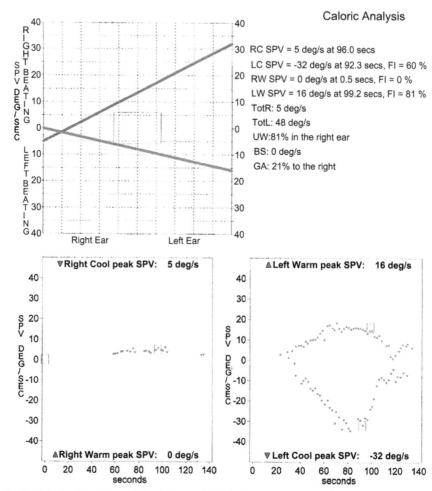

Fig. 8. Caloric stimulation of the left ear yielded robust response. Caloric stimulation of the right ear yielded poor responses (5 degrees with cold water stimulation and 0 degrees with warm water stimulation). The vestibular response asymmetry was calculated at 81%.

WHAT IS THE BEST NEXT STEP IN MANAGEMENT IF NONDESTRUCTIVE PROCEDURES FAIL IN CONTROLLING VERTIGO?

When conservative medical management and nondestructive procedures fail to control vertigo, the treating otologist needs to consider neural or labyrinthine destructive procedures to ablate all residual vestibular function in the hope of controlling the ongoing vestibulopathy. These procedures are grouped into chemical labyrinthectomy using IT-Gent injections, or surgical procedures, such as transcanal labyrinthectomy (TCL), TML, and selective vestibular nerve section (VNS).

Chemical Labyrinthectomy

IT-Gent use in the treatment of MD was introduced in the 1970s and popularized in the mid-1990s.[38,39] Gentamicin is a selective vestibulotoxic aminoglycoside antibiotic that

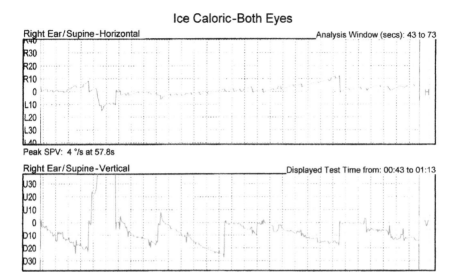

Fig. 9. Ice calorics responses. Note the residual left beating nystagmus when right ear irrigation was performed, which suggested the presence of residual functional vestibular fibers
on the side that underwent vestibular nerve section.

causes apoptotic cell death of the vestibular dark cells, resulting in partial or complete
ablation of peripheral vestibular function.[40,41] Its cochleotoxic effects vary considerably, and hearing deterioration occurs in 13% to 35% of patients.[42]

The therapeutic effect of gentamicin depends on host-dependent and host-
independent factors. Host-dependent factors such as round window permeability,
diffusion along the scala tympani, and genetic susceptibility to aminoglycosides affect
the biologic response seen with IT-Gent perfusion. Furthermore, host-independent
factors, such as dosage and method and technique of administration, may influence
the bioavailability and pharmacokinetics of gentamicin.

Advocates of vestibular ablation using IT-Gent cite the avoidance of surgery and
general anesthesia, and the absence of surgical complications such as meningitis,
facial paralysis, cerebrospinal fluid leak, among others. Nevertheless, many physicians are reluctant to use IT-Gent in people with serviceable hearing because of its
unpredictable effects on hearing.

When hearing is poor, IT-Gent is a reasonable option that offers effective vertigo
control with minimal morbidity. If failed, a TML can be offered.

A recent meta-analysis[42] reviewed 27 published reports between 1978 and 2002
using 5 different administration methods: multiple daily dosages, weekly dosing technique, low-dose technique, continuous microcatheter delivery, and the titration
method. The titration technique (daily or weekly until onset of nystagmus, hearing
loss, or resolution of vertigo) resulted in the highest complete and effective vertigo
control rate (81.7% and 96.3% respectively). The incidence of hearing loss ranged
between 23.7% with the low-dose method and 34.7% with the multiple daily dosage
method. The incidence of profound hearing loss (6%) was similar in all 5 methods.
When comparing degree of vestibular ablation with complete vertigo control and incidence of hearing loss, the complete ablation of vestibular function resulted in 92.1%
vertigo control and 36.7% incidence of hearing loss, whereas partial vestibular

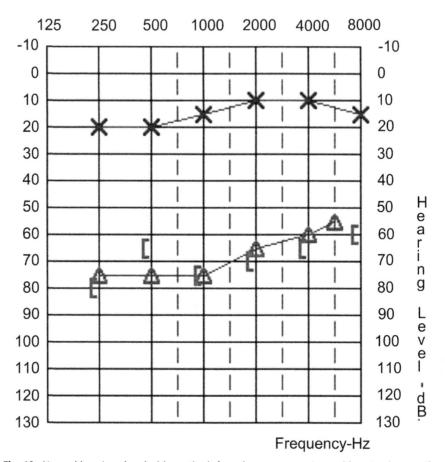

Fig. 10. Normal hearing thresholds on the left and severe sensorineural hearing loss on the right ear. The WDS for the right ear (not shown) is 24%.

ablation resulted in 74.8% vertigo control and 24.8% incidence of hearing loss. Hence, although complete ablation was more effective in controlling vertigo, the incidence of hearing loss increased.

VNS and Labyrinthectomy

Selective sectioning of the vestibular nerve can be performed via several approaches: translabyrinthine (TLVNS), retrolabyrinthine (RLVNS), retrosigmoid (RSVNS), middle fossa (MFVNS), and combined retrolabyrinthine-retrosigmoid (RRVNS). A labyrinthectomy can be performed via the TML or TCL approach.

The transcanal approach is typically performed under local anesthesia in medically frail individuals who cannot undergo a procedure under general anesthesia.

Rosenberg and colleagues[43] showed that vertigo control was achieved in 95%, 90%, and 92% of patients who had RLVNS, RSVNS, and RRVNS respectively. In the 47 patients who were studied, hearing levels improved in 34%, remained the same in 32%, and worsened in 34%.

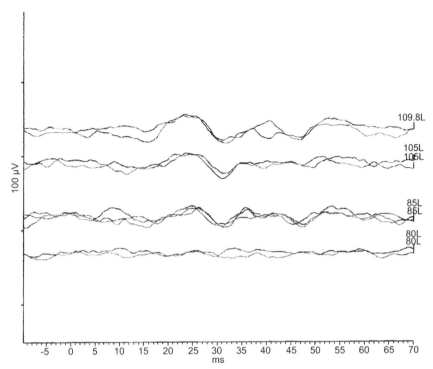

Fig. 11. Absent VEMP response on the right side, indicating severe saccular dysfunction.

By reviewing their results in 143 patients who underwent a modified RLVNS (a portion of the cochlear nerve was sectioned to ablate the cochleovestibular fibers), Nguyen and colleagues[44] showed that vertigo control (cured or improved) was obtained in 92%, hearing remained unchanged or improved in two-thirds of patients, and the percentage of patients with severe disability decreased from 42% before surgery to 7% following the RLVNS.

WHAT INFLUENCES THE SURGEON'S DECISION IN SELECTING THE TYPE OF DESTRUCTIVE SURGICAL PROCEDURE?

A national survey of the preferred surgical approach showed that 77% performed RSVNS, 14% MFVNS, and 9% RLVNS.[21]

When contemplating a nerve section several factors should be considered in choosing the approach:

(1) Position of sigmoid sinus
- Far forward: RSVNS
- Posterior or lateral: RLVNS

(2) Status of residual hearing
- Pure tone average (PTA)>80 dB, WDS<20%: TLVNS, TML, or TCL

(3) Suspicion of cochleovestibular fibers
- MFVNS
- Retrosigmoid: internal auditory canal (IAC).

The most important factor in selecting the type of procedure is the status of the patient's residual hearing. If hearing is poor, TML is offered. If hearing is serviceable, selective VNS or chemical labyrinthectomy using IT-Gent is usually recommended.

Other factors may influence the type of approach. If the sigmoid is forward, a retrosigmoid approach may provide better exposure. If the sigmoid is posterior, retrolabyrinthine VNS may be preferable. If a cleavage plane is not well visualized, the posterior lip of the IAC is typically drilled away. In patients with suspected active residual cochleovestibular fibers (Ort cochleovestibular bundle of the inferior vestibular nerve) or vestibulofacial fibers (Rasmussen cochleofacial bundle of the superior vestibular nerve), a more laterally placed exposure of the fundus of the internal auditory canal via a middle fossa approach can provide better surgical exposure.[45,46] These fibers leave the vestibular nerve shortly after the main trunks exit the lamina cribrosa.

VNS VERSUS LABYRINTHECTOMY IN CONTROLLING VERTIGO, CHRONIC DISEQUILIBRIUM, AND THE RESULTANT QOL

Teufert and colleagues[47] reviewed their experience with 25 patients who underwent TML and 17 patients who had a TLVNS. In their series, 64% of patients having TML and 64.7% of those having TLVNS had MD, respectively. Class A and B vertigo control was achieved in 86% of the TML group and 88% of the TLVNS group. Despite comparable vertigo control, the resolution of the chronic imbalance and disequilibrium was seen in 82% of the TLVNS group and 52% of the TML group.

Diaz and colleagues,[48] using a disease-specific outcome questionnaire in 44 patients with MD who underwent a TML, showed that 98% of their patients reported an improvement in their overall QOL. The resultant hearing loss did not significantly affect their QOL.

VNS VERSUS INTRATYMPANIC PERFUSION OF GENTAMICIN

Colletti and colleagues[49] reviewed their results in 209 patients who underwent RSVNS and 24 patients who received IT-Gent. Gentamicin (80 mg/mL) was mixed with 8.4% buffer (26 mg per injection) and injected up to once per week for 6 weeks. Class A and B vertigo control were obtained in 95.8% and 75% of patients in the RSVNS and IT-Gent groups, respectively. In the IT-Gent group, hearing was significantly worse than in the RSVNS group. In the IT-Gent group, mean PTA decreased from 50.1 dB to 74.7 dB, and WDS decreased from 87% to 65%.

Kaylie and colleagues[50] compared their post-surgical vertigo control rate with IT-Gent. Class A and B vertigo control at 18 and 24 months was obtained in 100%, 82.8%, and 72.3% of patients who underwent a TML, VNS, and ESS respectively. Compared with IT-Gent, TML offered better vertigo control, VNS was similar, and ESS was less effective. Postoperative PTA and WDS worsened (PTA>15 dB and WDS>20%) in 11% of their patients who underwent ESS or VNS. They felt that these results were slightly better than hearing preservation rate following IT-Gent.

Two years following the TML, A.S. began complaining of a sensation of aural fullness, increasing subjective tinnitus and decreased subjective hearing in the contralateral ear. An audiogram showed moderate sensorineural hearing loss in the left ear. The WDS was 76%. Repeat MRI was normal. ECoG showed an increased SP/AP ratio in the left ear. An infectious and autoimmune workup was negative. She was diagnosed with bilateral MD. Her vertigo spells resolved following a course of oral prednisone and intratympanic dexamethasone. However, her hearing remained unchanged. She was given a hearing aid for the left ear and was encouraged to consider cochlear implantation and to learn speech reading. Approximately 4 months later, she had further worsening of her left-sided hearing loss, and substantial increase in her subjective tinnitus on the left side. An audiogram revealed severe left-sided sensorineural hearing loss **(Fig. 12)**. The WDS decreased to 36% in that ear. Another course of steroids failed to improve her hearing. She continued to use a hearing aid on that side with benefit limited to sound awareness. She had a cochlear implant evaluation 4 months later, and was deemed to be an appropriate candidate audiologically. A cochlear implant was placed on the side that had undergone labyrinthectomy (ie, the right side). She continued to be troubled by frequent vertigo spells and was offered an endolymphatic sac decompression (ie, without shunting) on the left side. She underwent the ESS, but unfortunately continued to experience biweekly vertigo and a constant sensation of disequilibrium. A VNG showed no caloric response in the labyrinthectomized side, and a minimal response (8 degrees slow component eye velocity) on the nonlabyrinthectomized side. Rotary chair testing indicated bilateral vestibular hypofunction with decreased gain, slight phase lead, and 18% to 20% asymmetry (weaker response for clockwise rotations). She underwent 4 months of vestibular rehabilitation, which helped with her chronic disequilibrium and overall QOL but did not significantly decrease

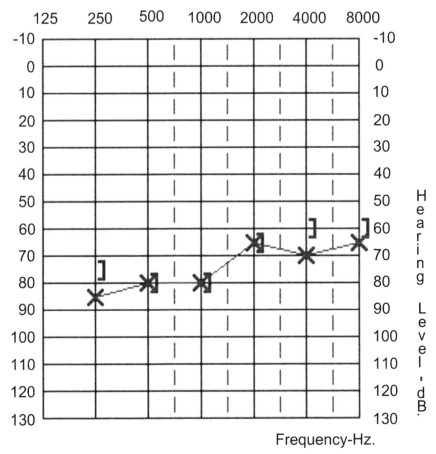

Fig. 12. Profound hearing loss on the right side and severe sensorineural hearing loss on the left side. The WDS for the left ear (not shown) is 36%.

the frequency of her vertigo spells. After several discussions, she was offered intramuscular streptomycin at 1 g intramuscularly twice a day. Her vertigo spells improved after a cumulative dose of 25 g. On her last follow-up, she described rare episodes of oscillopsia and continues to be free of vertigo spells.

WHAT ARE THE CHALLENGES IN THE DIAGNOSIS AND TREATMENT OF BILATERAL MD?

In this case, the contralateral ear involvement was delayed in time and is consistent with bilateral MD. This diagnosis can be further supported by increased SP/AP ratio on ECoG.

Role of Diagnostic Tests

In patients who develop bilateral disease at a short interval it is reasonable to consider entities that cause bilateral Ménière's-like symptoms. These entities can be infectious (otosyphilis),[5,18] neoplastic (bilateral endolymphatic sac tumors in a patient with Von-Hippel Lindau),[51] or immune mediated (Cogan syndrome).[6]

After several years following the initial presentation, it is reasonable to repeat the MRI. In patients with bilateral Ménière's syndrome secondary to immune-mediated symptoms, gado-MRI can evaluate for intralabyrinthine enhancement and is helpful in determining the stage of the inflammatory vestibulocochleitis. The initial enhancement seen at the acute labyrinthitis stage fades away during the subacute phase. The absence of fluid signal on T2-weighted images in the cochlea and labyrinth denotes a fibrous or osseous obliteration of the cochlear lumen. A computed tomography scan assists in determining whether this is caused by fibrous reaction or neo-ossification. Cochlear obliteration can be seen in 50% of cases with autoimmune or immune-mediated inner ear disease.[52]

Vertigo Control in Patients with Bilateral MD and Failed Medical Therapy

The risk of deafness and oscillopsia following complete bilateral cochleovestibular ablation renders the management of bilateral MD a challenging task. Although cochlear implantation provides an acceptable hearing rehabilitation for deafened individuals, the QOL and degree of disability resulting from severe bilateral vestibular hypofunction are severe.

Most physicians agree that a destructive procedure is contraindicated in the management of the second ear in patients with bilateral disease. Nevertheless, some physicians may offer nondestructive procedures for the second ear in patients with bilateral MD.

Shea and colleagues[53] showed good vertigo control in patients with bilateral MD using intramuscular streptomycin. All 11 patients treated in their series had complete vertigo control. One patient developed oscillopsia, and hearing worsened in 3 of 11 patients after treatment.

Hearing Rehabilitation Using Cochlear Implantation

In patients deafened by MD, cochlear implantation is a viable option for hearing restoration. Lustig and colleagues[54] showed improved auditory performance following implantation. A TML is not a contraindication for cochlear implantation. Using promontory stimulation testing in labyrinthectomized patients, investigators confirmed cochlear viability.[55] Reports of cochlear implantation in a labyrinthectomized ear yielded good auditory performance.[56]

Management of MD in an Only Hearing Ear

As with bilateral disease, MD in an only hearing ear is difficult to treat. A survey of 165 members of the American Neurotological Society showed that 99% of physicians recommended dietary modifications as a first-line therapy.[57] Only 39% of surveyed members offered oral corticosteroids as a first-line treatment, and 71% offered surgery for the only hearing ear when deemed appropriate.

SUMMARY

The diagnosis and treatment of MD continues to challenge many physicians. Current treatment strategies, ranging from non-destructive, function-preserving interventions to destructive, function-ablative procedures, are effective in controlling vertigo attacks. To date, no therapy has been shown to prevent the progressive cochlear dysfunction seen in MD. Nevertheless, current hearing rehabilitative strategies using acoustic or electric auditory stimulation help restore hearing to affected individuals. However, many patients continue to be disabled by the severe tinnitus and chronic imbalance that accompanies progressive disease.

REFERENCES

1. Ménière P. Maladies de l'oreille interne offrant les symptomes de la congestion cérébrale apoplectiforme. Gaz Méd de Paris 1861;16:88 [in French].
2. Arenberg IK, Balkany TJ, Goldman G, et al. The incidence and prevalence of Meniere's disease–a statistical analysis of limits. Otolaryngol Clin North Am 1980;13:597.
3. Stahle J, Stahle C, Arenberg IK. Incidence of Meniere's disease. Arch Otolaryngol 1978;104:99.
4. Committee on Hearing and Equilibrium guidelines for the diagnosis and evaluation of therapy in Meniere's disease. American Academy of Otolaryngology-Head and Neck Foundation, Inc. Otolaryngol Head Neck Surg 1995;113:181.
5. Pulec JL. Meniere's disease of syphilitic etiology. Ear Nose Throat J 1997;76:508.
6. Hughes GB, Barna BP, Kinney SE, et al. Clinical diagnosis of immune inner-ear disease. Laryngoscope 1988;98:251.
7. Cmejrek RC, Megerian CA. Obstructing lesions of the endolymphatic sac and duct mimicking Meniere's disease. Ear Nose Throat J 2004;83:753.
8. House JW, Doherty JK, Fisher LM, et al. Meniere's disease: prevalence of contralateral ear involvement. Otol Neurotol 2006;27:355.
9. Dornhoffer JL. Diagnosis of cochlear Meniere's disease with electrocochleography. ORL J Otorhinolaryngol Relat Spec 1998;60:301.
10. Ikeda M, Sando I. Paravestibular canaliculus in Meniere's disease. A histopathological study. Ann Otol Rhinol Laryngol Suppl 1985;118:11.
11. Masutani H, Nakai Y, Kato A. Microvascular disorder of the stria vascularis in endolymphatic hydrops. Acta Otolaryngol Suppl 1995;519:74.
12. Paparella MM. The cause (multifactorial inheritance) and pathogenesis (endolymphatic malabsorption) of Meniere's disease and its symptoms (mechanical and chemical). Acta Otolaryngol 1985;99:445.
13. Xenellis J, Morrison AW, McClowskey D, et al. HLA antigens in the pathogenesis of Meniere's disease. J Laryngol Otol 1986;100:21.
14. Yoo TJ, Yazawa Y, Tomoda K, et al. Type II collagen-induced autoimmune endolymphatic hydrops in guinea pig. Science 1983;222:65.

15. Clark SK, Rees TS. Posttraumatic endolymphatic hydrops. Arch Otolaryngol 1977;103:725.

16. Derebery MJ. Allergic and immunologic aspects of Meniere's disease. Otolaryngol Head Neck Surg 1996;114:360.

17. Shea JJ Jr, Ge X, Orchik DJ. Traumatic endolymphatic hydrops. Am J Otol 1995; 16:235.

18. Paparella MM. Pathogenesis of Meniere's disease and Meniere's syndrome. Acta Otolaryngol Suppl 1984;406:10.

19. Salt AN. Regulation of endolymphatic fluid volume. Ann N Y Acad Sci 2001;942: 306.

20. Merchant SN, Adams JC, Nadol JB Jr. Pathophysiology of Meniere's syndrome: are symptoms caused by endolymphatic hydrops? Otol Neurotol 2005;26:74.

21. Kim HH, Wiet RJ, Battista RA. Trends in the diagnosis and the management of Meniere's disease: results of a survey. Otolaryngol Head Neck Surg 2005; 132:722.

22. Gatland DJ, Billings RJ, Youngs RP, et al. Investigation of the physiological basis of summating potential changes in endolymphatic hydrops. Acta Otolaryngol 1988;105:218.

23. Ge X, Shea JJ Jr. Transtympanic electrocochleography: a 10-year experience. Otol Neurotol 2002;23:799.

24. Rauch SD, Zhou G, Kujawa SG, et al. Vestibular evoked myogenic potentials show altered tuning in patients with Meniere's disease. Otol Neurotol 2004;25:333.

25. Timmer FC, Zhou G, Guinan JJ, et al. Vestibular evoked myogenic potential (VEMP) in patients with Meniere's disease with drop attacks. Laryngoscope 2006;116:776.

26. Park HJ, Migliaccio AA, Della Santina CC, et al. Search-coil head-thrust and caloric tests in Meniere's disease. Acta Otolaryngol 2005;125:852.

27. Palomar-Asenjo V, Boleas-Aguirre MS, Sanchez-Ferrandiz N, et al. Caloric and rotatory chair test results in patients with Meniere's disease. Otol Neurotol 2006;27:945.

28. Santos PM, Hall RA, Snyder JM, et al. Diuretic and diet effect on Meniere's disease evaluated by the 1985 Committee on Hearing and Equilibrium guidelines. Otolaryngol Head Neck Surg 1993;109:680.

29. Silverstein H, Smouha E, Jones R. Natural history vs. surgery for Meniere's disease. Otolaryngol Head Neck Surg 1989;100:6.

30. Thirlwall AS, Kundu S. Diuretics for Meniere's disease or syndrome. Cochrane Database Syst Rev 2006;3:CD003599.

31. James AL, Burton MJ. Betahistine for Meniere's disease or syndrome. Cochrane Database Syst Rev 2001;1:CD001873.

32. Boleas-Aguirre MS, Lin FR, Della Santina CC, et al. Longitudinal results with intratympanic dexamethasone in the treatment of Meniere's disease. Otol Neurotol 2008;29:33.

33. Gottshall KR, Hoffer ME, Moore RJ, et al. The role of vestibular rehabilitation in the treatment of Meniere's disease. Otolaryngol Head Neck Surg 2005;133:326.

34. Quaranta A, Marini F, Sallustio V. Long-term outcome of Meniere's disease: endolymphatic mastoid shunt versus natural history. Audiol Neurootol 1998;3:54.

35. Telischi FF, Luxford WM. Long-term efficacy of endolymphatic sac surgery for vertigo in Meniere's disease. Otolaryngol Head Neck Surg 1993;109:83.

36. Kato BM, LaRouere MJ, Bojrab DI, et al. Evaluating quality of life after endolymphatic sac surgery: the Meniere's Disease Outcomes Questionnaire. Otol Neurotol 2004;25:339.

37. Brinson GM, Chen DA, Arriaga MA. Endolymphatic mastoid shunt versus endo-lymphatic sac decompression for Meniere's disease. Otolaryngol Head Neck Surg 2007;136:415.
38. Blakley BW. Clinical forum: a review of intratympanic therapy. Am J Otol 1997;18:520.
39. Nedzelski JM, Chiong CM, Fradet G, et al. Intratympanic gentamicin instillation as treatment of unilateral Meniere's disease: update of an ongoing study. Am J Otol 1993;14:278.
40. Forge A, Li L. Apoptotic death of hair cells in mammalian vestibular sensory epithelia. Hear Res 2000;139:97.
41. Nakagawa T, Yamane H, Shibata S, et al. Gentamicin ototoxicity induced apoptosis of the vestibular hair cells of guinea pigs. Eur Arch Otorhinolaryngol 1997;254:9.
42. Chia SH, Gamst AC, Anderson JP, et al. Intratympanic gentamicin therapy for Meniere's disease: a meta-analysis. Otol Neurotol 2004;25:544.
43. Rosenberg SI, Silverstein H, Hoffer ME, et al. Hearing results after posterior fossa neurectomy. Otolaryngol Head Neck Surg 1996;114:32.
44. Nguyen CD, Brackmann DE, Crane RT, et al. Retrolabyrinthine vestibular nerve section: evaluation of technical modification in 143 cases. Am J Otol 1992;13:328.
45. Green JD Jr, Shelton C, Brackmann DE. Middle fossa vestibular neurectomy in retrolabyrinthine neurectomy failures. Arch Otolaryngol Head Neck Surg 1992;118:1058.
46. Silverstein H, Jackson LE. Vestibular nerve section. Otolaryngol Clin North Am 2002;35:655.
47. Teufert KB, Berliner KI, De la Cruz A. Persistent dizziness after surgical treatment of vertigo: an exploratory study of prognostic factors. Otol Neurotol 2007;28:1056.
48. Diaz RC, LaRouere MJ, Bojrab DI, et al. Quality-of-life assessment of Meniere's disease patients after surgical labyrinthectomy. Otol Neurotol 2007;28:74.
49. Colletti V, Carner M, Colletti L. Auditory results after vestibular nerve section and intratympanic gentamicin for Meniere's disease. Otol Neurotol 2007;28:145.
50. Kaylie DM, Jackson CG, Gardner EK. Surgical management of Meniere's disease in the era of gentamicin. Otolaryngol Head Neck Surg 2005;132:443.
51. Megerian CA, Semaan MT. Evaluation and management of endolymphatic sac and duct tumors. Otolaryngol Clin North Am 2007;40:463.
52. Aftab S, Semaan MT, Murray GS, et al. Cochlear implantation outcomes in patients with autoimmune and immune-mediated inner ear diseases. Otol Neurotol 2010;31(8):1337–42.
53. Shea JJ, Ge X, Orchik DJ. Long-term results of low dose intramuscular strepto-mycin for Meniere's disease. Am J Otol 1994;15:540.
54. Lustig LR, Yeagle J, Niparko JK, et al. Cochlear implantation in patients with bilat-eral Meniere's syndrome. Otol Neurotol 2003;24:397.
55. Kartush JM, Linstrom CJ, Graham MD, et al. Promontory stimulation following lab-yrinthectomy: implications for cochlear implantation. Laryngoscope 1990;100:5.
56. Zwolan TA, Shepard NT, Niparko JK. Labyrinthectomy with cochlear implantation. Am J Otol 1993;14:220.
57. Peterson WM, Isaacson JE. Current management of Meniere's disease in an only hearing ear. Otol Neurotol 2007;28:696.

Infrequent Causes of Disequilibrium in the Adult

Marcello Cherchi, MD, PhD[a,b,]*

KEYWORDS

- Bilateral vestibular loss • Progressive supranuclear palsy
- Spinocerebellar ataxia • Mal de debarquement
- Vestibular paroxysmia • Episodic ataxia
- Psychogenic disequilibrium • Cervicogenic vertigo

This content focuses on some of the less common causes of dizziness in the adult. The diseases have been divided into the 2 broad categories of those causing chronic symptoms and those causing episodic symptoms. Presented here are the unusual causes of chronic disequilibrium in the adult, including bilateral vestibular loss, progressive supranuclear palsy, spinocerebellar ataxias, and mal de debarquement. Also discussed are the unusual causes of episodic disequilibrium in the adult, including psychogenic disequilibrium, vestibular paroxysmia, episodic ataxia, vestibular seizures, and cervicogenic vertigo.

BILATERAL VESTIBULAR LOSS
Epidemiology

Bilateral vestibular loss is uncommon. In some cases the cause is known. In other cases, the condition seems to be idiopathic. These patients tend to be older adults.

Pathophysiology

The percentage of idiopathic cases of bilateral vestibular loss varies from 21% to 51%.[1,2] Of the remaining cases, the most common etiology is ototoxicity, accounting for 17% to 66%,[1,3] with gentamicin being the most common ototoxic agent. Other causes include bilateral (usually sequential) vestibular neuritis and autoimmune inner ear disease. The underlying pathophysiology is either dysfunction of the peripheral

Disclosures: The author has nothing to disclose.

[a] Department of Neurology, Northwestern University Feinberg School of Medicine, 303 East Chicago Avenue, Ward 10-185, Chicago, IL 60611, USA
[b] Chicago Dizziness and Hearing, 645 North Michigan Avenue, Suite 410, Chicago, IL 60611-5800, USA
* Department of Neurology, Northwestern University Feinberg School of Medicine, 303 East Chicago Avenue, Ward 10-185, Chicago, IL 60611.
E-mail address: m-cherchi2@md.northwestern.edu

Otolaryngol Clin N Am 44 (2011) 405–414
doi:10.1016/j.otc.2011.01.011
0030-6665/11/$ – see front matter © 2011 Elsevier Inc. All rights reserved.

oto.theclinics.com

vestibular receptors (as in gentamicin ototoxicity) or dysfunction of the vestibular nerve (as in vestibular neuritis).

Typical Presentation

The common complaints are dizziness and oscillopsia ("jumpy vision" with each step or when driving in a car that goes over a bump). Patients will also be very dependent on their vision for maintaining balance, so falls will often result when trying to walk in the dark, or when closing the eyes in the shower. Depending on the cause, the chronology of symptoms is variable. In idiopathic cases, the development of symptoms may be insidious. In gentamicin ototoxicity, the onset of symptoms usually occurs within several weeks of starting intravenous gentamicin.

Physical Examination

Patients' gait and station will be obviously unsteady on physical examination. They fail unsighted tandem Romberg stance. On dynamic visual acuity testing, they typically lose 4 or more lines of visual acuity during active head rotation compared with acuity when the head is stationary. On fundoscopy, if the head is similarly oscillated, the retinae appear to move (rather than staying entirely steady).

Diagnostic Testing

The gold standard test for bilateral vestibular loss is rotary chair testing, which shows the combination of low vestibulo-ocular reflex (VOR) gain and increased phase lead (more so in the lower frequencies) on sinusoidal harmonic oscillation, and low response gains and time constants on step velocity testing. Vestibular evoked myogenic potentials are absent. Caloric responses, including those to ice water, are absent. Computerized dynamic posturography shows a constellation of abnormalities collectively referred to as a "vestibular" sensory pattern, as well as an "ankle dominant" pattern (especially in test conditions 4–6) on strategy analysis. Magnetic resonance imaging of the brain and internal auditory canals is usually normal, although when the etiology involves vestibular neuritis, there may be mild enhancement of the vestibular nerves on T1 post-contrast imaging (in contrast to vestibular schwannoma which enhances more intensely).

Treatment

Treatment is generally limited to physical therapy for vestibular rehabilitation. These patients can improve, but retain significant dependence on vision and proprioception for balance.

PROGRESSIVE SUPRANUCLEAR PALSY AND OTHER ATYPICAL PARKINSONISMS

Parkinson disease and the other parkinsonian disorders often involve disequilibrium at some point in the course of the disease. Idiopathic Parkinson disease is by far the most common pathology in this family of diseases, but will usually have come to the attention of a neurologist long before referral to a subspecialty clinic of balance disorders. The other diseases in this family include progressive supranuclear palsy (Steele-Richardson-Olszewski syndrome), multiple systems atrophy, corticobasal ganglionic degeneration, and dentatorubropallidoluysian atrophy. Of these, progressive supranuclear palsy (PSP) was selected for discussion because it often presents with disequilibrium early in the course of the disease and may elude diagnosis initially, or be misdiagnosed as idiopathic Parkinson disease.

Epidemiology

The prevalence of PSP has been estimated variably at 1.39 to 6.40 per 100,000. It is more common in men. The age of onset is usually in the fifth through seventh decades.

Pathophysiology

PSP is in a class of neurodegenerative diseases known as "tauopathies." Histopathologic studies demonstrate accumulation of abnormal tau protein seen as globose neurofibrillary tangles in the prefrontal cortex, globus pallidus, substantia nigra, and subthalamic nucleus.

Typical Presentation

By the time the diagnosis is made, symptoms have often been present for several years. Often the initial presentation will be a complaint of unsteadiness or falling, typically backward. Descending stairs sometimes poses a particular challenge. By the time of diagnosis, patients have usually developed some degree of dysphagia. Patients with PSP frequently seem to be oblivious to their deficits and consequently exhibit poor judgment regarding their ability to ambulate and to negotiate stairways. As the disease advances, patients become progressively immobilized and are eventually confined to a wheelchair, and then to a bed. The mean disease duration from the first onset of symptoms until death is 8.0 ± 4.1 years.[4] Patients usually die within approximately 5 years of being diagnosed,[5] with death typically resulting from the usual diseases affecting immobilized patients (aspiration, infections, thromboembolism, etc).

Physical Examination

There is usually axial hypertonia manifesting as truncal and neck stiffness (often with tonic hyperextension), although distracting maneuvers (such as having the patient open and close the hands) may be required to elicit this sign. The extremities usually have normal tone initially and lack the resting tremor of Parkinson disease, although as the disease advances, symmetric appendicular hypertonia may develop. Facies eventually become masked, although in contradistinction to Parkinson disease, the tone of the periorbital musculature tends to produce the appearance of a "frightened stare." Oculomotor examination shows obvious slowing of voluntary vertical saccades, although reflexive vertical saccades may initially be preserved; more subtle findings include convergence insufficiency and square wave jerks. Later in the disease, horizontal saccades are also affected. Cognitive evaluation reveals a mild to moderate dementia with apathy and executive dysfunction.

Diagnostic Testing

Videonystagmography corroborates and quantifies the clinical oculomotor examination. Caloric responses are normal. Rotatory chair testing sometimes exhibits "hang-up" at the extremes of lateral gaze on optokinetic testing. Vestibular evoked myogenic potential amplitudes are often reduced out of proportion to age. Midbrain atrophy can be noted on MRI.

Treatment

Only symptomatic treatment is available. Medication for idiopathic Parkinson disease (such as carbidopa-levodopa [Sinemet]) may bring about a modest, transient therapeutic response that is never sustained.

SPINOCEREBELLAR ATAXIAS
Epidemiology

The spinocerebellar ataxias (SCAs) are rare and were originally referred to as autosomal dominant ataxias because of their mode of inheritance. They comprise a family of more than 20 diseases whose number continues to grow as more forms are recognized. The mutations for most of the SCAs involve trinucleotide repeat expansions, although some are point mutations.

Pathophysiology

The different SCAs produce different combinations of pathology in the cerebellum, pons, inferior olives, and spinal cord. The pathology in the cerebellum usually affects the Purkinje cells, although SCA3 (Machado-Joseph disease) is an exception in this respect.

Typical Presentation

Despite the distinct genetics of each of the SCAs, there is considerable overlap in the clinical presentation(s). The age of onset is in the third to fifth decade, although SCA6 can present as late as the seventh decade. Most of the diseases involve gradually progressive ataxia.

Physical Examination

Most SCAs exhibit a variety of cerebellar signs such as dysmetria, dysdiadochokinesia, and dysarthria. Oculomotor signs include saccadic dysmetria (both hypometria and hypermetria), poor smooth pursuit, and spontaneous nystagmus. In some of the SCAs (types 1 and 7), saccades are slow; SCA2 in particular has markedly slow horizontal saccades. The "spinal" component of the "spinocerebellar ataxias" often manifests as pyramidal tract signs such as hyperreflexia and pathologic reflexes (Babinski sign, Hoffman sign), although not all of the SCAs exhibit such findings.

Diagnostic Testing

The various types of SCAs generally cannot be distinguished on clinical examination alone; genetic testing is available. Occasionally one finds that a single patient has mutations of 2 or more SCAs. Imaging often demonstrates progressive cerebellar atrophy. There may also be atrophy of the pons, medulla, and cervical spinal cord.

Treatment

Treatment is supportive.

MAL DE DEBARQUEMENT
Epidemiology

Mal de debarquement (MDD) is rare, although its incidence is unknown. In about 95% of cases it affects middle-aged females (mean 49.3 years).[6] Migraine is a frequent comorbidity.

Pathophysiology

The pathophysiology is unknown, but most agree that this is not a purely peripheral vestibular etiology.

Typical Presentation

Most cases of MDD seem to be triggered by exposure to motion that is quite prolonged, typically 4 hours or more,[6] and consequently the history usually begins after a boat cruise or long train ride. The patient will usually say that the ride was uneventful in that it induced no motion sickness; immediately after disembarking, the patient has the feeling of "still being on the boat" or train. Although many healthy people may have this sensation for several hours after such a ride, in patients with MDD, the symptoms continue for 6 months to 10 years (mean 3.5 ± 2.5 years).[6] Patients will complain that they always feel as if they are in motion, typically describing a rocking or swaying sensation, although a notable exception is that this sensation completely disappears when they ride in a car or other vehicle. This is an important clue, as virtually no other form of disequilibrium *improves* when the patient is subjected to additional vestibular stimulation. Occasionally one sees patients who lack the initial prolonged exposure to motion, yet the history (including improvement with movement and response to benzodiazepines) is otherwise consistent with MDD. Such cases have migraine-associated vertigo as a differential diagnosis.

Physical Examination

The physical examination is usually entirely normal.

Diagnostic Testing

Diagnostic testing is normal. Occasionally electronystagmography (ENG) will show direction-changing positional nystagmus.[7]

Treatment

Because of the rarity of this disease, no systematic studies of its treatment have been conducted. Usually patients have some response to benzodiazepines such as clonazepam.

PSYCHOGENIC DISEQUILIBRIUM
Epidemiology

Disequilibrium exclusively owing to psychiatric factors is somewhat uncommon, although the epidemiology is difficult to assess because many patients with primary otologic and neurologic causes of disequilibrium may secondarily develop psychological enhancement of that symptom. The cases of purely psychogenic disequilibrium usually involve anxiety and panic disorders.

Pathophysiology

The mechanism by which psychiatric pathology causes disequilibrium is unknown.

Typical Presentation

Patients usually describe episodes of disequilibrium lasting several minutes, often accompanied by symptoms of nausea, shortness of breath, palpitations, and diaphoresis. They may or may not describe associated feelings of anxiety and/or panic.

Physical Examination

The physical examination is normal.

Diagnostic Testing

Purely psychogenic disequilibrium should be a diagnosis of exclusion. A screening otologic and neurologic workup should be undertaken to exclude nonpsychological etiologies.

Treatment

Anxiolytics and antidepressants are reasonable to try.

VESTIBULAR PAROXYSMIA
Epidemiology

Vestibular paroxysmia (VP) is uncommon, although its exact incidence is unknown. It is also referred to in the literature as "disabling positional vertigo."

Pathophysiology

VP is believed to result from episodic irritability of the vestibular nerve. In many cases this appears to be caused by radiographically demonstrable microvascular compression (typically by the superior cerebellar artery or an aberrant loop of another small branch artery).[8] In some cases, VP probably arises as a consequence of a lesion of the vestibular nerve by vestibular neuritis, or from a traction injury (as in head trauma). In other cases, the underlying pathophysiology is unknown.

Typical Presentation

Usually patients will experience a very disturbing first event consisting of extremely abrupt-onset disequilibrium (with no prodrome) that lasts a fraction of a second and then completely stops, with no residual symptoms. The disequilibrium itself may be perceived as a spin, as a "shove" in the lateral or anteroposterior direction, or as a drop. In some cases the disequilibrium lasts a few seconds, but rarely longer. The frequency of recurrence is variable; it can occur as frequently as multiple times per day, or as infrequently as only a few times per year. The episodes are dangerous insofar as they have no warning and are quite violent.

Physical Examination

Usually physical examination is normal. On video Frenzel oculography, there is sometimes a modest baseline nystagmus beating away from the side of the lesion. In some cases, hyperventilation induces (after a delay of 30 to 120 seconds) nystagmus beating toward the lesion; this pattern is believed to be attributable to an increased rate of tonic firing of the involved vestibular nerve that in turn is triggered by the change in acid-base balance resulting from hyperventilation.[9]

Diagnostic Testing

In some cases, there is a reduced caloric response or reduced vestibular myogenic potential on the involved side. Sometimes microvascular compression can be demonstrated by good-quality imaging. Prolonged latency of Wave II on electrophysiologic (auditory brainstem response) testing secondary to vascular compression of the distal vestibulocochlear nerve has also been described.[10]

Treatment

Therapy with oxcarbazepine or other antiepileptic medications can reduce the frequency of the episodes. Some patients are fortunate enough to have the episodes completely stop after such therapy is initiated. For medically refractory cases in which microvascular compression can be confidently identified, surgical intervention is sometimes considered.[10]

EPISODIC ATAXIA, TYPE 1
Epidemiology

Episodic ataxia type 1 (EA1) is rare. It is a dominantly inherited condition.

Pathophysiology

EA1 results from several different missense mutations on chromosome 12 affecting the gene that encodes the KCNA1 potassium channel. This potassium channel is highly expressed in the cerebellum, and it is presumed that its episodic dysfunction is responsible for the clinical manifestations of the disease.

Typical Presentation

Symptom onset may be during infancy, and symptoms typically resolve by young adulthood. Patients suffer from episodes of incoordination, abnormal movements, and slurred speech. Usually the episodes occur spontaneously, but sometimes they appear to be triggered by a physiologic stressor or after being startled. The episodes typically last seconds to minutes, although their frequency is quite variable.

Physical Examination

During an episode, patients exhibit appendicular cerebellar signs, but do not usually have nystagmus. Between episodes, patients may exhibit myokymia in the hands and periorbital musculature.

Diagnostic Testing

Genetic testing is available. Imaging is usually normal; specifically, there is no cerebellar atrophy.

Treatment

Patients sometimes have a modest response to acetazolamide. They may also respond to carbamazepine. For those patients whose episodes are reliably triggered by particular activities, avoidance of triggers is often adequate.

EPISODIC ATAXIA, TYPE 2

Epidemiology

Episodic ataxia type 2 (EA2) is rare. It is a dominantly inherited condition. Half of patients with EA2 have migraines.

Pathophysiology

EA2 results from several different mutations on chromosome 19 affecting the gene that encodes the α1A subunit of the CACNA1A calcium channel. This calcium channel is expressed in the cerebellar granular cells and Purkinje cells. A different mutation in this gene manifests as familial hemiplegic migraine.[11]

Typical Presentation

Patients usually present in the second decade with spontaneous episodes of truncal ataxia lasting for hours to days, often associated with vertigo, nausea, and vomiting.

Physical Examination

During an episode, patients exhibit truncal ataxia and spontaneous nystagmus. Between episodes patients may have gaze-evoked and rebound nystagmus,[12] and suppression of the vestibulo-ocular reflex, and some patients also develop spontaneous downbeating nystagmus. As the disease progresses, patients begin to exhibit subtle cerebellar signs even between attacks, resulting in a mild chronic ataxia.

Diagnostic Testing

Genetic testing is available. Imaging may demonstrate atrophy of the cerebellar vermis.

Treatment

Patients often have a good response to acetazolamide. They may also respond to carbamazepine.

VESTIBULAR SEIZURES
Epidemiology

Vestibular seizures are rare. The exact incidence is unknown.

Pathophysiology

Vestibular seizures, by definition, involve abnormal electrical activity (seizure) affecting those parts of the cerebral cortex believed to mediate vestibular sensation (superoposterior temporal cortex and temporoparietal junction). The rarity of this phenomenon is because seizure activity rarely remains restricted exclusively to the small area of vestibular cortex. Seizure activity will more commonly spread, and when it does, other sensory, motor, and cognitive symptoms will ensue, and the salience of these other symptoms tends to overshadow the vestibular symptoms.

Typical Presentation

Vestibular seizures typically start abruptly and last seconds to minutes.

Physical Examination

The physical examination is normal.

Diagnostic Testing

Electroencephalography may reveal abnormalities over the temporal or temporoparietal regions. Brain imaging should be performed to exclude focal anatomic lesions such as tumors and cortical strokes.

Treatment

Anti-epileptic medications are the treatment.

CERVICOGENIC VERTIGO
Epidemiology

Cervicogenic vertigo is uncommon, but probably also underreported. It should be noted that this is a controversial diagnosis. Clinicians are frequently confronted with patients who complain of neck symptoms and dizziness, and although a thorough workup usually reveals no abnormalities, logic suggests a relationship between neck pathology and imbalance. Cervicogenic vertigo is frequently suspected as a cause of imbalance in patients who have sustained a neck injury, but because such injuries frequently produce medico-legal disputes (such as litigation over a whiplash injury), symptom enhancement for secondary gain may cloud the picture, making this phenomenon difficult to study (see article by Gianoli and Soileau in this publication).

Pathophysiology

The pathophysiology of cervicogenic vertigo is poorly understood. Although torquing of or impingement upon a vertebral artery seems like an obvious mechanism, such impairment of circulation would typically result in a constellation of brainstem symptoms rather than simply isolated disequilibrium. Another proposed mechanism involves abnormalities of proprioception mediating head-on-body position or other somatosensory inputs.[9]

Typical Presentation

Often there is some inciting event, such as a neck injury, and patients are often in litigation with respect to that injury. After the inciting event, patients usually complain of disequilibrium that is episodic insofar as it is exacerbated by head-on-neck movements, although they may also complain of a component of milder chronic disequilibrium. They may describe the disequilibrium in different ways, typically using descriptors such as "floating," "drifting," or "rocking." In addition, patients usually have complaints such as neck pain, neck stiffness, or limited range of motion of the neck.

Physical Examination

Physical examination may reveal tension of neck muscles. Rarely, video Frenzel oculography will detect horizontal nystagmus when the head is maintained in a position rotated to one or the other side, and the eyes are maintained in a neutral position (with respect to the orbits).

Diagnostic Testing

Otologic, vestibular, and imaging studies are usually normal.

Treatment

Usually physical therapy directed at the neck and vestibular rehabilitation are the only available therapies.

REFERENCES

1. Rinne T, Bronstein AM, Rudge P, et al. Bilateral loss of vestibular function: clinical findings in 53 patients. J Neurol 1998;245(6–7):314–21.
2. Zingler VC, Cnyrim C, Jahn K, et al. Causative factors and epidemiology of bilateral vestibulopathy in 255 patients. Ann Neurol 2007;61(6):524–32.
3. Gillespie MB, Minor LB. Prognosis in bilateral vestibular hypofunction. Laryngoscope 1999;109(1):35–41.
4. O'Sullivan SS, Massey LA, Williams DR, et al. Clinical outcomes of progressive supranuclear palsy and multiple system atrophy. Brain 2008;131(Pt 5):1362–72.
5. Bower JH, Maraganore DM, McDonnell SK, et al. Incidence of progressive supranuclear palsy and multiple system atrophy in Olmsted County, Minnesota, 1976 to 1990. Neurology 1997;49(5):1284–8.
6. Hain TC, Hanna PA, Rheinberger MA. Mal de debarquement. Arch Otolaryngol Head Neck Surg 1999;125(6):615–20.
7. Brown JJ, Baloh RW. Persistent mal de debarquement syndrome: a motion-induced subjective disorder of balance. Am J Otolaryngol 1987;8(4):219–22.
8. Hufner K, Barresi D, Glaser M, et al. Vestibular paroxysmia: diagnostic features and medical treatment. Neurology 2008;71(13):1006–14.

9. Cherchi M, Hain TC. Provocative maneuvers for nystagmus. In: Eggers S, Zee D, editors. Vertigo and imbalance: clinical neurophysiology of the vestibular system. Amsterdam: Elsevier; 2009. p. 111–34.

10. Jannetta PJ, Moller MB, Moller AR. Disabling positional vertigo. N Engl J Med 1984;310(26):1700–5.

11. Vahedi K, Taupin P, Djomby R, et al. Efficacy and tolerability of acetazolamide in migraine prophylaxis: a randomised placebo-controlled trial. J Neurol 2002; 249(2):206–11.

12. Baloh RW. Episodic vertigo: central nervous system causes. Curr Opin Neurol 2002;15(1):17–21.

Vertebrobasilar Infarcts and Ischemia

Gail Ishiyama, MD[a],*, Akira Ishiyama, MD[b]

KEYWORDS

- Vertebrobasilar insufficiency • Cerebrovascular disease
- Vertigo • Transient ischemic attacks • Stroke
- Sudden deafness • Geriatric
- Human temporal bone and inner ear

A 72-year-old man presented with a history of episodic, spontaneous vertigo spells that has been increasing in frequency over the past 6 months. He describes the symptoms as the abrupt onset of spinning vertigo, associated with nausea, and at times associated with tingling in his face, perioral, lips, and fingers, and blurring of the vision. He has also had generalized weakness associated with these spells. The spontaneous vertigo spells last from seconds to several minutes in duration, and the tingling sensations and weakness last twenty minutes. The symptoms resolve completely between episodes. He has a history of long-standing bilateral high-frequency hearing loss, but he does not experience fluctuations in hearing, neither spontaneously nor associated with the vertigo spells. He has been treated for benign positional vertigo 4 months ago, and the positional vertigo improved after a modified Epley maneuver. However, he continues to experience spontaneous vertigo spells. His medical history is significant for coronary artery disease, hypertension, chronic obstructive pulmonary disease, high cholesterol, and seasonal allergies. He is a 2-pack per day smoker for most of his life.

VERTEBROBASILAR INSUFFICIENCY

The history and presentation of this patient who may present to a neurotology or otolaryngology clinic should alert the clinician to the possibility of vertebrobasilar ischemia, or cerebrovascular disease. Reasons for a heightened suspicion include (1) spontaneous vertigo spells that last a few minutes in duration (2) accompanying focal neurological symptoms including numbness and visual disturbance (3) risk factors of age, hyperlipidemia, hypertension, cardiovascular disease, and tobacco

[a] Division of Neurotology, UCLA School of Medicine, Reed Neurological Research Center, 710 Westwood Boulevard, Box 951769, Los Angeles, CA 90095, USA
[b] Division of Head and Neck Surgery, Department of Surgery, UCLA School of Medicine, 10833 LeConte Avenue, Los Angeles, CA 90095, USA
* Corresponding author.
E-mail address: gishiyama@mednet.ucla.edu

abuse. The recent worsening of symptoms should trigger an expedited workup, referral to experts in cerebrovascular disease, and in some cases such as transient ischemic attacks within the last 72 hours, hospitalization is warranted. In this review, the first section addresses the anatomy and vascular supply of the posterior cerebral circulation and inner ear, with particular attention to major branches and labyrinthine circulation. Topics addressed include the causes of cerebrovascular/vertebrobasilar ischemia and infarcts related to symptoms of vertigo and dizziness. The natural history of posterior circulation ischemic attacks and strokes is discussed. Particular stroke syndromes and their presentation are described in detail. The common presentation to the neurotologist of vertebrobasilar infarct or ischemia is discussed, as well as ways to identify and evaluate the patient at risk for stroke. Critical components and key questions of the clinical examination are addressed, and guidelines for direction of evaluation are presented. Lastly, the relationship between migraine, migrainous stroke, and migraine-related stroke are discussed.

BRIEF SUMMARY OF THE ANATOMY OF THE POSTERIOR CIRCULATION

The vertebrobasilar vascular system feeds the posterior region of the brain, which includes the brainstem, cerebellum, and inner ear. The vertebrobasilar system represents about 20% of cerebral blood flow.[1] When vertigo is the presenting symptom of a transient ischemic attack or cerebrovascular stroke, the cerebrovascular region involved is the vertebrobasilar system. Ischemic attacks in the anterior circulation, that is, carotid system, may present with lightheadedness, but will not present with rotational vertigo. Vertigo can result from ischemia of the inner ear, brainstem, or cerebellar structures served by the posterior circulation. Posterior circulation transient ischemic attacks (TIAs) and strokes represent about 20% of all TIAs and strokes.[2]

The vertebral arteries originate from the subclavian arteries, which branch from the thoracic aorta. The two vertebral arteries are only rarely the same size, and in 72% of subjects in an anatomic study, one vertebral artery is at least double the size of the other.[3] The vertebral artery is designated into 4 sections: V1, which includes the origin and is the extracranial prevertebral portion; V2, which is the extracranial foraminal or cervical artery; V3, which is the extracranial postforaminal artery at the atlanto-axial region; and V4, which is the intracranial artery and includes the junction with the basilar artery. The most common sites of stenosis are at V1 and V4, particularly at the origin of the vertebral artery as it comes off of the subclavian, and at the vertebrobasilar junction.

The posteroinferior cerebellar artery (PICA) is the largest branch of the vertebral artery. It generally originates 1 to 2 cm below the basilar artery, but in angiograms has been shown to sometimes originate below the level of the foramen magnum.[4] PICAs supply the lateral medulla including the vestibular nuclei and the posteroinferior cerebellum. The two vertebral arteries merge to form the midline basilar artery, which courses along the ventral surface of the pons. The basilar artery gives off penetrating median, paramedian, and short circumferential branches.

The largest circumferential branches are the anterior inferior cerebellar arteries (AICAs), which arise from the proximal third of the basilar artery. In addition to supplying the labyrinth, AICAs supply the lateral pontine tegmentum, brachium pontis, flocculus, and part of the anterior cerebellum. An AICA infarct typically involves the middle cerebellar peduncle.[5,6] There is often a close relationship between the PICA and ipsilateral AICA; if one PICA is hypoplastic, the ipsilateral AICA may be large, and the contralateral PICA small.[7]

The vascular anatomy of the inner ear has been studied in multiple species.[8] The inner ear consists of the auditory and vestibular end organs for hearing and balance, respectively. The vestibular labyrinth is composed of the 3 semicircular canals (SCCs) and 2 otolith organs, the saccule and utricle. The vestibular end organs are involved in sensing head movement and position; the cristae ampullares sense angular acceleration. The cristae ampullares contain vestibular hair cells that act as mechanoelectrical receptors, transducing the mechanical bending of the stereocilia bundle to an electrical transduction current. Inner ear vascular supply is provided by the internal auditory artery (also known as the labyrinthine artery), arising most commonly as a branch of the ipsilateral AICA. Within the internal auditory canal, the internal auditory artery branches into two arteries:

1. The common cochlear artery, which feeds most of the cochlea, and a branch, the posterior vestibular artery, which feeds the inferior saccule and posterior SCC
2. The anterior vestibular branch, which feeds the horizontal and anterior SCC, utricle, and a small portion of the saccule.

The labyrinthine arteries are end-arteries; they do not anastomose with other major arterial branches.[9] Therefore, if blood flow is interrupted for as little as 15 seconds, the auditory nerve fibers become unexcitable. By contrast, there are richer anastomoses in the brainstem and overlying territories in the cerebellum, and thus the inner ear appears to be more vulnerable to interruption of blood flow than the brainstem or cerebellum.

Age-related atrophy of inner ear structures may be secondary to relative ischemia, that is, microvascular ischemia, a well-studied phenomenon in human temporal bone studies.[10,11] There is a significant (11.7%) loss of spiral ligamental volume and a 32% loss of stria vascularis volume in subjects older than 60 years compared with those younger than 40 years.[12] In the aging Fisher rat, there is a significant age-related 75% decrease in blood flow in the capillaries of the posterior crista.[13] Cells in the inner ear, especially strial marginal cells and the auditory and vestibular hair cells, may be exceptionally vulnerable to ischemia because of the high volume density of mitochondria, which is associated with high energy demand.

Before dividing into the two posterior cerebral arteries (PCAs), the basilar artery gives off the superior cerebellar arteries (SCAs). The cerebellum is fed by the AICAs, PICAs, and SCAs with prominent anastomoses between these arterial arcades on the cerebellar surface. These arteries feed areas of the brainstem related to wakefulness and consciousness, and there is a high degree of collateralization in this critical area. By contrast, there is little significant collateralization within the inner ear. This fact may explain why vertebrobasilar insufficiency can present with isolated labyrinthine infarctions[14] and cochlear hearing loss.[6]

The cause of vertebrobasilar insufficiency or ischemia (VBI) is usually atherosclerotic disease of the subclavian, vertebral, or basilar arteries. However, clinicians should realize that it has been estimated that 1 in 5 posterior circulation infarcts is cardioembolic, and another 1 out of 5 occurs from intra-arterial emboli from extracranial and intracranial vertebral arteries.[15] Emboli will travel to the distal arterial branches, often causing isolated cerebellar infarction in the distribution of the superior cerebellar artery, AICA, or PICA. Therefore, patients with isolated cerebellar infarctions should be evaluated for an embolic source. The evaluation should include looking for a cardiac source of emboli, and assessment of the intracranial and extracranial vertebrobasilar arteries, including the origin of the vertebral artery. There may be a tendency for cardiac catheterization embolic events to involve the posterior vertebrobasilar system.[16]

The extracranial vertebral arteries are also susceptible to dissection, which refers to a tear in the arteries, involving the medial coat. Sudden neck movements such as neck manipulations, or trivial motions such as bending the neck back to take medications, can be the inciting event. There is a predilection for development of atherosclerotic plaques at sites with turbulent flow, such as bifurcation points and at the origin of arteries.[17]

By contrast, dissections usually occur in portions of extracranial arteries that are mobile rather than at the origins of arteries, for example, at the distal extracranial vertebral artery V3. The extracranial and intracranial vertebrobasilar system is well visualized using present-day noninvasive imaging modalities. There are heritable disorders of connective tissue disease, such as Ehlers Danlos type IV associated with arterial dissection, which can occur in multiple sites[18]; however, transient emboli often are not seen, and very small infarcts in communicating areas may not be seen on magnetic resonance imaging (MRI). Therefore, the diagnosis of a posterior circulation TIA or stroke is sometimes made on a clinical basis.

THE POSTERIOR CIRCULATION: MECHANISMS OF STROKE AND TRANSIENT ISCHEMIC ATTACKS

A large study of 407 consecutive patients with posterior circulation events, of whom 59% had strokes without TIA, 24% had TIAs then strokes, and 16% had only TIAs, demonstrated that embolism was the most common stroke mechanism.[19] A total of 40% of patients suffered embolic stroke, of whom 24% were cardiac, 14% intra-arterial, and 2% were combined cardiac and intra-arterial. In 32%, large artery atherosclerotic occlusive disease caused hemodynamic vertebrobasilar ischemia. Distal infarcts, that is, those within the PCA, SCA, and top of the basilar artery, had a high likelihood of cardiac or artery-to-artery embolism. Areas that commonly demonstrated stenosis (>50%) included the origin of the vertebral artery in 131 (32.2%), intracranial vertebral artery in 132 (32.4%), basilar artery in 109 (26.8%), and PCA in 38 (9.3%). Many patients (14%) had penetrating and branch artery disease, meaning disease of the branch artery without disease of the parent artery. Most PCA infarcts were embolic. Patients with cardiac emboli had a poorer prognosis than patients with other stroke mechanisms. Consistent with prior studies, lateral medullary strokes were most often caused by atherosclerotic vertebral artery disease (see later discussion on PICA territory infarcts). Hypertension was present in 61% and cardiac disease comorbidity was common (64% of those evaluated with thorough cardiac studies). For the neurotologist, the patient with cardiac emboli as the origin of posterior circulation stroke is not likely to present to the outpatient clinic, and more likely would present to the emergency department. However, of relevance to the physician called on to see a patient with acute vertigo in the emergency room, key differences that distinguish the cerebellar stroke may be the nystagmus (often gaze-evoked, direction changing) and subtle cerebellar signs such as eye movement abnormalities.

DIZZINESS, VERTIGO, AND VERTEBROBASILAR ISCHEMIA

The clinician must evaluate the category of dizziness when a patient complains of dizziness. Global cerebral hypoperfusion is likely to present with a sense of lightheadedness and an impending fainting sensation. Presyncopal lightheadedness is somewhat nonspecific and may arise from cardiac arrhythmias, orthostatic hypotension, or vasovagal reactions. In presyncopal lightheadedness, there is no sense of movement of the external environment. By contrast, vertigo, the sensation of movement of the environment, often in a rotational manner, is a common presentation of vertebrobasilar insufficiency. In the case of posterior circulation ischemia, the onset of vertigo is usually abrupt and spontaneous rather than position-induced, and there may be a flurry of spells within a few weeks' time. Vertebrobasilar ischemia is a common cause of vertigo in the aging population. Therefore, it is critical to distinguish whether the dizziness is vertigo or lightheadedness.

Important questions to ask the patient:

"Do you feel as if you are about to pass out?" This would be consistent with global hypoperfusion.

"If you are seated still when the dizziness occurs, do you feel as if the world is moving?" This would be consistent with true vertigo.

"How long is the actual vertigo spell, and is the onset abrupt or gradual?"

"How often do the spells occur, and is the frequency of the spells increasing?"

"Are the spells provoked by positional changes of the head?" This may indicate benign paroxysmal positional vertigo (BPPV), but any vertigo can be associated with sensitivity to head movement.

"Are there accompanying otological signs with the spells of vertigo, such as aural fullness, hearing loss, or tinnitus?" These may indicate Ménière's disease but can also be seen in basilar migraine and TIAs in the AICA distribution.

"Are there accompanying focal neurologic signs with the spells of vertigo, or in isolation?" (**Box 1**). These would indicate vertebrobasilar TIAs.

"Is it followed by a headache?" Note that this does not necessarily indicate migraine vertigo, because strokes, TIAs, dissections, and seizures are often characterized by headache.

"Is there a personal history of hypertension, hyperlipidemia, diabetes mellitus, cancer, coronary artery disease, peripheral vascular disease, migraines with aura or complicated migraine, strokes or TIAs in the past?"

"Is there a family history of the above risk factors, as well as hearing loss, dizziness, connective tissue diseases, or migraines?"

THE IMPORTANCE OF THE NEUROLOGIC EXAMINATION AND OF IMAGING EVALUATIONS OF THE VERTEBROBASILAR SYSTEM

Any patient presenting with vertigo or hearing loss should be evaluated for focal neurologic signs that localize to the brainstem. In addition, patients should be asked if they suffer from spells that would be consistent with vertebrobasilar ischemia. The authors

---

Box 1
Neurologic review of systems

Have you experienced any of the following symptoms? Please check yes or no and indicate if constant or in episodes.

1. Double vision, blurred vision, or blindness

2. Numbness of the face or extremities

3. Weakness in arms or legs

4. Clumsiness in arms or legs

5. Confusion or loss of consciousness

6. Difficulty with speech

7. Difficulty swallowing

8. Pain in neck or shoulder

typically include in the patient questionnaire a neurologic review of systems that localizes to the posterior circulation (see **Box 1**).[20]

On examination, the patient presenting with vertigo or hearing loss should be evaluated for:

1. Facial weakness (which in AICA and PICA infarcts can be peripheral or central)
2. Facial sensory loss: this can be tested using a cold tuning fork, pinprick, or testing the corneal reflex with a cotton tip
3. Eye movement abnormalities including skew deviation, diplopia, and nystagmus, because gaze-evoked nystagmus or down-beat nystagmus is typical in cerebellar infarct
4. The visual fields, as most PCA infarcts will exhibit a visual field cut
5. Crossed sensory loss, a key indicator for brainstem involvement, commonly seen as loss of facial sensation on the ipsilateral side, and loss of extremity sensation on the contralateral side
6. Horner syndrome, tested in darkness for an ipsilateral smaller pupil, because the anisocoria or asymmetry will be accentuated in darkness. Horner syndrome occurs when there is loss of sympathetic outflow. The sympathetic system is responsible for pupillary dilation and thus there is a miosis, or pupillary constriction in the ipsilateral pupil.
7. Limb ataxia, testing for cerebellar ataxia with finger-to-nose, finger-to-finger, and heel-to-shin movements
8. Gait ataxia, which will generally be exhibited by a wide-based gait or inability to walk
9. Head-thrust test, which can reveal catch-up saccades in purely peripheral disorders such as vestibular neuritis or gentamicin ototoxicity. However, it is also important to note that in cases of AICA infarct, the head-thrust test will demonstrate catch-up saccades in many cases.

Symptoms that may localize to a PICA infarct should be queried including hiccoughs, inability to swallow, facial sensory and motor loss, and limb ataxia. Hearing always should be tested at bedside in patients with vertigo, and when suspicious, a full diagnostic audiogram with or without auditory brainstem responses should be requested.

THE ROLE OF IMAGING

An important clinical point to be made is that in patients with large artery atherosclerosis as an etiologic mechanism of TIA are prone to recurrence or early progression to stroke.[21] In a large study of all consecutive cerebrovascular events (strokes and TIAs), events in the posterior (vertebrobasilar) circulation were more likely to be associated with significant stenosis (26.2%) than those in the anterior (carotid) circulation (11.5%).[22] Therefore, imaging studies in this group of patients with posterior circulation events would be high yield. Furthermore, patients with vertebrobasilar TIAs secondary to atherosclerosis are even more likely to suffer early recurrence of a vascular event or progress to a stroke than patients with symptomatic carotid stenosis.[23] Therefore, the possibility of vertebrobasilar TIA should be assessed with a stroke protocol MRI that includes assessment of the intracranial and extracranial anterior and posterior cerebrovasculature. In the past, the only way to assess posterior circulation accurately was to undertake a cerebral angiogram, an invasive procedure with risks.

Fortunately, there are now noninvasive means of imaging the posterior circulation using contrast-enhanced magnetic resonance angiography (MRA) and computed tomographic angiography (CTA). Contrast-enhanced MRA (CE-MRA) has good sensitivity and specificity for the detection of 50% to 99% vertebral or basilar stenosis, better than CTA, ultrasonography, and/or time-of-flight MRA.[24] The CE-MRA should image the great vessels from the aortic arch to the circle of Willis. In a large study of patients presenting with posterior events, 39 patients had both CE-MRA and CTA, with corroborating results in 35 patients. In only 4 cases out of 186 was it necessary to conduct intra-arterial subtraction angiography.[25] Previously it was necessary to conduct traditional angiography to evaluate the V1 segment, in particular the origin or take-off of the vertebral artery, as noncontrast MRA is not able to visualize the origin of the vertebral artery well. With the advent of CE-MRA and CTA, noninvasive means of visualizing this area are possible. In a large British study of consecutive patients with vertebrobasilar ischemia (N = 186), 39 patients (21%) were found to have stenosis. The V1 and V4 areas were the most common sites of stenosis (42.9% and 34.7%, respectively); of those in the V1 area, 12 of the 39 (31%) were at the origin of the vertebral, the most common single site of stenosis of the vertebral artery.[25]

In patients presenting with symptoms attributable to the posterior circulation, a vertebral artery dissection may also be the cause. In the study by Gulli and colleagues,[25] 8 of 216 consecutive patients with posterior circulation cerebrovascular events occurred secondary to vertebral artery dissection. With current modern techniques, vertebral dissections can also be evaluated using noninvasive imaging, CE-MRA, or CTA.

ACUTE VERTEBROBASILAR OCCLUSION: INTERVENTIONS ARE POSSIBLE AND IN SEVERE CASES MUST BE TIMELY

Acute vertebrobasilar occlusion occurs when there is an occlusive or complete blockage of the basilar artery. This entity carries an extremely high morbidity and mortality. In young patients, the cause can be cardiac emboli or progression from vertebral dissection. Dissections may occur with neck trauma, such as in car accidents with whiplash, cervical neck manipulations, or spontaneously with a higher incidence in migraineurs. Local atherothrombosis is more common in elderly patients. Early percutaneous treatment is associated with an improved outcome, with best results observed within a 4-hour interval and a recommended time period of less than 6 hours, although even with recanalization the mortality rate is between 35% and 75%. Without intervention, mortality rates are as high as 80% to 90%.[26]

Percutaneous interventions for vertebral artery stenosis are now possible. Noninvasive testing can identify vertebral artery stenosis, including Doppler studies identifying reversed vertebral artery blood flow. Endovascular treatment using coronary wires and drug-eluting stents have proved successful for vertebrobasilar stenosis in endovascular centers.[27] One study reported that drug-eluting stents may decrease the incidence of restenosis when compared with non–drug-eluting stents for treatment of vertebral artery origin (V1) stenosis.[28]

THE SIGNIFICANCE OF A PERIPHERAL VERSUS A CENTRAL CAUSE OF VERTIGO IN VERTEBROBASILAR INSUFFICIENCY

The classic teaching has been to distinguish peripheral from central causes of vertigo and to distinguish peripheral from central patterns of nystagmus. A commonly mistaken clinical assumption is that a peripheral cause of dizziness is secondary to inner ear disease, and therefore not secondary to cerebrovascular disease such as vertebrobasilar ischemia or posterior circulation syndromes. Common peripheral causes of vertigo include well-known otological entities such as Ménière's disease, vestibular neuritis, and BPPV. Dizziness and imbalance are common problems in older subjects, with a population-based study reporting a prevalence of 24% of persons older than 72 years having dizziness that occurred within the previous 2 months.[29] BPPV accounted for 39% of all cases of vertigo in the older population presenting to neurotology clinics.[30] Older individuals are also a well-known higher risk group for cerebrovascular disease and stroke. Thus, the presentation of an older patient with vertigo, including position-dependent vertigo, must address the possibility of a vascular event, in particular vertebrobasilar ischemia.

Labyrinthine infarct is a peripheral cause of vertigo, and vestibular testing will be read as "peripheral vestibular pathology with no signs of central involvement." However, labyrinthine infarct can be a warning of an impending anterior inferior cerebellar artery infarct, which may be secondary to basilar artery thrombosis.[14] When dizziness is accompanied by other neurologic symptoms and signs such as ataxia, sensory loss, visual loss, or unilateral Horner sign, the diagnosis of a brainstem infarct may be easily made. However, a transient ischemic attack in the vertebrobasilar system may present with isolated vertigo or hearing loss, and clinicians need to be aware of this scenario to intervene and reduce the risk of impending stroke. Even with regard to the common peripheral cause of brief vertigo spells, namely BPPV, 11 of 240 cases were secondary to vertebrobasilar insufficiency.[31] In fact, animal studies have demonstrated instability of the otoconia after an ischemic attack of the labyrinthine artery.

VERTIGO AS A PRESENTATION OF VERTEBROBASILAR INSUFFICIENCY

Dizziness is likely the most common presenting complaint among patients age 75 years and older in office practices,[32] and dizziness accounted for 2.5% of all emergency department presentations in the United States during the 10-year period from 1995 through 2004.[33] In that same study, it was noted that the rate of visits for vertigo and dizziness increased each year, increasing by 37% over the decade with a disproportionate increase in the older population. There was an increase of 67% in patients older than 65 years for emergency department visits for dizziness over the decade compared with an increase of 15% for those aged 45 to 64 years. This result may be attributable in part to the public recognition that vertigo can be a sign of a transient ischemic attack, stroke, or impending stroke.

Studies have demonstrated that isolated vertigo can be the presentation of vertebrobasilar ischemia, and in fact vertigo is the most common initial isolated symptom and sign of ischemia in the posterior circulation (see **Box 1**). It is critical that clinicians and emergency room physicians understand that transient vertebrobasilar ischemia, especially of the labyrinth, may not be evident on imaging studies. In a study of 42 patients with vertigo due to vertebrobasilar insufficiency, there was a high incidence of isolated episodes of vertigo: 62% had at least one isolated episode of vertigo, and in 19% the TIAs began with an isolated episode of vertigo.[34] The fact that these patients with vertebrobasilar insufficiency who had isolated vertigo attacks also reported associated focal neurologic symptoms such as loss of vision or generalized weakness suggests that the vertigo is secondary to transient vertebrobasilar ischemia. In the classic synopsis on vertebrobasilar insufficiency, Williams and Wilson[20] noted that vertigo was the initial symptom in 48% of patients (**Table 1**).

Besides vertigo, visual symptoms (eg, diplopia, visual illusions, visual field defects) are the most common symptoms seen in vertebrobasilar ischemia (**Table 2**).[34] Thus, cerebrovascular causes must always be considered in patients presenting with abrupt spontaneous vertigo, especially in the setting of vascular risk factors. Typically the vertigo in vertebrobasilar TIAs is abrupt in onset and usually lasts several minutes. When the vertigo is accompanied by other symptoms of brainstem ischemia

Table 1
Initial symptoms of vertebrobasilar insufficiency in 65 patients

Symptom	No. of Patients (%)
Vertigo	32 (48)
Visual hallucinations	7 (10)
Drop attacks or weakness	7 (10)
Visceral sensations	5 (8)
Visual field defects	4 (6)
Diplopia	3 (5)
Headaches	2 (3)
Other	5 (8)

Data from Williams D, Wilson TG. The diagnosis of the major and minor syndromes of basilar insufficiency. Brain 1962;85:741–74.

(eg, visual symptoms, drop attacks, extremity numbness, or dysarthria), one would assume that the vertigo derives from vertebrobasilar ischemia. Of note, older patients with Ménière's disease and delayed endolymphatic hydrops may present with spontaneous vertigo spells and "drop attacks," which are believed to originate in the otolith organs. These attacks, also known as Tumarkin's otolithic crisis, are characterized by a feeling of being pushed as if by an external force, and there is no loss of consciousness.[35] The care of patients with otolithic "drop attacks" would fall within the expertise of the otolaryngology community. This presentation is in contrast to vertebrobasilar ischemic drop attacks in which patients describe buckling of the knees and bilateral lower extremity weakness, with or without a loss of consciousness.[20] These symptoms were first described as a clinical entity by Kremer as being caused by brainstem dysfunction, without imaging or angiographic evidence.[36] The clinical description remains accurate: "folding up at the knees." Isolated episodes of vertigo

Table 2
Frequency of symptoms associated with vertigo in 42 patients with vertebrobasilar insufficiency

Symptom	No. of Patients (%)
Visual (diplopia, field defects, illusions)	29 (69)
Drop attacks	14 (33)
Unsteadiness, incoordination	9 (21)
Extremity weakness	9 (21)
Confusion	7 (17)
Headache	6 (14)
Hearing loss	6 (14)
Loss of consciousness	4 (10)
Extremity numbness	4 (10)
Dysarthria	4 (10)
Tinnitus	4 (10)
Perioral numbness	2 (5)

Data from Grad A, Baloh RW. Vertigo of vascular origin: clinical and ENG features in 84 cases. Arch Neurol 1989;46:281–4.

with abrupt onset lasting several minutes in duration more likely represent labyrinthine ischemia, and evidence for an AICA or vertebrobasilar stenosis should be investigated.

PATIENTS WITH VERTEBROBASILAR ISCHEMIA HAVE A VERY HIGH INCIDENCE OF STROKE RISK FACTORS

In a study of consecutive patients presenting to a large stroke center, the New England Medical Center Posterior Circulation Registry, the group of patients with extensive atherosclerotic disease involving the basilar artery had a very high incidence of stroke risk factors. Hypertension was present in 70% of these patients and coronary artery disease was present in 60%. In patients with posterior circulation disease, stroke risk factors with high incidence included hypertension (58%), smoking (42%), diabetes mellitus (24.7%), and hyperlipidemia (19%). Comorbidities of coronary artery disease (42%), and peripheral vascular disease (11%) were common. Other important (modifiable) lifestyle factors included alcohol abuse (13%), obesity (11%), and use of oral contraceptive pills (2%).[37]

Medical therapy in atherosclerotic disease should include lipid-lowering therapy. A recently published study demonstrated regression of stenosis after 6 months of statin lipid-lowering therapy in patients with intracranial arterial stenosis. Of note, there was a higher success rate with middle cerebral artery stenosis (59% of the 41 patients had regression) compared with basilar artery stenosis (38% of the 13 patients had regression).[38] Observational studies have reported rates of regression between 8% and 29%, and rates of progression as high as 9% to 33% in symptomatic intracranial stenosis.[39,40] However, the degree of regression of the stenosis was not correlated with the degree of lipid lowering, as there were no differences in lipid profiles among patients.[38] Of note, the study was characterized by a relatively small size, and there was no clear evidence for an improvement in clinical parameters associated with the regression of intracranial stenosis; thus, future studies are warranted.

MODIFIABLE RISK FACTORS AND NONINVASIVE MEDICAL INTERVENTIONS AIMED AT PREVENTING VERTEBROBASILAR STROKE PROGRESSION AND RECURRENCE

In a prospective study of 794 patients following first-time ischemic strokes of multiple types, the use of statins (multiple types were used including fluvastatin, pravastatin, simvastatin, and atorvastatin) was associated with a significantly lower rate of secondary stroke: 16% of those not receiving statins versus 7.6% of those receiving statins had a recurrent stroke.[41] Those receiving statins also had an overall improved survival rate. The mechanism is likely not merely lowering of cholesterol; other proposed mechanisms include antithrombotic, antioxidative, anti-inflammatory, vasodilatory, or plaque-stabilizing properties of statins. The evidence-based guidelines for the management of risk factors to prevent first stroke include treatment of hypertension to under 140/90 in nondiabetics, abstention from tobacco, and tightly controlled hypertension for diabetics (under 130/80 mm Hg).[42] The treatment of adults with diabetes with a statin to lower the risk of a first stroke is recommended. The treatment of dyslipidemia is recommended. In patients with elevated homocysteine levels, use of folic acid and B vitamins may be useful given their safety and low cost (Level of Evidence: C).

As has been noted, a subset of vertebrobasilar insufficiency patients with stenosis or large artery atherosclerosis carries a very high risk of early recurrence and progression to stroke. However, none of the aforementioned vascular risk factors identified patients with vertebrobasilar stenosis, and nothing in the history of these patients suggested significant vertebrobasilar stenosis. Therefore, all patients must be evaluated for imaging evidence of stenosis to detect these high-risk patients. Just as in symptomatic and asymptomatic significant carotid stenosis, symptomatic vertebrobasilar stenosis is now recognized as a major risk factor for stroke recurrence or progression.

BENIGN PAROXYSMAL POSITIONAL VERTIGO IS ALSO ASSOCIATED WITH VERTEBROBASILAR INSUFFICIENCY

BPPV is likely the most common cause of vestibular vertigo, and there is a markedly increased incidence of BPPV in older subjects. In a large cross-sectional neurotologic survey, the 1-year prevalence of BPPV in subjects older than 60 years was nearly 7 times higher than that of subjects 18 to 39 years old, and the cumulative incidence of BPPV reached almost 10% at the age of 80.[43] Although BPPV is a peripheral cause of vertigo spells, in a study of 240 consecutive patients with BPPV, 11 patients had typical symptoms of vertebrobasilar insufficiency.[31] The association between BPPV and vertebrobasilar ischemia may be because transient ischemia to the vestibular end organs causes otolithic degradation or loosening from the otolithic membrane. Ischemia of the utricular macula presumably causes the release of otoconia, which become displaced into the posterior semicircular canal. The superior labyrinth circulation is supplied by the anterior vestibular artery, and there is generally little or no collateralization. Following ischemia of the anterior vestibular artery, there may be ischemic necrosis of the utricular macula causing release of the overlying otoconia. Of note, circulation of the posterior SCC, which is the most common site of displaced otoconia, is supplied by the posterior vestibular artery and can be spared in even a complete infarction of the anterior vestibular artery. Inner ear microvascular ischemia is also believed to mediate the association between migraine and BPPV.[44] Therefore, in the evaluation of patients presenting with BPPV, the clinician should ask about symptoms related to vertebrobasilar insufficiency. Particular attention to these symptoms should be paid in the older patient with vascular risk factors.

THE NATURAL COURSE OF VERTEBRAL OR BASILAR ARTERY STENOSIS: A HIGH RISK OF EARLY RECURRENT STROKE

It is critical for the clinician to recognize the first vertebrobasilar TIA. Contrary to traditional beliefs, there appears to be a higher risk of stroke after vertebrobasilar TIAs than after carotid TIAs.[23,45] Furthermore, a meta-analysis has suggested that the risk of recurrent stroke is as high or higher for vertebrobasilar stroke as that for anterior (carotid) stroke.[45] Using CE-MRA and CTA when MRA could not be conducted (pacemaker or claustrophobia), Marquardt and colleagues[22] evaluated consecutive patients presenting with vertebrobasilar ischemia and large artery stenosis. In their study, of patients presenting with vertebrobasilar TIAs or stroke, 26% (37 of 141) had significant vertebral or basilar artery stenosis. Of the patients with vertebrobasilar TIAs and large artery stenosis (vertebral or basilar artery stenosis 50% or greater), there was a very high risk of 90-day recurrence of stroke (22%) and TIA or stroke (46%) despite medical management that included aspirin, a statin, and antihypertensive treatment. Of note, even in patients without large vessel stenosis, 21% had a posterior circulation event in the first 90 days following an event. Vertebrobasilar events were associated with multiple TIAs shortly before first seeking medical attention, especially among patients with vertebrobasilar stenosis. Lastly, and of interest, patients presenting with posterior circulation events with stenosis did not differ from those without stenosis with regard to treatable vascular risk factors, such as hypertension or hyperlipidemia.[22] Therefore, one cannot predict which patients are at higher risk for vertebrobasilar stenosis.

Gulli and colleagues[25] conducted a prospective study of consecutive patients presenting with posterior circulation stroke or TIA. For those with vertebrobasilar stenosis, the risk of recurrent stroke within 90 days after a first event (using history) was very high: 30.5% as opposed to 8.9% of those without stenosis ($P = .002$). The probability of recurrence was highest soon after the initial event and reached as high as 34% in the first month after the initial event. In addition, of the 216 patients with a posterior event, 19 (8.8%) had a posterior vertebrobasilar transient ischemic event in the 30 days prior. Those TIAs were visual field defect in 7 patients, focal weakness or sensory disturbance in 7, unsteadiness or ataxia in 7, and vertigo in 3. The traditional belief that posterior circulation strokes have a lower recurrent stroke risk is clearly not the case, and the presence of stenosis in the vertebrobasilar distribution is a strong independent predictor of future stroke risk.

Another significant predictor of stroke after TIA is the presence of any lesions on diffusion-weighted imaging (DWI) on MRI. In a study of 343 consecutive TIA patients, DWI imaging was positive in 40%. A total of 15 patients had strokes within 3 months, and all early strokes but one occurred in patients with DWI findings. The absolute risk of stroke after TIA was 1.5% at 7 days and 2.9% at 3 months. TIA patients with a positive DWI result are approximately 10 times more likely to have a TIA or stroke than those with a negative DWI.[46]

The bottom line is that vertebrobasilar insufficiency and posterior circulation events are highly likely to recur in patients with vertebrobasilar stenosis, apparently despite medical management. There are no reliable predictors to aid in identifying patients who have large artery atherosclerotic stenosis; therefore, all patients need to be evaluated promptly for stenosis to identify those at high risk for stroke recurrence. Preventive treatment must be timely. For patients with significant vertebrobasilar stenosis, interventional procedures may prevent recurrences, and thus assessment by a stroke or interventional neuroradiologist should be timely. Vertebral angioplasty or stenting may be indicated, and initial studies show low complication rates at centers.[47,48]

TERRITORIAL INFARCTIONS
AICA Territory Infarcts and Audiovestibular Symptoms

Several prior studies have noted the association of hearing loss and prolonged vertigo associated with AICA territory infarct.[5,49] A temporal bone histopathology study of a patient with AICA territory infarct reported a complete loss of the sensory epithelium of the cochlea and vestibular labyrinth indicative of labyrinthine infarct.[15,50] In a series of patients with AICA infarcts, 5 patients suffered abrupt onset of sensorineural hearing loss.[5] It is important for clinicians to realize that sudden deafness, tinnitus, or vertigo spells can occur as a TIA or infarct in the AICA distribution. Audiovestibular TIAs typically occur with an abrupt onset, last a minute to a few minutes, and may precede a stroke by a few days to a few months.

Lee and colleagues[51] conducted the largest and most complete study, including complete auditory and vestibular testing, of 82 consecutive documented AICA infarcts (**Table 3**). The most common and dominant symptom was acute spontaneous, prolonged vertigo lasting longer than 24 hours, with nausea and vomiting in 80 of 82 patients (98%). The most common presentation of inner ear dysfunction was combined prolonged vertigo and hearing loss in 49 of 82 (60%). Of those with combined auditory and vestibular infarct, 13 had brief transient spells of vertigo or hearing loss lasting a few minutes within the month prior to the infarct. Isolated

Table 3 Frequency of symptoms in 82 consecutive patients with AICA infarcts	
Symptom	No. of Patients (%)
Acute prolonged vertigo (>24 h)	80 (98)
Acute hearing loss	52 (63)
Limb dysmetria	55 (67)
Gait ataxia	52 (63)
Facial sensory loss	23 (28)
Facial weakness	23 (28)
Body sensory loss	5 (6)
Horner syndrome	3 (4)
Dysarthria	3 (4)
Eye motion limitation	2 (2)
Limb weakness	2 (2)

Data from Lee H, Kim JS, Chung E-J, et al. Infarction in the territory of anterior inferior cerebellar artery: spectrum of audiovestibular loss. Stroke 2009;40:3745–51.

vestibular infarction without cochlear involvement was rarer (5%), as was isolated cochlear infarction without vestibular involvement (3%). Electronystagmography (ENG) revealed caloric paresis in 53 of 82 (65%) patients, and nearly all had abnormal central vestibular eye movement findings on optokinetic or smooth pursuit tests, or deficits of the vestibulo-ocular reflex (96%).

Of importance, in a study by Lee and colleagues,[51] patients with prodromal audiovestibular disturbances had 5 times higher prevalence of severe basilar artery occlusive disease than those without prodromal audiovestibular disturbance (62% vs 13%, $P<.001$). Given the low incidence of pure auditory or pure vestibular loss, the investigators speculated that internal auditory artery ischemia seldom results in selective involvement of the anterior vestibular artery or main cochlear artery. Conversely, there is strong support for vascular ischemia or infarct if a patient presents with acute onset of combined auditory and vestibular loss.

In a study following 12 consecutive patients with AICA infarcts, sensorineural hearing loss was identified in 11 (92%). Four of the patients had brief spells of hearing loss and/or tinnitus lasting a few minutes in duration or isolated vertigo spells occurring from 1 day up to 2 months before the AICA infarct.[6] These patients may present to neurologists, neurotologists, or otolaryngology specialists. The key characteristics of the hearing loss or vertigo spells are the abrupt onset and duration of one to a few minutes. Of course, if there are accompanying neurologic complaints (eg, facial palsy, ataxia, diminished sensation), the suspicion for a cerebrovascular event is raised. However, the vertigo or hearing loss/tinnitus may be isolated events.

Audiological testing in 6 of these 12 patients was revealing for a cochlear site of hearing loss. One patient had normal hearing, 1 had retrocochlear hearing loss, and 4 had hearing loss too profound to determine the site. In 7 of 12 patients, there was variable recovery of some hearing. On vestibular testing, ENG showed an absent caloric response in 10 patients and a diminished caloric response in the other 2 patients, indicating a labyrinthine infarct in the vestibular horizontal SCC. In 11 of 12 patients, optokinetic and smooth pursuit abnormalities were also reported.

Because the labyrinthine artery has little or no collateralization with other arterial sources, the hearing loss in an AICA infarct would be predicted to be cochlear in etiology. In animal studies, the stria vascularis, spiral ligament, organ of Corti, and spiral ganglion cells are strikingly vulnerable to occlusion of AICA.[52] Furthermore, the cochlear nerve has abundant collateralization.[53] Therefore, it is likely that in most cases, hearing loss in an AICA TIA or infarct stems from injury to the cochlea itself. The vertigo may derive from the labyrinth (given caloric abnormalities) or the cerebellum and pons (given oculomotor abnormalities). However, because the cerebellum and pons have more collateralization, the labyrinth is more likely the source of vertigo in the early brief spells of spontaneous vertigo lasting a few minutes in duration.

The most common cause for an AICA infarct is thrombosis or atheromatous formation of the basilar artery, blocking the origin of the AICA as noted in conventional angiography.[54] A more recent study of 23 consecutive AICA infarcts determined that large artery atherosclerotic disease in the vertebrobasilar system was the main cause of stroke in 12 (52%) patients with coexisting large artery disease and a cardiac embolic source in 4 (17%).[55] The most common MRA abnormality reported by Lee and colleagues[6] was diffuse or focal stenosis near the AICA origin of the basilar artery (20%), and MRI areas of infarct were commonly the middle cerebellar peduncle (83%), anterior inferior cerebellum (46%), and lateral inferior pons (44%), with complete AICA infarction in 16%. Also, patients with basilar stenosis tended to have AICA and multiple posterior circulation infarcts. Lastly, whereas it was previously reported that AICA infarcts have a high incidence of neurologic deficits localizing to the pons, these deficits were relatively less frequent than expected: facial weakness (21%), facial sensory loss (28%), and body sensory loss (only 6%) (see **Table 3**). Only 2 of the 82 patients had the complete syndrome as described by Adams.[56]

AICA infarcts may also occur in the setting of vertebrobasilar dolichoectasia, an elongation and distension of the vertebrobasilar arteries. The basilar artery is most often affected but the intracranial vertebral arteries can also be involved. Hypertensive and diabetic older subjects are more likely to develop dolichoectasia.[57] Thrombus can form in areas of turbulent flow and then embolize distally. Episodic or progressive neurologic symptoms can occur. Episodic symptoms may indicate ischemia caused by thrombosis, which blocks the origin of smaller branches such as AICA, or can be artery to artery embolic phenomenon, whereas progressive neurologic symptoms are more likely secondary to direct compression.[58] Both etiological scenarios would be well visualized using noninvasive studies, namely CE-MRA or CTA.

Posterior Inferior Cerebellar Artery Syndrome or Lateral Medullary Infarction

The classic syndrome associated with an infarct in the PICA distribution or dorsolateral medullary infarct has been termed Wallenberg syndrome. Major symptoms include vertigo, nausea and vomiting secondary to vestibular nuclei, or posteroinferior cerebellum infarct; severe imbalance likely related to damage to the cerebellum or cerebellar tracts; ipsilateral facial numbness (cranial nerve V and nucleus); ipsilateral facial palsy (peripheral or central); crossed hemisensory loss, dysphagia, and dysphonia (nucleus ambiguus). In a large study of 33 consecutive patients presenting with PICA infarcts, vertigo was common (91%) as was hemibody sensory changes (94%) (**Table 4**).[59] The investigators noted rostral versus caudal groups of patients based on MRI findings, which correlated with symptom clustering. The rostral group had often severe dysphagia but only one patient had nystagmus in the primary position. In the caudal group, no patients had dysphagia prominently, and vertigo and gait ataxia were severe with nystagmus prominent in the primary position. Kim[60] conducted the largest study of pure lateral medullary infarction without cerebellar involvement in 130 consecutive patients (**Table 5**). The symptom clustering was similar, with

Table 4 Frequency of symptoms in 33 consecutive PICA (lateral medullary) infarcts	
Symptom	**No. of Patients (%)**
Vertigo/dizziness	30 (91)
Gait ataxia	29 (88)
Nausea and vomiting	24 (73)
Nystagmus	22 (67)
Horner sign	24 (73)
Dysphagia	20 (61)
Hoarseness	18 (55)
Facial sensory changes	28 (85)
Hemibody sensory changes	31 (94)
Mild central facial paresis (ipsilateral)	12 (36)
Mild hemiparesis	4 (12)

Data from Kim JS, Lee JH, Suh DC, et al. Spectrum of lateral medullary syndrome: correlation between clinical findings and magnetic resonance imaging in 33 subjects. Stroke 1994; 25(7):1405–10.

rostral lesion patients exhibiting severe dysphagia, facial paresis, and dysarthria more often than caudal, and severe gait ataxia and headache less often than caudal.

Using both MRA and conventional angiograms, vertebral artery disease was noted in 67% and PICA disease was noted in 10% of 123 patients. The high prevalence of

Table 5 Frequency of symptoms in 130 consecutive lateral medullary infarcts without cerebellar involvement	
Symptom	**No. of Patients (%)**
Sensory symptoms and signs	125 (96)
Gait ataxia	120 (92)[a]
Horner sign	114 (88)
Dysphagia	84 (65)[b]
Dysarthria	28 (22)[b]
Vertigo	74 (57)
Nystagmus	73 (56)
Limb ataxia	72 (55)
Nausea and vomiting	67 (52)
Headache	67 (52)[a]
Skew deviation of eyes	53 (41)
Diplopia	41 (32)
Hiccoughs	33 (25)
Facial palsy	27 (21)[b]

[a] More common or severe in caudal group.
[b] More common or severe in rostral group.
Data from Kim JS. Pure lateral medullary infarction: clinical-radiological correlation of 130 acute, consecutive patients. Brain 2003;126:1864–72.

vertebral artery disease in lateral medullary infarct had been reported in histopathological postmortem studies as well.[61] In Kim's study,[60] the cause of infarct was large vessel infarction in 50%, arterial dissection in 15%, small vessel infarction in 13%, and cardiac embolism in 5%. Caudal lesions were more likely secondary to dissection. In addition, isolated PICA pathology without vertebral artery pathology was more often secondary to cardioembolism.

While the majority of lateral medullary stroke patients exhibited other neurologic deficits localizing to the brainstem, there are case reports of lateral medullary infarctions which presented with only vertigo and gait ataxia, without limb ataxia on examination. In all 3 cases, there was strong lateropulsion (a prominent motor disturbance that causes a deviation toward the side of the lesion) toward the ipsilateral side, causing an inability to walk.[62] Clinicians may mistakenly diagnose this presentation as an inner ear disorder, as the lesion may be small and missed on MRI. A key clinical difference is that the very strong lateropulsion noted in lateral medullary strokes is of such severity that walking may be severely impaired or not possible,[63] whereas patients with peripheral vestibular lesions may fall or veer toward the lesioned side but are usually able to walk. Patients with lateral medullary stroke may also have a concomitant skew deviation or an ocular tilt with ipsilateral head tilt, skew deviation with the ipsilateral eye lower than the contralateral eye, and ocular torsion with the upper pole of the eye rotated toward the side of the lesion.[64]

Superior Cerebellar Artery Infarcts are Mainly Embolic

The dominant features of SCA infarcts are ipsilateral limb ataxia, vertigo, nystagmus, and cerebellar signs including dysarthria and gait ataxia. In a recent study, 60 patients with SCA infarcts demonstrated that embolism was the predominant stroke mechanism with artery to artery embolism from atherosclerotic vertebrobasilar artery disease in 20 of 60 patients (33%). Fourteen patients had a cardioembolic source (23%), and 10 patients had multiple lesions in SCA and other vertebrobasilar territories.[65] Previous studies had also demonstrated the predominance of cardiac embolism as a source in SCA infarcts, with one study reporting 12 out of 30[66] and another reporting 11 out of 30.[67]

Basilar Migraine and Migraine-Associated Vertebrobasilar Strokes

In 1961, Bickerstaff[68] described a variant of migraine that exhibited symptoms that localized to the posterior circulation. In describing the alteration of consciousness that occurs in basilar migraine, Bickerstaff noted that it was "curiously slow in onset" and that patients seemed to be in a deep sleep. It has been proposed that this occurs secondary to dysfunction of the brainstem tegmentum. Symptoms can include the following:

- Visual symptoms in both temporal and nasal fields of both eyes
- Dysarthria
- Vertigo
- Tinnitus
- Decreased hearing
- Diplopia
- Ataxia
- Bilateral paresthesias
- Bilateral pareses
- Decreased level of consciousness.

Olsson[69] conducted a prospective study of 50 patients with basilar migraine and documented low-frequency sensorineural hearing loss in more than half of these.

Cutrer and Baloh[70] described spells of migraine-associated vertigo and reported 30% of subjects having spells that last a few minutes to 2 hours, with 49% having spells lasting longer than 24 hours. It is evident that the symptoms in basilar migraine are similar to those of vertebrobasilar insufficiency. Furthermore, while the original report described young adolescent girls with basilar migraine, there is much evidence that basilar migraine can occur in the middle-aged or elderly. The role of vasoconstriction and microvascular ischemia in migraine and migrainous aura is complex. Migraineurs are reported to be sensitive to angiography, which can precipitate a migrainous attack. Migrainous aura may sometimes become permanent, and on evaluation it may be recognized that a stroke has occurred. The International Headache Society criteria for migrainous cerebral infarction are that: the patient exhibit one or more migrainous aura symptoms not fully reversible within 7 days and/or neuroimaging confirmation of ischemic infarction, and the present attack is typical of prior attacks, but neurologic deficits are not reversible within 7 days, and/or neuroimaging shows an infarct in the relevant area in a patient that meets criteria for migraine with neurologic aura.[71]

To complicate matters for determining etiology, there are many disorders associated with strokes and migraine headaches, including antiphospholipid syndrome, MELAS (mitochondrial myopathy, encephalopathy, lactic acidosis, and stroke) and CADACIL (cerebral autosomal dominant arteriopathy with subcortical infarcts and leukoencephalopathy). There is likely a predominance of vertebrobasilar strokes associated with migrainous stroke. Bogousslavsky and colleagues[72] reported 9 PCA infarcts and 2 brainstem and cerebellar strokes among 22 migrainous strokes.

Migraine with aura appears to be associated with a higher frequency of infarcts than those with common migraine. For these reasons, the use of tryptans is considered contraindicated in cases of basilar migraine. In the case of migraine with transient unilateral hearing loss and tinnitus, the authors recommend the use of verapamil as the first-line agent, and agree that tryptans would be relatively contraindicated.[73] In a large study of 18,725 subjects (9044 men and 968 women) based in Iceland with a median follow-up period of 25.9 years, current, active migraine with aura was associated with an increased risk for cardiovascular disease mortality (hazard ratio 1.27), and greater risk of mortality from stroke (hazard ratio 1.40). There was no increased risk for persons with migraine without aura or nonmigraine headache.[74] It is noted that the added risk is low compared with conventional modifiable risk factors including smoking, hyperlipidemia, and hypertension. Another study using data from the Women's Health Study, which included 27,860 women 45 years or older followed for a mean of 13.6 years, noted an association between women with active migraine with aura having twice the risk for hemorrhagic stroke (hazard ratio 2.25).[75] Further studies are needed to evaluate whether this finding is related to medication treatment for the migrainous aura or other comorbidity.

REFERENCES

1. Boyajian RA, Schwend RB, Wolfe MM, et al. Measurement of anterior and posterior circulation flow contributions to cerebral blood flow contributions to cerebral blood flow. An ultrasound-derived volumetric flow analysis. J Neuroimaging 1995; 5:1–3.
2. Cloud GC, Markus HS. Diagnosis and management of vertebral artery stenosis. QJM 2003;96:27–54.
3. Stopford JS. The arteries of the pons and medulla oblongata. J Anat Physiol 1916;50:130–64.

4. Margolis MT, Newton TH. The posterior inferior cerebellar artery. In: Newton TH, Potts DG, editors. Radiology of the skull and brain, vol. 2. St Louis (MO): CV Mosby; 1974. p.1710–74.

5. Matsushita K, Naritomi H, Kazui S, et al. Infarction in the anterior inferior cerebellar artery territory: magnetic resonance imaging and auditory brain stem responses. Cerebrovasc Dis 1993;3:206–12.

6. Lee H, Sohn SI, Jung DK, et al. Sudden deafness and anterior inferior cerebellar artery infarction. Stroke 2002;33(12):2807–12.

7. Stevens RB, Stillwell DL. Arteries and veins of the human brain. Springfield (IL): CC Thomas; 1969.

8. Nakashima T, Naganawa S, Sone M, et al. Disorders of cochlear blood flow. Brain Res Rev 2003;43:17–28.

9. Konishi T, Butler RA, Fernandez C. Effect of anoxia on cochlear potentials. J Acoust Soc Am 1961;33:349–55.

10. Johnsson LF, Hawkins JE. Vascular changes in the human ear associated with aging. Ann Otol Rhinol Laryngol 1972;81:364–76.

11. Wright CG, Schuknecht HF. Atrophy of the spiral ligament. Arch Otolaryngol 1972;96:16–21.

12. Ishiyama G, Tokita J, Lopez I, et al. Unbiased stereological estimation of the spiral ligament and stria vascularis volumes in aging and Ménière's disease using archival human temporal bones. J Assoc Res Otolaryngol 2007;8(1):8–17.

13. Lyon MF, Wanamaker HH. Blood flow and assessment of capillaries in the aging rat posterior canal crista. Hear Res 1993;67(1–2):157–65.

14. Kim JS, Lee H. Inner ear dysfunction due to vertebrobasilar ischemic stroke. Semin Neurol 2009;29:534–40.

15. Kim JS, Lopez I, Diparte PL, et al. Internal auditory artery infarction: clinicopathologic correlation. Neurology 1999;52:40–4.

16. Keilson GR, Schwartz WJ, Recht LD. The preponderance of posterior circulation circulatory events is independent of the route of cardiac catheterization. Stroke 1992;23:1358–9.

17. Wityk RJ, Caplan LR. Vertebrobasilar occlusive disease. In: Carter LD, Spetzler RF, editors. Neurovascular Surgery. New York (NY): McGraw-Hill; 1995. p. 359–82.

18. Schievink WI, Michels W, Piepgras DG. Neurovascular complications of heritable connective tissue disorders. Stroke 1994;25:889–903.

19. Caplan LR, Wityk RJ, Glass TA, et al. New England Medical Center Posterior Circulation Registry. Ann Neurol 2004;56:389–98.

20. Williams D, Wilson TG. The diagnosis of the major and minor syndromes of basilar insufficiency. Brain 1962;85:741–74.

21. Purroy F, Montaner J, Molina CA, et al. Patterns and predictors of early risk of recurrence after transient ischemic attack with respect to etiologic subtypes. Stroke 2007;38:3225–9.

22. Marquardt L, Kuker W, Chandratheva A, et al. Incidence and prognosis of ≥50% symptomatic vertebral or basilar artery stenosis: prospective population-based study. Brain 2009;132:982–8.

23. Flossmann E, Touze E, Giles MF, et al. The early risk of stroke after vertebrobasilar TIA is higher than after carotid TIA [abstract]. Cerebrovasc Dis 2006; 219(Suppl 4):6.

24. Khan S, Cloud G, Kerry S, et al. Imaging of vertebral artery stenosis: a systematic review. J Neurol Neurosurg Psychiatry 2007;78:1218–25.

25. Gulli G, Khan S, Markus HS. Vertebrobasilar stenosis predicts high early recurrent stroke risk in posterior circulation stroke and TIA. Stroke 2009;40:2732–7.
26. Kamper L, Rybacki K, Mansour M, et al. Time management in acute vertebrobasilar occlusion. Cardiovasc Intervent Radiol 2009;32:226–32.
27. Zavala-Alarcon E, Emmans L, Little R, et al. Percutaneous intervention for posterior fossa ischemia. A single center experience and review of the literature. Int J Cardiol 2008;127(1):70–7.
28. Ogilvy CS, Yang X, Natarajan SK, et al. Restenosis rates following vertebral artery origin stenting: does stent type make a difference? J Invasive Cardiol 2010;22(3): 119–24.
29. Tinetti ME, Williams CS, Gill TM. Dizziness among older adults: a possible geriatric syndrome. Ann Intern Med 2000;132(5):337–44.
30. Katsarkas A. Dizziness in aging: a retrospective study of 1194 cases. Otolaryngol Head Neck Surg 1994;110:296–301.
31. Baloh RW, Honrubia V, Jacobson K. Benign positional vertigo—clinical and oculographic features in 240 cases. Neurology 1987;37:371–8.
32. Lalwani AK. Vertigo, disequilibrium, and imbalance with aging. In: Jackler RK, Brackmann DE, editors. Neurotology. 2nd edition. St Louis (MO): Mosby-Year Book Inc; 2005. p. 533–9.
33. Kerber KA, Meurer WJ, West BT, et al. Dizziness presentations in U.S. emergency departments, 1995–2004. Acad Emerg Med 2008;15:744–50.
34. Grad A, Baloh RW. Vertigo of vascular origin: clinical and ENG features in 84 cases. Arch Neurol 1989;46:281–4.
35. Ishiyama G, Ishiyama A, Jacobson K, et al. Drop attacks in older patients secondary to an otologic cause. Neurology 2001;57:1103–6.
36. Kremer M. Sitting, standing and walking. Br Med J 1958;2:63–8.
37. Caplan LR. Posterior circulation disease: clinical findings, diagnosis and management. Cambridge (MA): Blackwell Science; 1996. Chapter 7.
38. Tan T-Y, Kuo Y-L, Lin W-C, et al. Effect of lipid-lowering therapy on the progression of intracranial arterial stenosis. J Neurol 2009;256:187–93.
39. Akins PT, Pilgrim TK, Cross DT III, et al. Natural history of stenosis from intracranial atherosclerosis by serial angiography. Stroke 1998;29:433–8.
40. Mazighi M, Tanasescu R, Ducrocq X, et al. Prospective study of symptomatic atherothrombotic intracranial stenoses: the GESICA study. Neurology 2006;66:1187–91.
41. Milionis HJ, Giannopoulos S, Kosmidou M, et al. Statin therapy after first stroke reduces 10-year stroke recurrence and improves survival. Neurology 2009;72: 1816–22.
42. Goldstein LB, Adams R, Alberts MJ, et al. Primary prevention of ischemic stroke: a guideline from the American Heart Association/American Stroke Association Stroke Council: cosponsored by the atherosclerotic Peripheral Vascular Disease Interdisciplinary Working Group; Cardiovascular Nursing Council; Clinical Cardiology Council; Nutrition, Physical Activity, and Metabolism Council; and the Quality of Care and Outcomes Research Interdisciplinary Working Group: the American Academy of Neurology affirms the value of this guideline. Stroke 2006;37:1583–633.
43. Von Brevern M, Radtke A, Lezius F, et al. Epidemiology of benign paroxysmal positional vertigo: a population-based study. J Neurol Neurosurg Psychiatry 2007;78:710–5.
44. Ishiyama A, Jacobson KM, Baloh RW. Migraine and benign positional vertigo. Ann Otol Rhinol Laryngol 2000;109:377–80.

45. Flossmann E, Rothwell PM. Prognosis of vertebrobasilar transient ischemic attack and minor stroke. Brain 2003;126:1940–54.
46. Calvet D, Touze E, Oppenheim C, et al. DWI lesions and TIA etiology improve the prediction of stroke after TIA. Stroke 2009;40:187–92.
47. Cloud GC, Crawley F, Clifton A, et al. Vertebral artery origin angioplasty and primary stenting: safety and restenosis rates in a prospective series. J Neurol Neurosurg Psychiatry 2003;74:586–90.
48. Hatano T, Tsukahara T, Ogino E, et al. Stenting for vertebrobasilar artery stenosis. Acta Neurochir Suppl 2005;94:137–41.
49. Oas JG, Baloh RW. Vertigo and the anterior inferior cerebellar artery syndrome. Neurology 1992;42:2274–9.
50. Hinojosa R, Kohut RI. Clinical diagnosis of anterior inferior cerebellar artery thrombosis: autopsy and temporal bone histopathology study. Ann Otol Rhinol Laryngol 1990;99:261–71.
51. Lee H, Kim JS, Chung E-J, et al. Infarction in the territory of anterior inferior cerebellar artery: spectrum of audiovestibular loss. Stroke 2009;40:3745–51.
52. Kimura R, Perlman HB. Arterial obstruction of the labyrinth. Part I. Cochlear changes. Ann Otol Rhinol Laryngol 1958;67:5–24.
53. Mazzoni A. Internal auditory artery supply to the petrous bone. Ann Otol Rhinol Laryngol 1972;81:13–21.
54. Caplan LR. Intracranial branch atheromatous disease. Neurology 1989;39: 1246–50.
55. Kumral E, Kisabay A, Atac C. Lesion patterns and etiology of ischemia in the anterior inferior cerebellar artery territory involvement: a clinical-diffusion weighted-MRI study. Eur J Neurol 2006;13(4):395–401.
56. Adams RD. Occlusion of the anterior inferior cerebellar artery. Arch Neurol Psychiatry 1943;49:765–70.
57. Schwartz A, Rauenberg W, Hennerici M. Dolichoectatic intracranial arteries: review of selected aspects. Cerebrovasc Dis 1993;3:273–9.
58. Smoker WR, Corbett JL, Gentry LR, et al. High resolution computed tomography of the basilar artery: vertebrobasilar dolichoectasia: clinical-pathologic correlation and review. AJNR Am J Neuroradiol 1986;7:61–72.
59. Kim JS, Lee JH, Suh DC, et al. Spectrum of lateral medullary syndrome: correlation between clinical findings and magnetic resonance imaging in 33 subjects. Stroke 1994;25(7):1405–10.
60. Kim JS. Pure lateral medullary infarction: clinical-radiological correlation of 130 acute, consecutive patients. Brain 2003;126:1864–72.
61. Fisher CM, Karnes WE, Kubik CS. Lateral medullary infarction: the pattern of vascular occlusion. J Neuropathol Exp Neurol 1961;20:323–79.
62. Kim JS. Vertigo and gait ataxia without usual signs of lateral medullary infarction: a clinical variant related to rostral-dorsolateral lesions. Cerebrovasc Dis 2000;10: 471–4.
63. Bjerner K, Silfverskold BP. Lateropulsion and imbalance in Wallenberg's syndrome. Acta Neurol Scand 1968;44:91–100.
64. Brandt T, Dieterich M. Skew deviation with ocular torsion: a vestibular brainstem sign of topographic diagnostic value. Ann Neurol 1993;33:528–34.
65. Kumral E, Kisabay A, Atac C. Lesion patterns and etiology of ischemia in superior cerebellar artery territory infarcts. Cerebrovasc Dis 2005;19(5):283–90.
66. Amarenco P, Levy C, Cohen A. Causes and mechanisms of territorial and non-territorial cerebellar infarcts in 115 consecutive patients. Stroke 1994;25:105–12.

67. Kase C, Norrving B, Levine S. Cerebellar infarction: clinical and anatomic observations in 66 cases. Stroke 1993;24:76–83.
68. Bickerstaff ER. Basilar artery migraine. Lancet 1961;1:15–7.
69. Olsson JE. Neurotologic findings in basilar migraine. Laryngoscope 1991;101:1–41.
70. Cutrer FM, Baloh RW. Migraine associated dizziness. Headache 1992;32:300–4.
71. International Headache Society classification and diagnostic criteria for headache disorders, cranial neuralgias, and facial pain. Cephalalgia 1988;8:27.
72. Bogousslavsky J, Regli F, Van Melle G. Migraine stroke. Neurology 1988;38:223–7.
73. Evans RW, Ishiyama G. Migraine with transient unilateral hearing loss and tinnitus. Headache 2009;49(5):756–8.
74. Gudmundsson LS, Scher AI, Aspelund T, et al. Migraine with aura and risk of cardiovascular and all cause mortality in men and women: prospective cohort study. BMJ 2010;341:c3966.
75. Kurth T, Kase CS, Schurks M, et al. Migraine and risk of haemorrhagic stroke in women: prospective cohort study. BMJ 2010;341:c3659.

Dizziness in the Elderly

Kamran Barin, PhD[a],*, Edward E. Dodson, MD[b]

KEYWORDS

- Disequilibrium of aging • Age-related dizziness
- Vestibular disorders • Falls in older adults

D.P. is an 82-year-old woman describing gradual onset of lightheadedness and imbalance over the past 2 to 3 years. She denies antecedent illness or injury, and states that these symptoms have been noticeably worse in the last 6 months. She reports one full-fall 2 months ago after getting out of her daughter's car in the grocery store parking lot and hitting her head, resulting in a laceration on her forehead requiring stitches. She states that she felt somewhat woozy on getting out of the car, tried to grab the car door but missed, and was unable to prevent her fall. She denies loss of consciousness, and afterward reported position-dependent vertigo, which was later diagnosed as benign paroxysmal positional vertigo. This condition was successfully treated by a local otolaryngologist. She reports near-falls daily, and finds that she steadies herself by holding onto walls and furniture while walking around her house. She expresses appropriate concern for falls and fall-related injury, and is worried about maintaining her independence, as she currently lives alone and has a daughter living nearby who assists her. She reports that her medical history is significant for hypertension, congestive heart failure, 2 "mini strokes," rheumatoid arthritis (affecting her knees, hips, and hands), incontinence, osteoporosis, and bilateral cataracts (scheduled for surgery next month). She indicates long-standing bilateral hearing loss, and denies changes in her hearing with the onset of her balance symptoms.

DIZZINESS IN THE ELDERLY

Dizziness is a broad term used to describe a variety of sensations such as vertigo, unsteadiness, lightheadedness, and similar symptoms. The prevalence of dizziness increases steadily with age.[1,2] Although debate is still ongoing about the underlying causes of this increase in prevalence, there is universal agreement on its devastating

[a] Balance Disorders Clinic, Department of Otolaryngology-Head & Neck Surgery, The Ohio State University Medical Center, 915 Olentangy River Road, Suite 4000, Columbus, OH 43212, USA
[b] Division of Otology, Neurotology, and Cranial Base Surgery, Department of Otolaryngology-Head & Neck Surgery, The Ohio State University Medical Center, 915 Olentangy River Road, Suite 4000, Columbus, OH, USA
* Corresponding author.
E-mail address: barin.1@osu.edu

Otolaryngol Clin N Am 44 (2011) 437–454
doi:10.1016/j.otc.2011.01.013
0030-6665/11/$ – see front matter © 2011 Elsevier Inc. All rights reserved.

oto.theclinics.com

consequences and high physical, emotional, and financial toll on the older population.[3–5]

It is estimated that about one-fourth to one-third of the population older than 65 years has experienced some form of dizziness.[6,7] The prevalence varies among different studies because of several factors such as the differences in the cutoff age of the participants, the type of symptoms for inclusion in the study, the duration and frequency of symptoms, and whether the sample was taken from community-dwelling seniors, primary care facilities, or from specialty clinics. For those older than 85, the number of adults with dizziness increases to about 50%.[1] Furthermore, the prevalence of these symptoms is greater for women.[8,9]

Older individuals who suffer from dizziness appear to be at significantly higher risk of accidental falls and consequent injuries.[10,11] It is estimated that about 30% of adults older than 65 will fall at least once per year, and about 50% of those will fall again.[12,13] The consequences of such falls are devastating. Falls are the leading cause of accidental death in persons older than 65 years, and are the number one reason for hospital admission for nonfatal falls in this population.[4,5] Fall-related injuries can lead to mobility restrictions, loss of independence, and even confinement to nursing facilities.[3,14] In addition to the physical and emotional costs, these injuries also carry a heavy financial burden, estimated at more than $19 billion in direct costs in year 2000 and rising steadily since.[15,16]

Several studies have established that older adults with a history of dizziness, imbalance, and similar symptoms are at a higher risk of falling.[10,11,17] However, the association between the two has not been as strong in other studies,[18,19] which is not surprising given that falls are complex phenomena involving neurological, biomechanical, and other factors. Therefore, fall risk factors can be greatly influenced by the study design and patient selection methods. In 2006, Rubenstein and Josephson[20] used a meta-analysis of 12 large studies, and determined balance disorders and dizziness as the second and third leading cause of falls in older persons, respectively. Vertigo, unsteadiness, and related symptoms also have an indirect effect on falls; it is well established that these symptoms in older individuals lead to fear of falling.[21–23] In turn, fear of falls is considered a strong predictor for those who will suffer one or more subsequent falls.[24,25]

The general topic of falls is too broad and is beyond the scope of this article. However, the strong association between falls and symptoms of dizziness and imbalance highlights the importance of understanding the causes of these symptoms and designing effective methods for managing them in the older population.

CAUSES OF DIZZINESS AND DISEQUILIBRIUM IN OLDER INDIVIDUALS

Although the causes of balance problems in the elderly are seemingly obvious, the substantial body of research in the past 2 or 3 decades suggests that the underlying reasons are far from simple or obvious. In some studies, no specific etiology could be identified to explain the symptoms of a large subset of the subjects.[26] The term *presbystasis* is used to describe this type of age-related disequilibrium that cannot be attributed to any known pathology.[26] On the other hand, other studies have been able to assign one or more diagnostic categories to the majority of the elderly patients suffering from dizziness.[27–29] These discrepancies have led some investigators to suggest that dizziness in the elderly should be viewed as a multifactorial geriatric syndrome involving many different symptoms and originating from many different sensory, neurologic, cardiovascular, and other systems.[6]

The underlying causes of dizziness and disequilibrium in older adults can be divided into 3 broad categories:

1. Age-related decline of acuity in the sensory and motor pathways as well as deterioration of integration mechanisms within the central nervous system. Loss of hair cells in the labyrinth is an example of such an age-related change in the sensory systems. These types of losses are considered a normal part of aging because they are so common in older adults. However, they are most likely caused by subtle pathologies, such as ischemia, that are highly prevalent in the elderly.
2. Pathologies that cause dizziness in any age group but become more prevalent in older individuals, either because the age-related changes noted above make the elderly more susceptible to these pathologies or because the cumulative probability of exposure to these pathologies increases with time. An example of such pathology is benign paroxysmal positional vertigo (BPPV), which can occur at any age but is far more common in the elderly because of the ongoing deterioration of the maculae of the otolith organs.
3. An assortment of environmental and lifestyle factors that increase the chance of dizziness and balance problems in the elderly. One such example is increased use of medications in the elderly, with many of the medications having the common side effect of dizziness (see article by Shoair and colleagues in this publication).

A different type of classification is often used to divide the risk factors for falls.[30] This classification involves causes that are intrinsic to the patients versus those that are extrinsic. For dizziness and balance problems, such a classification is more relevant when considering appropriate intervention methods, discussed later in this article. Here, each of the aforementioned 3 categories are discussed in detail.

AGE-RELATED DETERIORATION OF SENSORY AND MOTOR MECHANISMS

Human balance function depends on sensory inputs from the vestibular, proprioceptive, and visual systems as well as proper integration of those inputs in the central nervous system (CNS). Furthermore, control of movements requires the motor centers to accurately process the sensory information and transmit the necessary commands to the appropriate muscles. Both structural and functional deteriorations in all of these systems have been reported with increasing age.

Vestibular System

Age-related loss of hair cells has been documented within the cristae ampullares of the semicircular canals and the maculae of the saccule and utricle.[31,32] Earlier studies had indicated greater loss of hair cells in the semicircular canals and saccules, and a higher proportion of loss for type I versus type II hair cells.[33] More recent studies have used a counting method that is deemed to be less biased. These studies have confirmed age-related loss of hair cells in the labyrinth, but the affected sites and types of hair cells have differed somewhat from previous studies.[34]

Structural integrity of the vestibular nerve is also affected by age. The number of primary vestibular neurons within Scarpa's ganglion has been shown to decline by approximately 25% over one's life span.[35,36] Similarly, the study of brainstem specimens in different age groups has demonstrated a decrease in the number of secondary vestibular neurons within the vestibular nuclei.[37]

Age-related degeneration of peripheral and central vestibular structures is similar to that of the auditory system, and is most likely caused by subtle changes of blood flow to the inner ear.[37] Microvascular changes with aging have been reported in both human and animal studies.[38–40] Any decrease in blood flow can have profound effects because inner ear arteries lack anastomotic connections.

Age-related changes of the vestibular structures have been confirmed by vestibular function tests. For example, both longitudinal and cross-sectional studies have shown decrease in vestibulo-ocular reflex (VOR) gain during sinusoidal rotations.[41,42] This finding indicates that unlike pathologies that usually affect only one labyrinth, age-related changes of the vestibular pathways are more likely to mimic bilateral reduction of function. In addition, increase in the low-frequency phase for sinusoidal stimuli and decrease in the time constant for step velocity stimuli have been reported in older subjects.[43] These findings are consistent with deterioration of the velocity storage mechanism within the brainstem. A similar degradation of central vestibular pathways has been demonstrated for otolith-ocular responses during off-vertical axis rotations.[44]

Despite overwhelming evidence in support of age-related changes of peripheral and central vestibular structures, the relationship between those changes and complaints of dizziness and disequilibrium in the elderly is still uncertain. Several studies have demonstrated high prevalence of vestibular impairments in elderly individuals.[45,46] However, once patients with specific vestibular pathologies are removed from the sample, the contribution of age-related vestibular decline to balance impairment in the elderly is not as profound.[18,43] It is clear that additional studies are needed to examine the association of age-related changes in the vestibular pathways with symptoms of dizziness and disequilibrium in older adults.

Proprioceptive System

The proprioceptive sensors residing in muscles, joints, and tendons provide information regarding orientation of one body segment with respect to the others. Compared with the vestibular and visual inputs, these sensors have lower thresholds for motion detection and operate at significantly higher frequencies.[47,48] These sensors provide critical information regarding the point of contact with the ground, which can be extrapolated to detect orientation and movement of the body. Proprioceptive cues from the neck also play an important role in detecting head orientation and in providing a stable platform for the vestibular and visual receptors.

The proprioceptive system undergoes several age-related changes. Vibration and touch thresholds decline in older individuals, adversely affecting tactile information arising from the feet at their contact point with the ground.[49] Similarly, the ability to detect the position and direction of joint movements declines with age.[50]

Several studies have demonstrated a decrease in postural stability when proprioceptive input is altered in such a way that it provides inaccurate information regarding orientation.[51] Horak and colleagues[52] compared the performance of patients with severe neuropathy with age-matched controls, and demonstrated that the performance of control subjects became similar to that of patients with neuropathy for test conditions in which proprioceptive input was altered. Therefore, it is not surprising that reduction of vibration and tactile sensation at the ankle and knee joints has been associated with increased risk of falls in the elderly.[53]

The role of neck proprioception on postural control has been studied using vibration of neck muscles.[54–56] Prolonged unilateral vibration of neck muscles during in-place stepping caused subjects to rotate about a vertical axis away from the side of vibration.[54] Using a similar type of neck vibration during locomotion, Deshpande and Patla[55] demonstrated reduced sensitivity of neck proprioception in older adults. This observation is an important one because as noted before, age-related decline of the vestibular system usually involves bilateral reduction of function. In younger patients who suffer from bilateral vestibular loss, the neck receptors play an important role as substitutes for the vestibular system.[57] This mode of compensation may not be available in the elderly because of the reduced neck proprioception.

Visual System

The visual system undergoes significant age-related changes. In addition to visual acuity, several other visual functions such as depth perception, accommodation, contrast sensitivity, and dark adaptation decline with age.[58] Depth perception and contrast sensitivity have been shown to be the most important visual impairments that contribute to falls.[59] These impairments affect the ability of older adults to accurately judge distances and to avoid obstacles.

Age-related changes in static visual acuity as measured with stationary subjects and stationary targets have been studied extensively.[58,60] The association between reduced static visual acuity and balance problems in the elderly is still in dispute.[59] Deterioration of dynamic visual acuity, in which either the target or the subject is moving, has also been documented in older individuals.[61] Of interest, patients with acute unilateral and bilateral vestibular lesions also exhibit impaired dynamic visual acuity and complain of blurred vision during head movements.[62] The coexistence of this impairment in the elderly and in patients with known balance disorders may explain some of the symptoms in older adults.

It has been shown that reliance on visual input increases with age.[63] For example, when subjects were exposed to moving visual surrounds, older subjects were affected more and produced greater postural sway.[64] While both older and younger subjects were able to adapt to moving visual stimuli, this adaptation required significantly more time for older individuals.[65] In addition, postural sway of older subjects who were presented with spatially inaccurate visual stimuli was significantly greater than the sway response of younger subjects.[51]

Motor System

Sensory information regarding orientation and movement of the body is processed by the motor centers, and appropriate commands are transmitted to a select group of skeletal muscles to preserve balance and maintain upright postural stability. The most notable effect of aging on the motor system relates to changes in the characteristics of muscle.[66] Muscle strength has been shown to be 20% to 40% lower in the 70- to 80-year-old age group compared with that of young adults. This reduction in muscle strength is related to decreases in the number and size of muscle fibers as well as changes in the central motor command centers.[67] Similarly, the speed by which the muscles can be contracted declines with age.[68] These and other similar age-related changes in skeletal muscles may prevent older individuals from exerting adequate force and reacting quickly to postural disturbances.[69]

Similar changes occur in the eye muscles, which can lead to age-related decline of oculomotor function. Fast eye movements or saccades are only modestly affected by aging. Saccade latency has been shown to increase with age, but other saccade parameters such as peak velocity or accuracy are not significantly affected.[42] The gain of slow tracking eye movements or smooth pursuit also declines substantially with age, especially for higher velocity target movements.[70] The ability to suppress vestibular nystagmus by fixation accordingly declines, as the tracking and fixation mechanisms share many neural pathways.[42] Finally, the gain of reflexive optokinetic responses is also reduced in older individuals, mainly for high-velocity surround movements.[42]

Although changes of the eye muscles may have an effect on the decline of oculo-motor responses, aging of central structures (discussed in the next section) appears to have a substantially greater role in age-related control of eye movements.[42] These changes have profound effects on the perception of orientation and balance, because they influence the sensory input from the visual system.

Central Integration Mechanisms

The brainstem, cerebellum, and higher cortical structures within the CNS all undergo age-related degenerative changes. These include decrease in the number of neurons, loss of myelination, decrease in the number of Purkinje cells, and other neuronal changes.[71] Age-related degeneration of central structures is likely to affect integration of information from different sensory mechanisms and to interfere with accurate perception of orientation and motion.

A few examples of impaired sensory integration have been mentioned previously. Over-reliance on the visual system, even when it is providing erroneous spatial information, is an example of how prioritization of inputs from different sensory mechanisms can be affected in older individuals.[51,63] Another example is the faulty integration of optokinetic and vestibular inputs that can lead to deterioration of dynamic visual acuity.[61] **Fig. 1** illustrates that subtle age-related reduction in both the VOR and optokinetic gains can result in an image not remaining stationary on the retina, thereby causing blurred vision during head movements. This type of deterioration in visual-vestibular interaction has been documented in older individuals.[42]

One manifestation of impaired sensory integration in the elderly is related to the time required for adaptation following changes to the balance control mechanisms. For example, when proprioceptive input was modulated by vibration of different muscles in the lower leg, there were no significant age-related differences in lower-level reflexes.[72] However, older individuals failed to adapt to the reintroduction of accurate proprioceptive cues as quickly as did younger subjects. Similar age-related differences in adaptation time were noted previously when subjects were exposed to moving visual stimuli.[65] These observations have profound and troubling implications for older individuals with regard to recovery and compensation after diseases that involve the balance system.

Pathologic Causes of Dizziness

Although age-related changes in the sensory and motor systems do play a role in the high prevalence of dizziness among the elderly, they are no longer considered the most prominent contributors. In contrast to earlier research, most of the studies in the past two decades have been able to identify one or more specific pathologies as the underlying cause of symptoms.[26,29,45,73] None of these pathologies was unique to the elderly. That is, the same diseases are responsible for causing dizziness in both younger and older individuals.[29] These pathologies become more prevalent in older individuals either because the age-related changes already noted make the elderly more susceptible to them or because the cumulative probability of exposure to them increases with time.

In a recent study of elderly patients seen in primary care settings, the major cause of dizziness in more than 80% of the patients was ascribed to 1 of 3 categories[73]:

1. Cardiovascular (including cerebrovascular)
2. Peripheral vestibular
3. Psychiatric diseases.

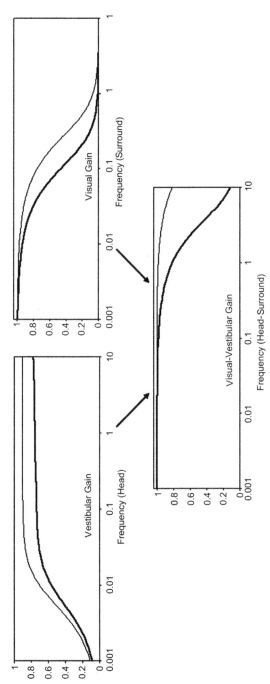

Fig. 1. Vestibular gain defined as the ratio of slow-phase eye velocity to head velocity, visual (optokinetic) gain defined as the ratio of eye velocity to surround velocity, and visual-vestibular interaction gain defined as the ratio of eye velocity to combined head-visual surround velocity for younger (*thin line*) and older (*thick line*) adults. Both the vestibular and visual gains for older individuals represent a subtle decline caused by age-related changes. When the visual-vestibular interaction gain is significantly less than 1, the images will not remain stationary on the retina and will appear blurry. The data are theoretical and do not represent the exact responses. (*Data from* AudiologyOnline presentation by Zapala (2010). Available at: http://www.audiologyonline.com/ceus/recordedcoursedetails.asp?class_id516469.)

In 8% of patients no clear cause was identified, and "all other causes" were attributed to 11% of the patients. Two or more contributing causes were identified in 70% of the patients. Adverse medication effects were the leading secondary cause. The results of this study were similar to those of previous studies with respect to the disease categories, but the prevalence of peripheral vestibular diseases was significantly lower than for other studies. This study was based on the patient population seen in primary care facilities, and did not include formal assessment of vestibular function.[29,45]

Dizziness is one of the primary symptoms in more than 60 diseases.[74] All of them should be considered in the differential diagnosis of older dizzy patients; however, the prevalence of some of the diseases is far greater in the elderly.

Among the peripheral vestibular disorders, BPPV is by far the most common finding. In one study, almost 40% of patients older than 70 years were diagnosed with BPPV.[29] In some cases, BPPV was secondary to other diseases such as a previous peripheral vestibular disorder or diabetes. Late-onset Ménière's disease, vestibular neuritis, and other otologic diseases do occur in the elderly but they are not as common. The authors' own clinical experience suggests that some older patients who present with a sudden onset of symptoms are experiencing decompensation rather than a new vestibular lesion. These patients usually have a history of long-standing previously compensated peripheral vestibular disease.

Among the non-vestibular causes of dizziness, cardiovascular and cerebrovascular diseases are common in the elderly.[73] Atherosclerotic narrowing of the blood vessels can lead to ischemic events and produce symptoms similar to either peripheral vestibular or central lesions, depending on the affected sites.[71] Vertebrobasilar insufficiency (VBI), which is a common cause of dizziness in the elderly, is an example of this type of disorder[75] (see article by Ishiyama and Ishiyama in this publication). Other diseases in this category include those that reduce cardiac output such as arrhythmia, heart valve failure, and congestive heart failure.

Some neurologic disorders such as Parkinson disease are also more prevalent in the elderly, but are not considered a major cause of isolated dizziness. Similarly, metabolic and endocrine disorders can cause dizziness with about the same frequency in younger and older adults.

Finally, the impact of psychiatric disorders, including cognitive impairments, should be considered in the elderly. Sloane and colleagues[76] compared the prevalence and characteristics of psychiatric diseases between older patients having chronic dizziness with age-matched and sex-matched controls. More than 37% in the chronic dizziness group had a psychiatric diagnosis. Although psychiatric diseases rarely were considered the primary cause of dizziness, they were common as a contributing factor to dizziness in the elderly. In this study, anxiety and depression were the most common findings, similar to results from other studies that have examined psychogenic aspects of chronic dizziness in patients of all age groups.[77] One psychogenic factor that is specific to the elderly is increased fear of falls. It has been shown that fear of falling is an important risk factor for actual falls.[24,25]

Environmental and Lifestyle Causes of Dizziness

In addition to age-related changes and pathological factors that affect balance mechanisms, several lifestyle and environmental factors can contribute to disorientation and sense of imbalance. The most prominent of these factors is the adverse effects of medications. Several studies have linked use of CNS-acting medications to increased risk of falls in the elderly.[78] Furthermore, adverse medication effects have been considered the leading secondary cause of dizziness.[73] Benzodiazepines, antidepressants, and anticonvulsants have been the most commonly implicated classes of medication.[79] However, there is considerable debate about the methodological efficacy of studying drug effects in risk populations. Nonetheless, ototoxic and vestibulotoxic effects of some medications such as aminoglycosides or chemotherapeutic agents are well known. The use of medication is usually unavoidable. However, careful review of the necessity, dosage, drug interactions, and possible alternatives can greatly reduce the dizziness side effects of these medications.

Another factor in this category relates to vision correction. In general, poor vision contributes to disorientation. Regular eye examinations and using correct prescription glasses can greatly improve this deficit. As the visual acuity for both distance and near vision decreases with age, more adults are required to wear multifocal lenses for vision correction. The use of these lenses has been associated with disorientation and increased chance of contact with surrounding objects, especially when performing a secondary task.[80] Advising patients to wear single-focal lenses during outdoor activities may greatly reduce the chance of falling.[81]

The aforementioned is a partial list of environmental and lifestyle factors that can influence a patient's sense of balance. Careful attention to these and other similar factors combined with patient education and simple corrective measures may alleviate the symptoms without extensive medical intervention.

DIAGNOSIS OF DIZZINESS IN OLDER INDIVIDUALS

As noted, dizziness in younger and older individuals can be caused by the same diseases. Therefore, the diagnostic process is the same regardless of age. It includes a careful and detailed history, a thorough physical examination, and targeted laboratory tests. There are several excellent articles, including some in this issue, that cover diagnosis of dizzy patients in detail. Here the authors focus only on the issues that are specific or particularly relevant to the elderly.

History

As is the case with dizziness in any age group, a case history should include a thorough description of the patient's current and previous medical conditions, medication use, social environment, and family risk factors. An accurate description of the symptoms, their time course, and precipitating events is essential in identifying the underlying cause. These symptoms include vertigo, unsteadiness, presyncope, and other less well-defined sensations such as lightheadedness.[74] **Table 1** is a summary of the most likely causes for dizziness in the elderly. It is not a comprehensive list but rather is based on the prevalence of different pathologies in older adults.

Physical Examination

Physical examination is particularly important in the evaluation of dizziness in the elderly because in some settings such as nursing homes, extensive laboratory tests may not be available or convenient.[82] A typical physical examination consists of neurologic, neurotologic, and general medical examination.[83] **Table 2** summarizes different systems evaluated during a typical physical examination for dizziness.

The Dix-Hallpike maneuver and its variations are highly useful because of the increased prevalence of BPPV in the elderly. The test procedures may have to be modified if the patient is frail, or has neck or back problems. For example, it is not necessary to move the patient vigorously, as the canaliths are moved by gravity and not by the acceleration of the body. Nor is it necessary to extend the patient's neck excessively, as most patients can induce their symptoms by simply turning in bed.

Table 1
Common causes of dizziness in the elderly for different types of symptoms

Symptom	Subtype	Likely Cause	Comments
Vertigo	Position-induced	BPPV	If nystagmus does not match BPPV, consider central pathologies. If induced by neck rotation, consider cervical vertigo
	Acute-onset persistent with neurologic signs	Stroke	Acute ischemia involving vestibular structures can mimic vestibular neuritis
		Tumors	
		Degenerative diseases	
	Acute-onset persistent without neurologic signs	Labyrinthitis	Differential diagnosis is based on presence of hearing loss
		Vestibular neuritis	
	Recurrent with no neurologic signs	Ménière's disease	Late-onset Ménière's is possible but not common. Migraines lack progressive auditory symptoms. Transient ischemic attacks should be considered in patients with vascular risk factors
		Migraine	
Disequilibrium	Acute or rapidly progressive	Stroke	Autoimmune or postinfectious diseases should also be considered. May include severe oculomotor abnormalities
	Worse in the absence of other sensory inputs	Bilateral vestibular loss	Usually includes history of ototoxicity. Hearing loss or oscillopsia may be present
	Worse in the absence of vision with numbness/weakness	Proprioception and somatosensory loss	Often associated with peripheral neuropathy associated with metabolic disorders, diabetes, or renal failure
	With bradykinesia, rigidity, tremor	Parkinson disease	Frontal lobe or other basal ganglia disorders
	With speech disorder, lack of coordination, intention tremor	Cerebellar lesions	The imbalance is usually the same with or without vision
	Isolated disequilibrium, gait difficulty, lightheadedness	Disequilibrium of aging	Often accompanied by borderline diffuse central findings but no other specific complaints
Presyncope	With blood pressure drop on standing	Postural hypotension	Associated with reduced blood volume, autonomic disorders, or chronic use of hypertension medications
	Abnormal cardiac examination	Heart valve disease	When 24-h electrocardiogram is abnormal, indicates transient arrhythmia
		Arrhythmia	
	Induced by fear or anxiety	Vasovagal attacks	Decline in heart rate and blood pressure leads to decrease in cerebral blood flow
Lightheadedness, nonspecific	Associated with fear, anxiety, depression	Psychogenic	Often accompanied by autonomic symptoms

Data from Baloh R. Dizziness in older people. J Am Geriatr Soc 1992;40(7):713–21; and Kerber K. Dizziness in older people. In: Eggers SD, Zee DS, editors. Vertigo and imbalance: clinical neurophysiology of the vestibular system: Elsevier; 2010. p. 9, 491–501.

Table 2
Common components of physical examination

System	Examination	Comments
Vestibular	Dix-Hallpike	May require special accommodations for patients who are frail or have neck or back problems
	Head impulse	When positive, almost always indicates a peripheral vestibular lesion. When negative, does not rule out peripheral lesions
	Spontaneous nystagmus	Use Frenzel lenses to eliminate fixation
	Pneumatic otoscopy/Valsalva	Look for horizontal nystagmus in perilymph fistula or torsional/vertical nystagmus in superior canal dehiscence
	Hearing	Use tuning forks
Vision	Static visual acuity	Check both monocular and binocular vision
	Dynamic visual acuity	Look for significant drop in visual acuity during head movements
Proprioception	Temperature/pain/vibration	Check for neuropathies
Motor (musculoskeletal)	Muscle tone/strength	Lower extremity weakness is a fall risk factor
	Gait	Check tandem walking for different abnormal patterns
	Postural stability/sensory integration	Romberg test with eyes open and closed while standing on a solid surface or foam
	Coordination	Past-pointing, heel-knee, or similar tests
Oculomotor	Gaze motility/nystagmus	Look for restricted range of motion and nystagmus
	Saccade/tracking	Assess both accuracy and velocity of both slow and fast eye movements
Cardiovascular	Orthostatic drop in blood pressure	Look for drop of greater than 20 mm Hg in systolic blood pressure or drop of greater than 10 mm Hg in diastolic blood pressure on standing
	Irregular heart rhythm	Can be intermittent
Psychogenic	Cognition	Questionnaire-based assessment such as Mini-Mental State Examination
	Anxiety	Questionnaire-based assessment such as Beck Anxiety Inventory. Hyperventilation test can be helpful
	Depression	Questionnaire-based assessment such as Geriatric Depression Scale
	Handicap	Questionnaire-based assessment such as Dizziness Handicap Inventory

Data from multiple sources including: Kerber K. Dizziness in older people. In: Eggers SD, Zee DS, editors. Vertigo and imbalance: clinical neurophysiology of the vestibular system: Elsevier; 2010. p. 9, 491–501; and Jacobson G, McCaslin D, Grantham S, et al. Significant vestibular system impairment is common in a cohort of elderly patients referred for assessment of falls risk. J Am Acad Audiol 2008;19(10):799–807.

The safety and comfort of the test can be improved by having additional assistants to help with positioning of the patient. Finally, in cases of severe neck or back problems, specialized equipment may be needed to safely perform the procedure.

Another useful test is the head impulse test.[84] A positive test, characterized by catch-up saccades following horizontal head impulses or thrusts, almost always indicates peripheral vestibular pathology.[85] The test is also helpful in confirming bilateral vestibular loss when caloric testing is bilaterally weak. Again, the procedure can be modified for the elderly to minimize neck problems by reducing the amplitude of the head thrust while maintaining its relatively high velocity.

Laboratory Tests

Laboratory tests may become necessary after taking a thorough history and performing a complete physical examination. Typical laboratory tests for dizziness include vestibular function tests, auditory tests, imaging tests, cardiovascular tests and, less commonly, endocrinological tests. It is important to recognize that normal limits for many of the laboratory tests are ill-defined for older individuals.[83] In fact, it is not clear whether one should consider age-related changes of balance function a normal phenomenon. Therefore, it is best to use these tests judiciously in the elderly, because some perceived abnormal findings may prove to be of little help in the ultimate diagnosis and management of the patient. This section provides a brief review of laboratory test findings that are specific to the elderly.

Vestibular function tests

The most commonly used vestibular function test is videonystagmography (VNG) or electronystagmography (ENG). It includes tests of oculomotor function (saccade, tracking, optokinetic), tests of gaze stabilization (gaze, spontaneous nystagmus, static position), tests of VOR (caloric), and specialized tests (Dix-Hallpike maneuver and its variations, pressure/fistula).

In the saccade test, saccade latencies increase with age, but other parameters such as accuracy or peak velocity are not significantly affected.[42] Some abnormalities in the saccade test, such as abnormal latencies, may be caused by poor visual acuity; this is a particular issue with VNG because patients are usually unable to wear corrective glasses during the test. Also, most of the saccade parameters are sensitive to drug effects.

In the tracking test the gain, defined as the ratio of eye to target velocities, decreases with age, especially for higher frequencies.[70] Similarly, slow-phase velocity of nystagmus in the optokinetic test decreases for higher velocity stimuli. Again, the effects of poor vision and medications should be considered in interpretation of the results.

In gaze stabilization tests, one should recognize that end-point nystagmus begins at lower off-center gaze positions and is more common in the elderly. End-point nystagmus is a normal occurrence characterized by intermittent mild nystagmus when the eyes are directed at extreme gaze positions, and should not be mistaken for abnormal gaze-evoked nystagmus. Also, square-wave jerk nystagmus with fixation seems to be common in the elderly, and is considered part of normal aging by some investigators.[86] Therefore, the frequency of square waves and the patient's age should be considered before deciding the clinical significance of the finding. However, the age-adjusted normal limit for this finding is not readily available.

In the caloric test, bilateral caloric weakness is common in older patients. Although the finding may represent age-related reduction of vestibular function in some patients, in many others it is a false-positive finding that reflects poor temperature transfer from the external auditory canal to the labyrinth. The latter group demonstrates normal rotary chair results that indicate normal VOR function.[87] No other age-related changes have been observed in other caloric test parameters.[41]

In the Dix-Hallpike maneuver and its variations, the issues are the same as those discussed earlier for the bedside tests. That is, safety precautions must be taken to deal with frailty and neck or back problems in the elderly, regardless of whether the test is performed as part of the VNG/ENG battery or separately.

In rotation tests, older asymptomatic individuals show reduced VOR gain and increased phase lead, mainly in low frequencies. These findings represent age-related decline in vestibular function and loss of velocity storage mechanisms in the vestibular nuclei.[41,43] Rotary chair testing can be helpful in older adults to clarify the results of caloric tests.

Vestibular-evoked myogenic potentials (VEMP) are based on short-latency muscle responses typically recorded from the neck muscles (cervical VEMP) or from the eye muscles (ocular VEMP) in response to loud clicks or tone bursts. The use of this test to evaluate the otolith organs and the inferior portion of the vestibular nerve is becoming more common. Several recent studies have demonstrated that both cervical and ocular VEMP parameters are affected by age.[88–92] All of the studies consistently demonstrate that VEMP amplitudes decline while VEMP thresholds increase with age. The response rates also are shown to decrease in older adults. Some studies have described age-related changes in VEMP latencies whereas others have not.[90–92] One complicating factor in the elderly is the reduced ability to maintain high levels of muscle contraction, perhaps due to age-related loss of muscle tone or use of muscle relaxants. This factor can affect VEMP amplitude and threshold, and should be considered in interpreting the results. As more clinical applications for VEMP testing are identified in all age groups, the role of the test in evaluating older adults is also emerging.

Dynamic posturography consists of two separate tests: the motor coordination test (MCT), in which postural sway is measured in response to sudden translation or rotation of the support base, and the sensory organization test (SOT), in which postural sway is measured under different visual and proprioceptive conditions.[41,69] In one study, MCT parameters did not change with age except for latency (reaction time), which showed modest increase with age.[69] In SOT, there was a significant increase in postural sway when visual and proprioceptive inputs were altered.[41] Dynamic posturography is not a diagnostic test, although its results can help to identify inappropriate sensory integration and to design more effective exercise programs for the elderly.

Other tests

Magnetic resonance imaging (MRI) and computed tomography (CT) are imaging modalities that are used to identify structural abnormalities in the brain of dizzy patients. Their applications are the same in both younger and older individuals, but there are a few areas of particular interest in the elderly. Imaging studies, MRI in particular, can help with identifying white matter lesions. Although the significance of small lesions is in doubt, larger white matter enhancements have been associated with a variety of balance-related symptoms in the elderly.[83]

Magnetic resonance angiography (MRA) and other tests such as Doppler ultrasound can help in identifying the vascular origin of dizziness, which is a common finding in the elderly. Unfortunately, some of the other common causes such as transient ischemia may not produce distinguishable findings in imaging studies.

Tests of cardiovascular function such as electrocardiography or Holter monitoring can identify constant and intermittent cases of arrhythmia. Cardiovascular causes of dizziness are also common in the elderly.

MANAGEMENT OF DIZZINESS IN OLDER INDIVIDUALS

Management of dizziness involves a medical, rehabilitative or, in rare cases, surgical approach. Physical therapy, either as the primary mode of management or in conjunction with other management modalities, appears to be an effective approach in reducing dizziness in older adults (see article by Alrwaily and Whitney in this publication). The approach is most appropriate when the underlying cause is vestibular-related or when the cause is nonspecific.[50] However, physical therapy is a worthwhile option for other causes of dizziness in the elderly. Exercise therapy may include vestibular rehabilitation, strength training, fitness training, and other carefully planned exercises. In addition to the traditional outpatient approach to therapy, home-based and group exercise programs can be very effective.[50]

If the cause of dizziness is BPPV, simple and effective methods such as canalith repositioning or liberatory maneuvers are available (see article by Cho and White in this publication). Again, the same precautions that are necessary in performing diagnostic maneuvers must be considered when administering therapeutic procedures.

When other specific pathologies are identified, there is usually an established management protocol. For example, initial treatment of Ménière's disease includes low-salt diet, diuretics, and possibly vestibular suppressants (see article by Semaan and Megerian in this publication). Further treatment may require shunt surgery, vestibular nerve section, or transtympanic gentamicin injections. However, management approaches that rely on central compensation mechanisms for their therapeutic effect, such as vestibular nerve section or gentamicin therapy, must be used cautiously in the elderly. As discussed earlier, compensation mechanisms deteriorate with age and may not provide effective recovery following those procedures.

Management of cerebrovascular and cardiovascular causes of dizziness usually involves controlling the underlying risk factors. Similarly, psychogenic causes of dizziness can be addressed by managing contributing factors such as anxiety or depression.

SUMMARY

Dizziness is a common and potentially serious complaint among the elderly. Left untreated, it can lead to falls and serious injuries. When possible, a multidisciplinary approach with an integrated strategy is more effective in the diagnosis and management of dizziness because the underlying causes often span multiple systems.

REFERENCES

1. Jönsson R, Sixt E, Landahl S, et al. Prevalence of dizziness and vertigo in an urban elderly population. J Vestib Res 2004;14(1):47–52.
2. Neuhauser H, von Brevern M, Radtke A, et al. Epidemiology of vestibular vertigo: a neurotologic survey of the general population. Neurology 2005;65(6):898–904.
3. Tinetti M, Williams C. Falls, injuries due to falls, and the risk of admission to a nursing home. N Engl J Med 1997;337(18):1279–84.
4. Kannus P, Parkkari J, Koskinen S, et al. Fall-induced injuries and deaths among older adults. JAMA 1999;281(20):1895–9.
5. "Falls among older adults: an overview". Available at: http://www.cdc.gov/HomeandRecreationalSafety/Falls/adultfalls.html. Accessed August 14, 2010.
6. Tinetti M, Williams C, Gill T. Dizziness among older adults: a possible geriatric syndrome. Ann Intern Med 2000;132(5):337–44.

7. Sloane P, Baloh R. Persistent dizziness in geriatric patients. J Am Geriatr Soc 1989;37(11):1031–8.
8. Neuhauser H. Epidemiology of vertigo. Curr Opin Neurol 2007;20(1):40–6.
9. Maarsingh O, Dros J, Schellevis F, et al. Dizziness reported by elderly patients in family practice: prevalence, incidence, and clinical characteristics. BMC Fam Pract 2010;11:2.
10. Graafmans W, Ooms M, Hofstee H, et al. Falls in the elderly: a prospective study of risk factors and risk profiles. Am J Epidemiol 1996;143(11):1129–36.
11. O'Loughlin J, Boivin J, Robitaille Y, et al. Falls among the elderly: distinguishing indoor and outdoor risk factors in Canada. J Epidemiol Community Health 1994;48(5):488–9.
12. Rubenstein L, Josephson K. The epidemiology of falls and syncope. Clin Geriatr Med 2002;18(2):141–58.
13. King M, Tinetti M. Falls in community-dwelling older persons. J Am Geriatr Soc 1995;43(10):1146–54.
14. Alexander B, Rivara F, Wolf M. The cost and frequency of hospitalization for fall-related injuries in older adults. Am J Public Health 1992;82(7):1020–3.
15. Stevens J, Corso P, Finkelstein E, et al. The costs of fatal and non-fatal falls among older adults. Inj Prev 2006;12(5):290–5.
16. "Costs of falls among older adults". Available at: http://www.cdc.gov/HomeandRecreationalSafety/Falls/fallcost.html. Accessed August 14, 2010.
17. Stel V, Pluijm S, Deeg D, et al. A classification tree for predicting recurrent falling in community-dwelling older persons. J Am Geriatr Soc 2003;51(10):1356–64.
18. Whitney S, Marchetti G, Schade A. The relationship between falls history and computerized dynamic posturography in persons with balance and vestibular disorders. Arch Phys Med Rehabil 2006;87(3):402–7.
19. Moreland J, Richardson J, Goldsmith C, et al. Muscle weakness and falls in older adults: a systematic review and meta-analysis. J Am Geriatr Soc 2004;52(7):1121–9.
20. Rubenstein L, Josephson K. Falls and their prevention in elderly people: what does the evidence show? Med Clin North Am 2006;90(5):807–24.
21. Burker E, Wong H, Sloane P, et al. Predictors of fear of falling in dizzy and non-dizzy elderly. Psychol Aging 1995;10(1):104–10.
22. Perez-Jara J, Enguix A, Fernandez-Quintas J, et al. Fear of falling among elderly patients with dizziness and syncope in a tilt setting. Can J Aging 2009;28(2):157–63.
23. Holmberg J, Karlberg M, Harlacher U, et al. Experience of handicap and anxiety in phobic postural vertigo. Acta Otolaryngol 2005;125(3):270–5.
24. Delbaere K, Crombez G, Vanderstraeten G, et al. Fear-related avoidance of activities, falls and physical frailty. A prospective community-based cohort study. Age Ageing 2004;33(4):368–73.
25. Li F, Fisher K, Harmer P, et al. Fear of falling in elderly persons: association with falls, functional ability, and quality of life. J Gerontol B Psychol Sci Soc Sci 2003;58(5):P283–90.
26. Belal A, Glorig A. Dysequilibrium of ageing (presbyastasis). J Laryngol Otol 1986;100(9):1037–41.
27. Lawson J, Fitzgerald J, Birchall J, et al. Diagnosis of geriatric patients with severe dizziness. J Am Geriatr Soc 1999;47(1):12–7.
28. Sloane P. Evaluation and management of dizziness in the older patient. Clin Geriatr Med 1996;12(4):785–801.

29. Katsarkas A. Dizziness in aging: the clinical experience. Geriatrics 2008;63(11): 18–20.
30. Bueno-Cavanillas A, Padilla-Ruiz F, Jiménez-Moleón J, et al. Risk factors in falls among the elderly according to extrinsic and intrinsic precipitating causes. Eur J Epidemiol 2000;16(9):849–59.
31. Rosenhall U, Rubin W. Degenerative changes in the human vestibular sensory epithelia. Acta Otolaryngol 1975;79(1/2):67–80.
32. Richter E. Quantitative study of human Scarpa's ganglion and vestibular sensory epithelia. Acta Otolaryngol 1980;90(3/4):199–208.
33. Merchant S, Velázquez-Villaseñor L, Tsuji K, et al. Temporal bone studies of the human peripheral vestibular system. Normative vestibular hair cell data. Ann Otol Rhinol Laryngol Suppl 2000;181:3–13.
34. Ishiyama G. Imbalance and vertigo: the aging human vestibular periphery. Semin Neurol 2009;29(5):491–9.
35. Ishiyama A, Lopez I, Ishiyama G, et al. Unbiased quantification of the microdissected human Scarpa's ganglion neurons. Laryngoscope 2004;114(8):1496–9.
36. Lopez I, Ishiyama G, Tang Y, et al. Estimation of the number of nerve fibers in the human vestibular endorgans using unbiased stereology and immunohistochemistry. J Neurosci Methods 2005;145(1/2):37–46.
37. Tang Y, Lopez I, Baloh R. Age-related change of the neuronal number in the human medial vestibular nucleus: a stereological investigation. J Vestib Res 2001;11(6):357–63, 2001–2.
38. Lyon M, Davis J. Age-related blood flow and capillary changes in the rat utricular macula: a quantitative stereological and microsphere study. J Assoc Res Otolaryngol 2002;3(2):167–73.
39. Lyon M, Wanamaker H. Blood flow and assessment of capillaries in the aging rat posterior canal crista. Hear Res 1993;67(1/2):157–65.
40. Johnsson L, Hawkins J. Vascular changes in the human inner ear associated with aging. Ann Otol Rhinol Laryngol 1972;81(3):364–76.
41. Peterka R, Black F, Schoenhoff M. Age-related changes in human vestibuloocular reflexes: sinusoidal rotation and caloric tests. J Vestib Res 1990;1(1): 49–59, 1990–1.
42. Kerber K, Ishiyama G, Baloh R. A longitudinal study of oculomotor function in normal older people. Neurobiol Aging 2006;27(9):1346–53.
43. Baloh R, Enrietto J, Jacobson K, et al. Age-related changes in vestibular function: a longitudinal study. Ann N Y Acad Sci 2001;942:210–9.
44. Furman J, Redfern M. Effect of aging on the otolith-ocular reflex. J Vestib Res 2001;11(2):91–103.
45. Jacobson G, McCaslin D, Grantham S, et al. Significant vestibular system impairment is common in a cohort of elderly patients referred for assessment of falls risk. J Am Acad Audiol 2008;19(10):799–807.
46. Katsarkas A. Dizziness in aging: a retrospective study of 1194 cases. Otolaryngol Head Neck Surg 1994;110(3):296–301.
47. Fitzpatrick R, McCloskey D. Proprioceptive, visual and vestibular thresholds for the perception of sway during standing in humans. J Physiol 1994;478(Pt 1):173–86.
48. Behm D, Bambury A, Cahill F, et al. Effect of acute static stretching on force, balance, reaction time, and movement time. Med Sci Sports Exerc 2004;36(8): 1397–402.
49. Wiles P, Pearce S, Rice P, et al. Vibration perception threshold: influence of age, height, sex, and smoking, and calculation of accurate centile values. Diabet Med 1991;8(2):157–61.

50. Sturnieks D, St George R, Lord S. Balance disorders in the elderly. Neurophysiol Clin 2008;38(6):467–78.
51. Peterka R, Black F. Age-related changes in human posture control: sensory organization tests. J Vestib Res 1990;1(1):73–85, 1990–1.
52. Horak F, Dickstein R, Peterka R. Diabetic neuropathy and surface sway-referencing disrupt somatosensory information for postural stability in stance. Somatosens Mot Res 2002;19(4):316–26.
53. Lord S, Clark R, Webster I. Physiological factors associated with falls in an elderly population. J Am Geriatr Soc 1991;39(12):1194–200.
54. Bove M, Courtine G, Schieppati M. Neck muscle vibration and spatial orientation during stepping in place in humans. J Neurophysiol 2002;88(5):2232–41.
55. Deshpande N, Patla A. Postural responses and spatial orientation to neck proprioceptive and vestibular inputs during locomotion in young and older adults. Exp Brain Res 2005;167(3):468–74.
56. Patel M, Fransson P, Karlberg M, et al. Change of body movement coordination during cervical proprioceptive disturbances with increased age. Gerontology 2010;56(3):284–90.
57. Malmström E, Karlberg M, Fransson P, et al. Cervical proprioception is sufficient for head orientation after bilateral vestibular loss. Eur J Appl Physiol 2009;107(1): 73–81.
58. Lord S, Clark R, Webster I. Visual acuity and contrast sensitivity in relation to falls in an elderly population. Age Ageing 1991;20(3):175–81.
59. Lord S. Visual risk factors for falls in older people. Age Ageing 2006;35(Suppl 2): ii42–5.
60. Haegerstrom-Portnoy G, Morgan MW. Normal age-related vision changes. In: Rosenbloom AA, Morgan MV, editors. Vision and aging. St Louis (MO): Butterworth-Heinemann; 2007. p. 31–48.
61. Ishigaki H, Miyao M. Implications for dynamic visual acuity with changes in aged and sex. Percept Mot Skills 1994;78(2):363–9.
62. Schubert M, Herdman S, Tusa R. Vertical dynamic visual acuity in normal subjects and patients with vestibular hypofunction. Otol Neurotol 2002;23(3): 372–7.
63. Poulain I, Giraudet G. Age-related changes of visual contribution in posture control. Gait Posture 2008;27(1):1–7.
64. Borger L, Whitney S, Redfern M, et al. The influence of dynamic visual environments on postural sway in the elderly. J Vestib Res 1999;9(3):197–205.
65. O'Connor K, Loughlin P, Redfern M, et al. Postural adaptations to repeated optic flow stimulation in older adults. Gait Posture 2008;28(3):385–91.
66. Larsson L, Ramamurthy B. Aging-related changes in skeletal muscle. Mechanisms and interventions. Drugs Aging 2000;17(4):303–16.
67. Faulkner J, Larkin L, Claflin D, et al. Age-related changes in the structure and function of skeletal muscles. Clin Exp Pharmacol Physiol 2007;34(11):1091–6.
68. Roos M, Rice C, Vandervoort A. Age-related changes in motor unit function. Muscle Nerve 1997;20(6):679–90.
69. Peterka R, Black F. Age-related changes in human posture control: motor coordination tests. J Vestib Res 1990;1(1):87–96, 1990–1.
70. Moschner C, Baloh R. Age-related changes in visual tracking. J Gerontol 1994; 49(5):M235–8.
71. McPherson D, Whitaker S, Wrobel B. DDX: Disequilibrium of aging. In: Goebel JA, editor. Practical management of the dizzy patient. Philadelphia: Lippincott Williams & Wilkins; 2008. p. 297–344.

72. Quoniam C, Hay L, Roll J, et al. Age effects on reflex and postural responses to propriomuscular inputs generated by tendon vibration. J Gerontol A Biol Sci Med Sci 1995;50(3):B155–65.
73. Maarsingh O, Dros J, Schellevis F, et al. Causes of persistent dizziness in elderly patients in primary care. Ann Fam Med 2010;8(3):196–205.
74. Drachman D. A 69-year-old man with chronic dizziness. JAMA 1998;280(24): 2111–8.
75. Baloh R. Dizziness in older people. J Am Geriatr Soc 1992;40(7):713–21.
76. Sloane P, Hartman M, Mitchell C. Psychological factors associated with chronic dizziness in patients aged 60 and older. J Am Geriatr Soc 1994;42(8):847–52.
77. Eckhardt-Henn A, Breuer P, Thomalske C, et al. Anxiety disorders and other psychiatric subgroups in patients complaining of dizziness. J Anxiety Disord 2003;17(4):369–88.
78. Ganz D, Bao Y, Shekelle P, et al. Will my patient fall? JAMA 2007;297(1):77–86.
79. Agostini J, Tinetti M. Drugs and falls: rethinking the approach to medication risk in older adults. J Am Geriatr Soc 2002;50(10):1744–5.
80. Menant J, St George R, Sandery B, et al. Older people contact more obstacles when wearing multifocal glasses and performing a secondary visual task. J Am Geriatr Soc 2009;57(10):1833–8.
81. Haran M, Cameron I, Ivers R, et al. Effect on falls of providing single lens distance vision glasses to multifocal glasses wearers: VISIBLE randomised controlled trial. BMJ 2010;340:c2265.
82. Domínguez M, Magro J. Bedside balance testing in elderly people. Curr Aging Sci 2009;2(2):150–7.
83. Kerber K. Dizziness in older people. In: Eggers SD, Zee DS, editors. Vertigo and imbalance: clinical neurophysiology of the vestibular system. Philadelphia: Elsevier; 2010. p. 9 491–501.
84. Aw S, Halmagyi G, Black R, et al. Head impulses reveal loss of individual semi-circular canal function. J Vestib Res 1999;9(3):173–80.
85. Newman-Toker D, Kattah J, Alvernia J, et al. Normal head impulse test differentiates acute cerebellar strokes from vestibular neuritis. Neurology 2008;70(24 Pt 2): 2378–85.
86. Square wave jerks (SWJ). Available at: http://www.dizziness-and-balance.com/ practice/nystagmus/SWJ.htm. Accessed August 14, 2010.
87. Barin K. Interpretation and usefulness of caloric testing. In: Jacobson G, Shepard N, editors. Balance function assessment and management. San Diego (CA): Plural Publishing; 2008. p. 229–52.
88. Janky K, Shepard N. Vestibular evoked myogenic potential (VEMP) testing: normative threshold response curves and effects of age. J Am Acad Audiol 2009;20(8):514–22.
89. Tseng C, Chou C, Young Y. Aging effect on the ocular vestibular-evoked myogenic potentials. Otol Neurotol 2010;31(6):959–63.
90. Nguyen K, Welgampola M, Carey J. Test-retest reliability and age-related charac-teristics of the ocular and cervical vestibular evoked myogenic potential tests. Otol Neurotol 2010;31(5):793–802.
91. Brantberg K, Granath K, Schart N. Age-related changes in vestibular evoked myogenic potentials. Audiol Neurootol 2007;12(4):247–53.
92. Lee S, Cha C, Jung T, et al. Age-related differences in parameters of vestibular evoked myogenic potentials. Acta Otolaryngol 2008;128(1):66–72.

Medication-Related Dizziness in the Older Adult

Osama A. Shoair, BS, Abner N. Nyandege, MS,
Patricia W. Slattum, PharmD, PhD*

KEYWORDS

- Dizziness • Adverse drug event • Medication-related dizziness
- Older adult

KEY POINTS

- Dizziness is highly prevalent among patients aged 65 years and older and is associated with multiple risk factors such as comorbid diseases and medications.
- The consequences of dizziness affect patients' health and quality of life and create an enormous economic burden on the health care system.
- For physicians to manage dizziness appropriately in older adults, it is crucial to assess the possible underlying causes of dizziness that will facilitate accurate clinical decision making.
- Performing a medication history and review are important for adjusting the medication regimen to help prevent or resolve medication-related dizziness.

Mrs K. J. is a pleasant, articulate 79-year-old woman describing episodic vertigo and chronic lightheadedness that began approximately 2 years ago without any antecedent illness or injury. She states that the vertigo occurs without warning, lasting 15 to 30 minutes at each occurrence, and resolves completely with no residual symptoms. She has noted tightness in her chest, numbness and tingling in her lips and hands, grayed vision, and clammy sweating during these episodes. She denies associated auditory symptoms. She reports that she had 4 such episodes in the past year. Her symptoms of lightheadedness occur daily and seem slightly worse on transitioning from supine to sitting or sitting to standing position. She feels reasonably well when she first begins her morning routine but reports a foggy, disconnected feeling by midmorning, which persists until evening before gradually improving. She denies falls but reports near-falls 2 to 3 times per week. She lives alone following the death of her husband last year and becomes

Geriatric Pharmacotherapy Program, Department of Pharmacotherapy and Outcomes Science, Virginia Commonwealth University, 410 North 12th Street, Box 980533, Richmond, VA 23298-0533, USA
* Corresponding author.
E-mail address: pwslattum@vcu.edu

Otolaryngol Clin N Am 44 (2011) 455–471
doi:10.1016/j.otc.2011.01.014
0030-6665/11/$ – see front matter © 2011 Elsevier Inc. All rights reserved.

tearful and slightly agitated when expressing concerns for her own future in light of these symptoms. Her medical history is significant for hypertension, peripheral neuropathy affecting her legs below the knee, depression, anxiety, and seasonal allergies. Her medication list includes hydrochlorothiazide, propranolol, diazepam, meclizine, calcium and vitamin D supplements, fish oil, and garlic tablets.

MEDICATION-RELATED DIZZINESS

Dizziness is highly prevalent among adults aged 65 years and older in primary care or family practice settings, with estimates of greater than 30% in community-dwelling older adults and a higher prevalence in women than men.[1–3] A study of emergency department (ED) visits (1993–2005) from the National Hospital Ambulatory Medical Care Survey (NHAMCS) is in agreement with these facts from studies conducted in single institutions. From a total of 9472 dizziness cases sampled over this period, the study demonstrated that dizziness is an extremely common ED symptom that preferentially affects older adults and a greater proportion of women.[4] From an epidemiologic standpoint, it can be hypothesized that the incidence of dizziness-associated complications are expected to increase in the future based on the increasing US population projections for persons aged 65 years and older. According to the US Census Bureau, it is projected that 20% of Americans will be aged 65 years and older by 2030, and by 2050, this age group is projected to increase to 88.5 million from 38.7 million in 2008. Similarly, the 85 years and older population is expected to increase to 19 million by 2050 from 5.4 million in 2008.[5]

Although dizziness seems to increase with aging, normal aging is not the cause of dizziness but other factors associated with aging make older adults more susceptible to dizziness.[6] Comorbid conditions, drug-related problems (due in part to altered pharmacokinetics and pharmacodynamics), polypharmacy, larger number of doses of medications per day, low body weight, and a history of adverse drug reactions predispose older adults to dizziness.[7–11]

Pharmacokinetics describes the relationship between the dose of the drug administered and the resulting drug concentrations achieved in the systemic circulation. Aging is generally characterized by changes in all pharmacokinetic processes including absorption, distribution, metabolism, and excretion,[10] although the most clinically important changes are those affecting hepatic and renal drug elimination. Hepatic metabolism may be reduced in older adults, particularly for drugs metabolized primarily by oxidative pathways. Impaired renal function with aging results in reduced renal clearance for drugs eliminated by the kidneys.[10] Altered pharmacokinetics with aging increases the risk of adverse drug events (ADEs), such as dizziness in older adults.

Pharmacodynamics describes the relationship between drug concentrations in the systemic circulation and drug response. Aging also affects pharmacodynamics through several mechanisms including altered concentrations of the drug at the receptor, altered interactions between the drug and its receptor, and changes in homeostatic regulation. Pharmacodynamic changes often result in increased sensitivity to medications, especially for drugs acting on the central nervous system (CNS).[10,12] Altered pharmacodynamics can also contribute to increased risk of ADEs, such as dizziness in older adults.

Polypharmacy refers to the use of multiple medications and/or the administration of more medications than is clinically indicated, representing unnecessary drug use.[13] Polypharmacy is associated with higher risk of ADEs, inappropriate use of medications, nonadherence, geriatric syndromes, and mortality in older adults.[13,14] In addition, ADEs can result from prescriber-related factors such as therapeutic duplication, that is, prescriptions for one patient initiated by more than one prescriber, increasing the risk of uncoordinated care.[15]

There is a wide range of consequences associated with dizziness, and these may significantly affect the quality of life and health care burden.[16,17] For example, Cigolle and colleagues[18] performed a cross-sectional study to examine the prevalence of geriatric conditions among older adults (eg, dizziness) and the association of these conditions with activities of daily living dependency (eg, cognitive impairment contributing to dependency for bathing and dressing). In this study, data were obtained from the year 2000 from the Health and Retirement Study, a biennial longitudinal health interview survey of a cohort of adults aged 50 years or older in the United States. The results showed a strong and significant association, suggesting that geriatric conditions are associated with disability.[18]

Considerable progress has been made in the clinical setting to describe and define dizziness and its potential causes. Dizziness is a common symptom reported by older patients during physician visits.[19] Dizziness is an obscure multifactorial symptom associated with various diseases affecting the sensory organs, the CNS, or both. It may also be induced by processes outside the CNS or sensory organs, such as cardiovascular diseases, or by medications.[20] Dizziness is a complex and subjective complaint.[21] In fact, difficulty in diagnosing dizziness in older adults in family practice and in specialty practice settings has been reported. The term dizziness can describe many different sensations that can be categorized by subtypes. These subtypes include vertigo, presyncope, disequilibrium, and nonspecific dizziness.[6] In a medical chart audit study, it was recommended that documentation of selected key quality indicators in the management of dizziness could improve clinical diagnosis.[22]

Medication-related dizziness can be difficult to diagnose, especially in older persons, in whom it can masquerade as a geriatric syndrome.[11] Geriatric syndromes are difficult to define, but they are characterized as symptoms with multifactorial causes, which become more common with aging and are in fact often mistaken for normal aging.[23] Shared risk factors may lead to geriatric syndromes. The common geriatric syndromes associated with high degree of morbidity include incontinence, falls, pressure ulcers, delirium, and functional decline.[23] Dizziness is considered by some geriatricians to meet the definition of a geriatric syndrome.[11] ADEs in older patients often present as nonspecific symptoms or geriatric syndrome indicators, such as cognitive impairment or falls. Falls may be related to osteoarthritis, poor visual acuity, and/or prescription medication affecting balance. Discovering the underlying cause may be challenging.[24] Similarly, other health issues associated with dizziness are often multifactorial.[25] Involvement of cardiovascular, neurologic, sensory, and psychological domains, as well as medication-related ADEs suggest that dizziness may be a geriatric syndrome.[22] Results from a cross-sectional study of ED visits for dizziness from the NHAMCS database support these associations. The study showed that the following diagnoses were at least twice as likely among patients presenting with dizziness: otovestibular, cerebrovascular, metabolic, and cardiovascular disorders.[4]

Because dizziness in the elderly may be more serious than in any other age group, accurate diagnosis and appropriate intervention are crucial.[19] The key component in the evaluation and general management of dizziness in older adults is patient history. A complete medication history is considered critical to the evaluation.[6] Similarly, Salles and colleagues[26] suggest that an interdisciplinary treatment approach to minimize contributive causes of dizziness in the elderly is to adjust the medication regimen. Medication history should include prescription medications, over-the-counter medications, herbal medicines, and nutraceuticals, as well as recreational drugs (including smoking and alcohol).[27] Common drug categories implicated in dizziness in older adults are listed in **Table 1**.[19,28,29]

A recent report examining the epidemiology of central vertigo and dizziness indicated that of the 13 causes of central vertigo reviewed in this study, medication-related dizziness was not considered or discussed in detail.[30] Perhaps, the omission was because of the paucity of the published literature associating medication and dizziness or because medications are simply considered the least consequential factor associated with dizziness. Yet, according to the US Food and Drug Administration (FDA) safety information data contained in the Adverse Event Reporting System (AERS) database, between the years 2004 and 2009, dizziness was reported to be associated with a wide variety of medications. The authors' preliminary analysis identified more than 70,000 reports.[31] Because AERS reporting is voluntary, it has been suggested that there is a high degree of under-reporting,[32] and thus the actual number of cases of medication-associated dizziness may be even more than in the records document.

Table 1
Medications that often cause dizziness in older adults

Class of Medication	Possible Mechanism
α_1-Adrenergic antagonists	Orthostatic hypotension
Alcohol	Hypotension, osmotic effects
Aminoglycosides	Ototoxicity
Anticonvulsants	Orthostatic hypotension, cerebellar dysfunction
Antidepressants	Orthostatic hypotension
Anti-Parkinson medication	Orthostatic hypotension
Antipsychotics	Orthostatic hypotension
β-Blockers	Hypotension or bradycardia
Calcium channel blockers	Hypotension, vasodilation
Class 1a antiarrhythmics	Torsades de pointes
Digitalis glycosides	Hypotension
Diuretics	Volume contraction, vasodilation
Narcotics	CNS depression, torsades de pointes
Oral sulfonylurea	Hypoglycemia
Vasodilators	Hypotension, vasodilation
Anticoagulants	Bleeding complications
Antidementia agents	Bradycardia, syncope
Antihistamines: sedating	Torsades de pointes
Antirheumatic agents	Vestibular disturbance
Anti-infectives: anti-influenza agents, antifungals (oral), quinolones	Torsades de pointes
Antithyroid agents	Bone marrow toxicity
Anxiolytics	CNS depression
Attention-deficit/hyperactivity disorder agents	Cardiac arrhythmias
Cholesterol-lowering agents	Hypotension
Bronchodilators	Hypotension
Skeletal muscle relaxants	Central anticholinergic effects
Urinary and gastrointestinal antispasmodics	Central anticholinergic effects

Data from Refs.[19,28,29]

In fact, Kroenke and colleagues,[33] in an earlier review on the frequency of various causes of dizziness, generally categorized medication-related causes as other causes, accounting for only 16% of the causes of dizziness. The other causes of dizziness included anemia and metabolic causes (eg, hypoglycemia, hyperglycemia, electrolyte disturbances, thyroid disease).[33] This possible underestimation is not consistent with findings from the most recent cross-sectional diagnostic study describing subtypes of dizziness in older adult patients in a primary care setting assessing the contributory causes of dizziness.[34] In this study, 417 older adult patients in the Netherlands, aged 65 to 95 years, who consult their family physician for persistent dizziness, underwent a comprehensive evaluation by a panel of specialists. It was found that an ADE was considered to be the most common minor contributory cause of dizziness (23%).[34] In contrast to the results from the study by Kroenke and colleagues,[33] the conclusion drawn from this study was that medications are a significant cause of dizziness in some patients.

This article provides an overview of the available literature regarding medication-related dizziness in adults aged 65 years and older.

LITERATURE SEARCH STRATEGY

We searched MEDLINE/PubMed to identify potential studies of drug-induced dizziness in older adults for inclusion in this review. The search strategy included all articles published between January 1996 and June 2010, and used various MeSH terms, including dizziness, combined with one of the following search terms at a time: pharmaceutical preparations, psychotropic drugs, histamine antagonists, benzodiazepines, cholinergic antagonists, antihypertensive agents, anticonvulsants, hypnotics and sedatives, and polypharmacy. Additional articles were also obtained by searching databases such as CINAHL and PsycINFO and by manually reviewing the bibliographies of retrieved articles. Relevant English-language articles that studied adults aged 65 years and older were included. All studies were required to have medications as a predictor variable and dizziness as an outcome variable. Articles in foreign languages, including Chinese and German, were excluded. Relevant articles were selected by reviewing the abstracts to ensure that the inclusion and exclusion criteria were met.

We identified a total of 364 potential citations, of which, 105 were selected after applying the aforementioned inclusion and exclusion criteria. Ninety-four articles were found to be irrelevant to this review after further scrutiny. The following were excluded: studies that focused on relationships between dizziness and other outcomes not related to the objective of this article, case studies and case series, studies only assessing efficacy of drugs and not their safety/tolerability, studies of investigational drugs, studies of drug assays and pharmacokinetic evaluation, phase 1 clinical studies, and studies focusing on drug use, rather than dizziness, as a predictor for falls and fractures. A total of 11 unique original research studies and systematic reviews were found to be suitable for conducting this review, which we organized by the class of medication: antihypertensives, benzodiazepines, hypnotics, anxiolytics, and antiepileptics.

ANTIHYPERTENSIVE DRUGS

Antihypertensive drug use among older adults is common.[35] According to one study, the proportion of persons reporting treatment of hypertension increased with age and was highest (49.6%) among those aged 65 years and older who reported treatment for the condition in 2003. Generally, women were more likely than men to report treatment of hypertension.[35] **Box 1** provides a list of all FDA-approved antihypertensive medications available at present.[36] Of the adverse effects associated with antihypertensives, dizziness is more frequent among users than nonusers of these drugs.[19] Further information from the FDA[36] indicates that dizziness is a common side effect associated with the classes of medications listed in **Box 1**, except for calcium channel blockers and renin inhibitors.

Several other studies investigated in detail the potential association between antihypertensive medication use and dizziness in older adults. Hale and colleagues[37] performed a prospective study to evaluate CNS effects in older subjects using antihypertensive drugs. In this study, older adult participants were first screened on an annual basis for undetected medical disorders, and those in whom medical disorders were detected were referred to private physicians for 2 years of follow-up care. Findings from this study showed that dizziness was identified significantly more often in women than in men and may be dose related. This trend was particularly observed among women using propranolol, diuretics alone, and diuretics in combination with another antihypertensive agent such as hydralazine, reserpine, or clonidine. Clearly, this information seems to suggest that use of multiple medications (polypharmacy) contributes to the frequency of episodes of dizziness observed among women.[37] This finding is in agreement with that from a study by Hussain and colleagues,[38] which showed that the occurrence of adverse drug reactions to antihypertensive drugs was high among women and was greatly increased among those on combination therapy compared with monotherapy. However, for men, propranolol was the only antihypertensive drug associated with a significant increase in episodes of dizziness.[37]

Cleophas and colleagues[39] tested whether using the combination of a β-blocker with a negative chronotropic calcium channel blocker (amlodipine, diltiazem, or mibefradil) would cause intolerable side effects in 335 patients (aged 18–75 years) with chronic stable angina pectoris. This study was a 10-week, double-blind,

---

Box 1
A list of all of the FDA-approved medications available now to treat hypertension

Types of high–blood-pressure medicines

Angiotensin-converting enzyme inhibitors

β-Blockers

Calcium channel blockers

Peripherally acting α-adrenergic blockers

Angiotensin II antagonists

Vasodilators

Centrally acting α-adrenergics

Diuretics

Renin inhibitors

Combination medicines[a]

[a] An example of the combination medicines is amlodipine besylate and atorvastatin calcium (Caduet), containing an antihypertensive and a lipid-lowering agent. Combination medicines also include products containing more than 1 antihypertensive.

Data from US Food and Drug Administration, Office of Women's Health. High blood pressure—medicines to help you. Available at: http://www.fda.gov/forconsumers/byaudience/forwomen/ucm118594.htm. Accessed July 30, 2010.

parallel-group comparison of amlodipine 5 and 10 mg, diltiazem 200 and 300 mg, and mibefradil 50 and 100 mg treatment added to stable (baseline) β-blocker treatment. Serious symptoms of dizziness occurred in 14% of the patients, resulting in their withdrawal from therapy: 19 patients were on mibefradil (8 on low dose, 11 on high dose), 4 patients were on diltiazem (1 on low dose, 3 on high dose), and 9 patients were on amlodipine (4 on low dose, 5 on high dose).[39] Doses of diltiazem in this trial were low compared with the doses used in standard practice in the United States. It was observed that low-dose diltiazem caused fewer symptoms of dizziness, and fewer patient withdrawals were observed among low-dose mibefradil users. Therefore, these data suggest that patients in the United States (with higher dose standards) might experience more pronounced symptoms or higher incidence of dizziness with this combination of medications and doses.

On the other hand, Ko and colleagues[40] studied the adverse cardiovascular effects of β-blockers individually (carvedilol, metoprolol, bisoprolol, and bucindolol) in comparison with placebo. In this study, the investigators analyzed randomized trials on β-blockers in patients with heart failure and systolic dysfunction. The analysis included 9 trials involving 14,594 patients, with follow-up periods ranging from 6 to 24 months. The results showed that β-blocker use was associated with a significant relative increase in reported dizziness (relative risk, 1.37; 95% confidence interval [CI], 1.09–1.71) and an absolute increase with a risk of 57 per 1000 cases (95% CI, 11–104). The results further indicated that the increased risk of dizziness was accompanied by hypotension because β-blockers lower blood pressure by various mechanisms. In addition, the study assessed withdrawal from therapy owing to dizziness in 7789 patients from 4 trials. Overall, the investigators concluded that most patients in this study did not experience cardiovascular adverse effects (including dizziness) because the trials under review enrolled healthier and relatively fewer female and older adult patients.[40]

Angiotensin-converting enzyme (ACE) inhibitors have also been associated with dizziness.[36] Blakley and Gulati[41] illustrated the use of a practical new technique that may be useful in identifying groups of medications associated with dizziness. The patient group for this study included those who had electronystagmography at the Health Sciences Centre, Winnipeg, Canada. The mean age of the study group of 102 dizzy patients was 60 (±16) years, and these patients were taking a total of 173 drugs in 22 categories. ACE inhibitors were shown to be associated with dizziness. However, a similar association was not found with other antihypertensive agents. In general terms, the results indicate that antihypertensive drug use is more common in dizzy patients and that the pattern of drug use in dizzy patients is different from that of non-dizzy patients. In other words, dizzy patients take more medications, and the dizziness they experience may be attributed to polypharmacy.[41]

Ensrud and colleagues[42] performed a cross-sectional examination of the prevalence and correlates of postural hypotension, postural dizziness, and associated risk factors, including medical conditions, medications, and physical findings, in 9704 patients. The patients were non-black, ambulatory women, aged 65 years and older, living in a general community setting, participating in the multicenter Study of Osteoporotic Fractures. Of the risks identified, use of medications, specifically diuretics (odds ratio [OR], 1.15; 95% CI, 1.03–1.28), was associated with postural dizziness. However, these associations were only age-adjusted and might have been confounded by other covariates or risk factors.[42]

Finally, in an Oslo Health Study by Tamber and Bruusgaard,[43] a multipurpose health survey was conducted to explore the association between dizziness and factors such as self-reported diseases and medicines used. Results from the self-administered questionnaire showed increased likelihood of faintness or dizziness with use (weekly or more frequent use) of blood pressure medications (OR, 1.27; 95% CI, 1.11–1.45). However, the investigators did not provide the details of the type of high–blood-pressure medication used, making it unclear which particular class or classes of antihypertensives are directly associated with dizziness.[43]

BENZODIAZEPINES AND RELATED DRUGS

Benzodiazepines and related drugs (BZDs/RDs) are another group of medications commonly used in persons aged 65 years or older.[44,45] The likelihood of BZDs/RDs causing adverse events is high, and caution is advised.[45] Of particular interest, dizziness has been reported from a non-randomized clinical study by Puustinen and colleagues.[46] The primary objective of the study was to describe the relationship between long-term use of BZDs/RDs and health, functional abilities, and cognitive function in patients aged 65 years and older, who were admitted to 2 acute care hospitals in Finland. The association between BZDs/RDs and dizziness was established after adjusting for the confounding variables of gender and the number of medications with CNS effects. Moreover, these findings were observed following long-term use of these agents, and the effect of dizziness tended to be related to the number of BZDs/RDs used. Unfortunately, the investigators did not report detailed data supporting these observations. Furthermore, the investigators noted that the use of BZDs/RDs, even concomitantly with other BZDs/RDs, was common and long-standing in this frail population under study,[46] suggesting that the side effects experienced are likely to be attributed to polypharmacy.

SEDATIVE HYPNOTICS AND OTHER DRUGS

There is a paucity of data regarding drug-related dizziness caused by sedative hypnotics; only 2 studies were identified in the literature. First, medications other than antihypertensives were studied by Tamber and Bruusgaard.[43] This study showed an increased likelihood of faintness or dizziness between the use (weekly or more frequent use) of sedatives (adjusted OR, 1.60; 95% CI, 1.34–1.92), tranquilizers (OR, 1.61; 95% CI, 1.26–2.04), and other medications or prescriptions (OR, 1.35; 95% CI, 1.23–1.49). In this study, women reported faintness or dizziness more often than men in age-adjusted multivariate analyses. For cutoff points of dizziness (any trouble, a little troubled, or quite a lot and extremely troubled), an increasing number of medications used (1–6) was associated with an increasing likelihood of faintness or dizziness. Again, polypharmacy seems to play a role in causing dizziness. Surprisingly and in contrast to other reports, prevalence of dizziness was not observed to increase with age. In fact, on multivariate analysis there was no difference in cutoff points of dizziness between participants aged 75 or 76 years and those aged 30 years. The investigators noted, however, that because the study was based on self-reports, it might be influenced by recall bias, affecting the interpretation of the results.[43]

The second study is a meta-analysis to quantify and compare the potential benefits and risks of short-term treatment with sedative hypnotics in older people with insomnia, who are otherwise free of psychiatric or psychological disorders.[47] The meta-analysis included randomized, double-blind, controlled trials of any pharmacologic treatment of insomnia (including agents such as antihistamines, benzodiazepines, zolpidem, zopiclone, and zaleplon) for at least 5 consecutive nights; 24 studies (involving 2417 participants) with extractable data met the inclusion and exclusion criteria. Results showed that of the adverse effects identified, psychomotor-type side effects, such as dizziness or loss of balance, were reported in 13 studies (1016 participants) and were more common after treatment with a sedative than placebo, although the results were not statistically significant (OR, 2.25; 95% CI, 0.93–5.41; P = .07).[37] The investigators noted, however, that interpretation of the data must take into account that all sedatives or all benzodiazepines were grouped together for analysis, irrespective of differences in half-life, potency, or dose, and that a potential source of variability exists because the participants in the studies were from different settings. Although modest clinical benefits were observed with the use of sedative hypnotics, the added risk of adverse events may not justified these benefits, particularly in the vulnerable older adult population.[47]

ANXIOLYTIC DRUGS

There is also a paucity of data regarding anxiolytic medications and related dizziness. However, available evidence suggests that anxiolytic agents are associated with dizziness in older adult patients. Hale and colleagues[48] conducted a study to determine if the use of antianxiety agents is associated with more frequent complaints of CNS symptoms of dizziness, fainting, and blackout spells in an ambulatory older adult population. These participants were enrolled in the Dunedin Program (Dunedin, Florida). The results showed that 3 benzodiazepines (chlordiazepoxide, diazepam, and flurazepam) accounted for 87.2% and 79.8% of all anxiolytic drugs used by men and women, respectively. For women, statistically significant increases in reports of dizziness were observed in users of anxiolytic drugs compared with controls, although not observed in men. When reports of CNS symptoms were analyzed by individual drugs, few significant associations were found. Only users of diazepam reported a higher prevalence of dizziness than controls, probably because of the pharmacokinetic characteristics of diazepam in older adults taking multiple doses.[48] Diazepam accumulation is extensive and its washout is slow, and active compounds are present 2 weeks after the last dose.[49] However, the observed association of anxiety-related dizziness should be interpreted with caution. Dizziness may be a manifestation of anxiety itself, and therefore, the symptom may simply reflect the underlying condition being treated rather than the side effects of medications.[48]

Additional investigations from the study by Ensrud and colleagues[42] found that anxiety and/or sleeping medications taken at least once weekly (OR, 1.43; 95% CI, 1.26–1.62) were also associated with postural dizziness. However, the association was only age-adjusted, and thus, the strength of association obtained might be confounded by other possible risk factors of postural dizziness.

ANTIEPILEPTIC DRUGS

Epilepsy among older persons in the United States is common,[50] requiring frequent use of antiepileptic drugs. In addition, these drugs are commonly used off-label to treat conditions such as neuropathic pain and diabetic neuropathy, neuromuscular disorders, and behavioral disturbances in Alzheimer's disease and other psychiatric disorders.[51–53] In fact, it has been reported that the frequency of antiepileptic drug use is even greater in patients residing in long-term care facilities, ranging from 10% to 12%.[54] Dizziness is one of the most common adverse effects reported in clinical trials of antiepileptic medications, and it may occur even at therapeutic doses.[55] A summary of the side effects of the commonly used antiepileptic drugs is provided in **Table 2**. In particular, barbiturates, carbamazepine, felbamate, gabapentin, lamotrigine, levetiracetam, phenytoin, tiagabine, topiramate, valproic acid, zonisamide, and oxcarbazepine are reported to be associated with dizziness in older adults, and the dizziness is dose-dependent.[53] This list agrees with a recent study performed by the Agency for Healthcare Research and Quality (AHRQ) on the Effective Health

Table 2
Side effects of antiepileptic drugs

Drug (Brand Name)	Side Effects
Phenytoin (Dilantin, Phenytek)	Dizziness, ataxia, diplopia, slurred speech, decreased coordination, confusion, gum hyperplasia
Carbamazepine (Carbatrol, Equetrol, Tegretol, Tegretol XR)	Dizziness, diplopia, ataxia, vertigo
Valproic acid (Depakene, Stavzor)	Dizziness, nausea, diarrhea, vomiting, dyspepsia, weight gain, tremor, drowsiness, ataxia
Gabapentin (Neurontin)	Somnolence, dizziness, ataxia, weight gain, peripheral edema, fatigue, sedation
Pregabalin (Lyrica)	Somnolence, dizziness, ataxia, dry mouth, confusion, diarrhea, diplopia, blurred vision
Lamotrigine (Lamictal)	Somnolence, dizziness, ataxia, confusion, nausea, diplopia, sedation, headache
Topiramate (Topamax)	Somnolence, dizziness, ataxia, psychomotor slowing, anemia
Zonisamide (Zonegran)	Somnolence, dizziness, anorexia, nausea, irritability, sedation, confusion, headache, psychosis
Oxcarbazepine (Trileptal)	Somnolence, dizziness, diplopia, fatigue, nausea, vomiting, ataxia, abnormal vision, abdominal pain, tremor, dyspepsia, abnormal gait
Levetiracetam (Keppra, Keppra XR)	Somnolence, asthenia, infection, dizziness
Tiagabine (Gabitril)	Dizziness, asthenia, somnolence, nausea, nervousness/irritability, tremor, abdominal pain, impaired attention
Primidone (Mysoline)	Dizziness, sedation, ataxia, confusion, depression
Felbamate (Felbatol)	Insomnia, dizziness, sedation, headache
Rufinamide (Banzel)	Headache, dizziness, fatigue, somnolence, convulsion, diplopia, tremor, nystagmus
Lacosamide (Vimpat)	Headache, dizziness, diplopia, ataxia, fatigue, tremor, somnolence, blurred vision

Data from Refs.[53,55]

Adapted from Thompson D, Takeshita J, Thompson T, et al. Selecting antiepileptic drugs for symptomatic patients with brain tumors. J Support Oncol 2006;4(8):411–6.

Care Program for Epilepsy assessing the untoward side effects (including dizziness) associated with antiepileptic drugs.[56] However, the AHRQ report was general and included patients of all ages. Dose-dependent side effects are also demonstrated in the study by Thompson and colleagues,[57] in which dose reduction for older adults was recommended for valproic acid, gabapentin, and pregabalin.

Older adults may be particularly vulnerable to medications that compromise balance because of a variety of factors,[55] such as polypharmacy[58] and pharmacodynamic changes.[59] Pharmacodynamic changes at the organ system level involve age-related impairment of homeostatic mechanisms resulting in an exaggerated response to a drug.[59] Fife and Sirven[55] summarized the findings of primarily randomized controlled trials on the incidence of dizziness, gait imbalance, or ataxia in patients taking antiepileptic drugs compared with those taking placebo. In contrast to the study results by Thompson and colleagues,[57] primidone was included and was significantly associated with dizziness. According to the study by Fife and Sirven,[55] primidone and phenytoin are more likely to cause dizziness or imbalance than other antiepileptic drugs. The investigators noted, however, that the direct effects of antiepileptic drugs on balance are seriously under-studied, and they suggested that prospective trials are needed to better understand these effects.[57] Also, in the study by Ensrud and colleagues,[42] antiepileptic medication use was associated with postural dizziness (OR, 1.25; 95% CI, 1.03–1.53).

CONCLUSIONS AND RECOMMENDATIONS

Evidence from the available literature clearly implicates medications as a risk factor for dizziness in the older adult population. Use of 3 or more medications (polypharmacy) for all classes considered is associated with increased risk of dizziness. The association between polypharmacy and dizziness is also suggested in a cross-sectional diagnostic study of community-dwelling older adult patients.[34] This study found that the use of drugs in older adults was high: 33% of the dizzy patients used more than 5 drugs.[34] Kao and colleagues[25] made similar observations.

This review found that there is a paucity of available literature reporting detailed studies on medication-related dizziness. In fact, most studies have focused on cardiovascular and CNS agents, and there is insufficient or a complete lack of studies on other classes of medications. Alarmingly, in 2007, the top 5 therapeutic classes of prescribed drugs purchased by Medicare beneficiaries aged 65 years and older (ranked by total expense) were metabolic, cardiovascular, CNS, and gastrointestinal agents and hormones.[60,61] Of these top 5 therapeutic classes, metabolic and gastrointestinal agents are also associated with dizziness and are presented in **Table 1**. On this basis, the risk of medication-related dizziness may be underestimated. In fact, this limitation has been noted by Maarsingh and colleagues,[34] who suggested that the varying rates in reports of medication-related dizziness can possibly be explained by the fact that previous investigators may have underestimated the contribution of drugs as a cause of dizziness in older adults, because the reports studied only a small selection of all drugs potentially causing dizziness.[34]

It is crucial for physicians in clinical practice to have as much information as possible to make appropriate clinical decisions in the management of dizziness in the older adult population. Effective and safe patient care is challenging, especially for the vulnerable older population. As Salles and colleagues[26] suggest, one of the goals for successfully managing dizziness in older adults is to identify and reduce the risk factors of chronic dizziness to minimize physical, psychological, and social morbidity.[26] Dizziness must be carefully investigated to establish the possible cause and hence the appropriate intervention. To this end, the most important tools available to help the physician reach a diagnosis are patient history, clinical examination, and follow-up care.[19] Patients should be asked about details of their medication history; medical history, specifically systemic disorders that interfere with cerebral blood supply (such as vasculitis), which may produce vertigo due to either focal brainstem involvement or diffuse cerebral ischemia; description of the nature of the dizziness, including sensation, frequency, and duration; and any associated symptoms such as hearing loss, tinnitus, nausea and vomiting, and cranial nerve deficits. It is also important to determine the relationship between dizziness and position and motion.[6,26] The 10 instruments available to quantify functional effects of dizziness are listed in **Table 3**. These tools have been validated for use in older adults for detecting patient burden due to dizziness.[66,72]

Table 3
Standardized instruments for evaluating the severity and effect of dizziness on quality of life

Instrument or Tool	Domains	Items (n)	Scalability
Dizziness Handicap Inventory[62]	Activities that bring on or worsen dizziness, effect of symptoms on daily activities, emotional effect of dizziness (isolation, depression, fear)	25	1 overall scale (range, 0–50) and 3 subscales (functional, emotional, and physical)
Dizziness Handicap Inventory Short Form[63]	Activities that bring on or worsen dizziness, effect of symptoms on daily activities, emotional effect of dizziness (isolation, depression, fear)	13	1 scale (range, 0–13)
UCLA Dizziness Questionnaire[64]	Frequency and severity of dizziness, effect on daily activities and quality of life, fear of becoming dizzy	5	Not reported
Vertigo-Dizziness-Imbalance Questionnaire[65]	Characterization of dizziness and associated symptoms, effect on quality of life	36	2 scales: symptoms (range, 0–100) and health-related quality of life (range, 0–100)
DiNA[66]	Identify the priorities of older adults with dizziness, evaluate psychometric properties of dizziness	18 quantitative items except 1: presumed etiology	Likert scale 1–6, yes/sometimes/no, other predefined answers
Vestibular Disorders of Daily Living Scale[67]	Effects of vertigo and balance disorders on independence and on routine activities of daily living	28	4 scales: total scale (range, 1–8), functional subscale (range, 1–5), ambulation subscale (range, 1–8), and instrumental subscale (range, 1–10)
Activities-specific Balance Confidence[68]	Assess balance confidence in daily activities	16	0–100 response continuum
Vertigo Handicap Questionnaire[69]	Handicap of restriction activity, social anxieties, fears about vertigo, severity of vertigo attacks	22	5-point Likert verbal scale (range, 0–4)
Dizzy Factor Inventory[70]	Symptom factors, obvious responses of significant others to the dizzy, activity level	44	5-point Likert verbal scale (range, 0–5)
Vertigo Symptom Scale[71]	Acute attack of vertigo scale, vertigo of short duration, somatization scale, autonomic symptom scale	27	6-point Likert verbal scale (range, 0–5)

Abbreviations: DiNA, dizziness needs assessment; UCLA, University of California, Los Angeles.
Adapted from Sloane PD, Coeytaux RR, Beck RS, et al. Dizziness: state of the science. Ann Intern Med 2001;134(9 Pt 2):823–32.

Discontinuation of medications in older adults who are on complex drug regimens to manage multiple chronic diseases can be challenging, particularly when multiple prescribers are involved. Centrally-acting medications generally require slow tapering rather than an abrupt discontinuation to avoid withdrawal symptoms. This requirement is also true with β-blockers. Determining a specific medication-related cause for dizziness can, therefore, take time because changes are made to the medication regimen and symptoms are followed over time. Interestingly, most medication discontinuations or reductions do not result in adverse outcomes for older patients.[73]

Pharmacologic treatment with drugs such as meclizine (Antivert) is often recommended to manage dizziness in older adults.[74] Caution is advised, however, when prescribing meclizine for older adults. Meclizine is problematic because it is an antihistamine medication with anticholinergic properties.[75,76] Anticholinergic medications may contribute to adverse effects, including dizziness, confusion, memory impairment, falls, dry mouth, dry eyes, urinary incontinence, and constipation.[76,77] Because the anticholinergic adverse effects of meclizine include dizziness, the cumulative anticholinergic burden needs to be considered in deciding whether to prescribe this medication, because older adults may also be taking medications that are highly anticholinergic for incontinence and other conditions. Moreover, changes in sensitivity to anticholinergic medications have been associated with aging.[76] Because meclizine is available over the counter as Marezine (cyclizine), it is important to provide older patients with appropriate counseling regarding dose and frequency of use.

In addition, prescribing cascades involving anticholinergic drugs should be avoided. A prescribing cascade occurs when a medication is prescribed to treat the side effects of another medication.[78] Using meclizine to treat medication-related dizziness is an example of a prescribing cascade. Alternatives to the medication possibly contributing to dizziness should be considered before adding other medications. When anticholinergic medications such as meclizine are determined to be necessary, the minimum dose possible should be prescribed. Dose reduction may sometimes ameliorate the anticholinergic effects.[79] Overall, the management of a medication regimen requires careful risk-benefit assessment.

In conclusion, medication-related dizziness is an important consideration in older adults. Attention should be paid to older adult patients who are particularly prone to ADEs caused by polypharmacy, the changes in pharmacokinetics and pharmacodynamics, and the burden of comorbid conditions. However, more detailed investigations are needed to confidently assess the effects of specific medications on dizziness. The current evidence provides prescribers with some guidance on managing the potential effect of medications on patients presenting with dizziness. It is anticipated that the number of older adult patients presenting with conditions such as dizziness, possibly related to polypharmacy, will likely increase in the future as medication use increases in the expanding older adult population.

ACKNOWLEDGMENTS

The editors gratefully acknowledge Dr Perry D. Taylor's facilitation with this article.

REFERENCES

1. Colledge NR, Wilson JA, Macintyre CC, et al. The prevalence and characteristics of dizziness in an elderly community. Age Ageing 1994;23(2):117–20.
2. Stevens KN, Lang IA, Guralnik JM, et al. Epidemiology of balance and dizziness in a national population: findings from the English Longitudinal Study of Ageing. Age Ageing 2008;37(3):300–5.

3. Maarsingh OR, Dros J, Schellevis FG, et al. Dizziness reported by elderly patients in family practice: prevalence, incidence, and clinical characteristics. BMC Fam Pract 2010;11:2.

4. Newman-Toker DE, Hsieh YH, Camargo CA Jr, et al. Spectrum of dizziness visits to US emergency departments: cross-sectional analysis from a nationally representative sample. Mayo Clin Proc 2008;83(7):765–75.

5. U.S. Census Bureau. National population projections, released August 2008. 2008. Available at: http://www.census.gov/population/www/projections/2008projections.html. Accessed July 30, 2010.

6. Eaton DA, Roland PS. Dizziness in the older adult, part 1. Evaluation and general treatment strategies. Geriatrics 2003;58(4):28–30, 33–6.

7. Hayes BD, Klein-Schwartz W, Barrueto F Jr. Polypharmacy and the geriatric patient. Clin Geriatr Med 2007;23(2):371–90, vii.

8. Catania PN. Risk factors for drug-related problems in elderly ambulatory patients. Home Care Provid 1998;3(1):20–1, 24.

9. Hanlon JT, Lindblad CI, Hajjar ER, et al. Update on drug-related problems in the elderly. Am J Geriatr Pharmacother 2003;1(1):38–43.

10. Corsonello A, Pedone C, Incalzi RA. Age-related pharmacokinetic and pharmacodynamic changes and related risk of adverse drug reactions. Curr Med Chem 2010;17(6):571–84.

11. Tinetti ME, Williams CS, Gill TM. Dizziness among older adults: a possible geriatric syndrome. Ann Intern Med 2000;132(5):337–44.

12. Hilmer SN, McLachlan AJ, Le Couteur DG. Clinical pharmacology in the geriatric patient. Fundam Clin Pharmacol 2007;21(3):217–30.

13. Hajjar ER, Cafiero AC, Hanlon JT. Polypharmacy in elderly patients. Am J Geriatr Pharmacother 2007;5(4):345–51.

14. Hohl CM, Dankoff J, Colacone A, et al. Polypharmacy, adverse drug-related events, and potential adverse drug interactions in elderly patients presenting to an emergency department. Ann Emerg Med 2001;38(6):666–71.

15. Vinks TH, de Koning FH, de Lange TM, et al. Identification of potential drug-related problems in the elderly: the role of the community pharmacist. Pharm World Sci 2006;28(1):33–8.

16. Neuhauser HK, Radtke A, von Brevern M, et al. Burden of dizziness and vertigo in the community. Arch Intern Med 2008;168(19):2118–24.

17. Tinetti ME, Williams CS, Gill TM. Health, functional, and psychological outcomes among older persons with chronic dizziness. J Am Geriatr Soc 2000;48(4): 417–21.

18. Cigolle CT, Langa KM, Kabeto MU, et al. Geriatric conditions and disability: the Health and Retirement Study. Ann Intern Med 2007;147(3):156–64.

19. Sloane PD, Coeytaux RR, Beck RS, et al. Dizziness: state of the science. Ann Intern Med 2001;134(9 Pt 2):823–32.

20. Katsarkas A. Dizziness in aging: the clinical experience. Geriatrics 2008;63(11):18–20.

21. Kroenke K, Lucas CA, Rosenberg ML, et al. Causes of persistent dizziness. A prospective study of 100 patients in ambulatory care. Ann Intern Med 1992; 117(11):898–904.

22. Kwong EC, Pimlott NJ. Assessment of dizziness among older patients at a family practice clinic: a chart audit study. BMC Fam Pract 2005;6(1):2.

23. Inouye SK, Studenski S, Tinetti ME, et al. Geriatric syndromes: clinical, research, and policy implications of a core geriatric concept. J Am Geriatr Soc 2007;55(5): 780–91.

24. Hamilton HJ, Gallagher PF, O'Mahony D. Inappropriate prescribing and adverse drug events in older people. BMC Geriatr 2009;9:5.
25. Kao AC, Nanda A, Williams CS, et al. Validation of dizziness as a possible geriatric syndrome. J Am Geriatr Soc 2001;49(1):72–5.
26. Salles N, Kressig RW, Michel JP. Management of chronic dizziness in elderly people. Z Gerontol Geriatr 2003;36(1):10–5.
27. Samy HM, Hamid MA. Dizziness, vertigo, and imbalance. emedicine neurootology 2010. Available at: http://www.emedicine.medscape.com. Accessed August 4, 2010.
28. Lexi-Drugs. Lexi-Comp, Inc. Available at: http://online.lexi.com/crlsql/servlet/crlonline. Accessed August 4, 2010.
29. Arizona Center for Education and Research on Therapeutics (CERT). Available at: http://www.azcert.org/medical-pros/drug-lists/drug-lists.cfm. Accessed August 4, 2010.
30. Karatas M. Central vertigo and dizziness: epidemiology, differential diagnosis, and common causes. Neurologist 2008;14(6):355–64.
31. U.S. Food and Drug Administration. Adverse Event Reporting System (AERS). Available at: http://www.fda.gov/Drugs/GuidanceComplianceRegulatoryInformation/Surveillance/AdverseDrugEffects/default.htm. Accessed August 3, 2010.
32. U.S. Food and Drug Administration. MedWatch: the FDA safety information and adverse event reporting program. Available at: http://www.fda.gov/Safety/MedWatch/default.htm. Accessed August 3, 2010.
33. Kroenke K, Hoffman RM, Einstadter D. How common are various causes of dizziness? A critical review. South Med J 2000;93(2):160–7 [quiz: 168].
34. Maarsingh OR, Dros J, Schellevis FG, et al. Causes of persistent dizziness in elderly patients in primary care. Ann Fam Med 2010;8(3):196–205.
35. Miller GE, Zodet M. Trends in the pharmaceutical treatment of hypertension, 1997 to 2003. Research findings No. 25. Rockville (MD): Agency for Healthcare Research and Quality; 2006. Available at: http://meps.ahrq.gov/mepsweb/data_files/publications/rf25/rf25.pdf. Accessed August 4, 2010.
36. U.S. Food and Drug Administration, Office of Women's Health. High blood pressure—medicines to help you. Available at: http://www.fda.gov/forconsumers/byaudience/forwomen/ucm118594.htm. Accessed July 30, 2010.
37. Hale WE, Stewart RB, Marks RG. Central nervous system symptoms of elderly subjects using antihypertensive drugs. J Am Geriatr Soc 1984;32(1):5–10.
38. Hussain A, Aqil M, Alam MS, et al. A pharmacovigilance study of antihypertensive medicines at a South Delhi hospital. Indian J Pharm Sci 2009;71(3):338–41.
39. Cleophas TJ, van der Sluijs J, van der Vring JA, et al. Combination of calcium channel blockers and beta-blockers for patients with exercise-induced angina pectoris: beneficial effect of calcium channel blockers largely determined by their effect on heart rate. J Clin Pharmacol 1999;39(7):738–46.
40. Ko DT, Hebert PR, Coffey CS, et al. Adverse effects of beta-blocker therapy for patients with heart failure: a quantitative overview of randomized trials. Arch Intern Med 2004;164(13):1389–94.
41. Blakley BW, Gulati H. Identifying drugs that cause dizziness. J Otolaryngol Head Neck Surg 2008;37(1):11–5.
42. Ensrud KE, Nevitt MC, Yunis C, et al. Postural hypotension and postural dizziness in elderly women. The Study of Osteoporotic Fractures. The Study of Osteoporotic Fractures Research Group. Arch Intern Med 1992;152(5):1058–64.

43. Tamber AL, Bruusgaard D. Self-reported faintness or dizziness – comorbidity and use of medicines. An epidemiological study. Scand J Public Health 2009;37(6): 613–20.

44. Bartlett G, Abrahamowicz M, Tamblyn R, et al. Longitudinal patterns of new benzodiazepine use in the elderly. Pharmacoepidemiol Drug Saf 2004;13(10): 669–82.

45. Bogunovic OJ, Greenfield SF. Practical geriatrics: use of benzodiazepines among elderly patients. Psychiatr Serv 2004;55(3):233–5.

46. Puustinen J, Nurminen J, Kukola M, et al. Associations between use of benzodiazepines or related drugs and health, physical abilities and cognitive function: a non-randomised clinical study in the elderly. Drugs Aging 2007;24(12): 1045–59.

47. Glass J, Lanctot KL, Herrmann N, et al. Sedative hypnotics in older people with insomnia: meta-analysis of risks and benefits. BMJ 2005;331(7526):1169.

48. Hale WE, Stewart RB, Marks RG. Antianxiety drugs and central nervous system symptoms in an ambulatory elderly population. Drug Intell Clin Pharm 1985; 19(1):37–40.

49. Salzman C, Shader RI, Greenblatt DJ, et al. Long v short half-life benzodiazepines in the elderly. Kinetics and clinical effects of diazepam and oxazepam. Arch Gen Psychiatry 1983;40(3):293–7.

50. Leppik IE, Birnbaum A. Epilepsy in the elderly. Semin Neurol 2002;22(3): 309–20.

51. Rogawski MA, Loscher W. The neurobiology of antiepileptic drugs for the treatment of nonepileptic conditions. Nat Med 2004;10(7):685–92.

52. Roane DM, Feinberg TE, Meckler L, et al. Treatment of dementia-associated agitation with gabapentin. J Neuropsychiatry Clin Neurosci 2000;12(1):40–3.

53. Lackner TE. Strategies for optimizing antiepileptic drug therapy in elderly people. Pharmacotherapy 2002;22(3):329–64.

54. Cloyd JC, Lackner TE, Leppik IE. Antiepileptics in the elderly. Pharmacoepidemiology and pharmacokinetics. Arch Fam Med 1994;3(7):589–98.

55. Fife TD, Sirven J. Antiepileptic drugs and their impact on balance. Aging Health 2005;1:147–55.

56. Agency for Healthcare Research and Quality (AHRQ). Effective Health Care Program. Evaluation of effectiveness and safety of antiepileptic medications in patients with epilepsy (Evidence-Based Practice Center Systematic Review Protocol, 2010.). Available at: http://www.effectivehealthcare.ahrq.gov/ehc/products/159/463/EpilepsyCERProtocol6%252024%252010%2520docx-1%2520cmw%2520Posting.pdf. Accessed August 13, 2010.

57. Thompson D, Takeshita J, Thompson T, et al. Selecting antiepileptic drugs for symptomatic patients with brain tumors. J Support Oncol 2006;4(8):411–6.

58. Agostini JV, Han L, Tinetti ME. The relationship between number of medications and weight loss or impaired balance in older adults. J Am Geriatr Soc 2004; 52(10):1719–23.

59. Jackson SH. Pharmacodynamics in the elderly. J R Soc Med 1994;87(Suppl 23): 5–7.

60. Soni A. Expenditures for the top five therapeutic classes of outpatient prescription drugs, Medicare beneficiaries, age 65 and older, 2007. Statistical brief #280. Rockville (MD): Agency for Healthcare Research and Quality; 2010. Available at: http://www.meps.ahrq.gov/mepsweb/data_files/publications/st280/stat280.pdf. Accessed August 13, 2010.

61. Ruckenstein MJ, Staab JP. The basic symptom inventory-53 and its use in the management of patients with psychogenic dizziness. Otolaryngol Head Neck Surg 2001;125(5):533–6.
62. Jacobson GP, Newman CW. The development of the dizziness handicap inventory. Arch Otolaryngol Head Neck Surg 1990;116(4):424–7.
63. Tesio L, Alpini D, Cesarani A, et al. Short form of the dizziness handicap inventory: construction and validation through Rasch analysis. Am J Phys Med Rehabil 1999;78(3):233–41.
64. Honrubia V, Bell TS, Harris MR, et al. Quantitative evaluation of dizziness characteristics and impact on quality of life. Am J Otol 1996;17(4):595–602.
65. Prieto L, Santed R, Cobo E, et al. A new measure for assessing the health-related quality of life of patients with vertigo, dizziness or imbalance: the VDI questionnaire. Qual Life Res 1999;8(1–2):131–9.
66. Kruschinski C, Klaassen A, Breull A, et al. Priorities of elderly dizzy patients in general practice: findings and psychometric properties of the "Dizziness Needs Assessment" (DiNA). Z Gerontol Geriatr 2010;43(5):317–23.
67. Cohen HS, Kimball KT. Development of the vestibular disorders activities of daily living scale. Arch Otolaryngol Head Neck Surg 2000;126(7):881–7.
68. Powell LE, Myers AM. The Activities-specific Balance Confidence (ABC) Scale. J Gerontol A Biol Sci Med Sci 1995;50(1):M28–34.
69. Yardley L, Putman J. Quantitative analysis of factors contributing to handicap and distress in vertiginous patients: a questionnaire study. Clin Otolaryngol Allied Sci 1992;17(3):231–6.
70. Hazlett RL, Tusa RJ, Waranch HR. Development of an inventory for dizziness and related factors. J Behav Med 1996;19(1):73–85.
71. Yardley L, Masson E, Verschuur C, et al. Symptoms, anxiety and handicap in dizzy patients: development of the vertigo symptom scale. J Psychosom Res 1992;36(8):731–41.
72. Duracinsky M, Mosnier I, Bouccara D, et al. Working Group of the Societe Francaise d'Oto-Rhino-Laryngologie (ORL). Literature review of questionnaires assessing vertigo and dizziness, and their impact on patients' quality of life. Value Health 2007;10(4):273–84.
73. Iyer S, Naganathan V, McLachlan AJ, et al. Medication withdrawal trials in people aged 65 years and older: a systematic review. Drugs Aging 2008;25:1021–31.
74. Eaton DA, Roland PS. Dizziness in the older adult, part 2. Treatments for causes of the four most common symptoms. Geriatrics 2003;58(4):46, 49–52.
75. Rudd KM, Raehl CL, Bond CA, et al. Methods for assessing drug-related anticholinergic activity. Pharmacotherapy 2005;25(11):1592–601.
76. Rudolph JL, Salow MJ, Angelini MC, et al. The anticholinergic risk scale and anticholinergic adverse effects in older persons. Arch Intern Med 2008;168(5):508–13.
77. Mintzer J, Burns A. Anticholinergic side-effects of drugs in elderly people. J R Soc Med 2000;93(9):457–62.
78. Gill SS, Mamdani M, Naglie G, et al. A prescribing cascade involving cholinesterase inhibitors and anticholinergic drugs. Arch Intern Med 2005;165(7):808–13.
79. Lieberman JA 3rd. Managing anticholinergic side effects. Prim Care Companion J Clin Psychiatry 2004;6(Suppl 2):20–3.

Vestibular Rehabilitation of Older Adults with Dizziness

Muhammad Alrwaily, PT, MS[a], Susan L. Whitney, PT, PhD[a,b,c],*

KEYWORDS

• Vestibular rehabilitation • Elderly • Dizziness • Vertigo

Poor balance is common in older adults (65 years and older),[1] often leading to accidents and falls, and significant disability. Approximately 30% of the community-dwelling older adults in developed countries fall, with 10% to 20% falling twice or more each year.[2–6] Tinetti and colleagues[5] reported that 10% of those who fall sustain a serious injury, including hip fractures, dislocation, and head trauma. Nine of 10 patients who sustain hip fracture from falling are age 65 years or older. Twenty percent of patients who fall and sustain hip fracture die within 1 year.[7] Patients who fall more than twice a year are considered frequent fallers.[5,8] Older adults who fall often develop pain and a low level of confidence in their activities of daily living.[9] A lack of balance confidence may negatively affect functional abilities in everyday life and cause the older adult to change behavior to avoid falling. A change in balance confidence may result in restrictions of mobility and an increase in dependence on others.[3]

Loss of balance resulting in falls in older adults has been linked to dizziness.[10] Dizziness is a well-known problem in the elderly, with a reported prevalence of dizziness in 13% to 38% of older adults depending on the population studied (see article by Barin and Dodson in this publication).[11–13] Dizziness significantly affects older adults and is more common in women than men.[12] Sloane and colleagues[11] studied the prevalence of dizziness severe enough to require a physician's consultation or the necessity of medication and found that about 30% of community-dwelling adults experience such dizziness. In people older than 65 years of age, dizziness was found to affect

[a] Department of Physical Therapy, University of Pittsburgh, 6035 Forbes Tower, Pittsburgh, PA 15260, USA
[b] Department of Otolaryngology, University of Pittsburgh, 6035 Forbes Tower, Pittsburgh, PA 15260, USA
[c] King Saud University, Riyadh, Saudi Arabia
* Corresponding author. Department of Physical Therapy, University of Pittsburgh, 6035 Forbes Tower, Pittsburgh, PA 15260.
E-mail address: whitney@pitt.edu

Otolaryngol Clin N Am 44 (2011) 473–496
doi:10.1016/j.otc.2011.01.015
0030-6665/11/$ – see front matter © 2011 Elsevier Inc. All rights reserved.

functional ability in activities of daily living (ADL), which was significantly associated with reduced quality of life both physically and psychologically and with worsening of cognitive status.[13–15] Dizziness is also associated with fear and increased risk of falling.[10,16–19] People complaining of dizziness have more locomotor and mental disorders than those who are not dizzy.[14,20] These worsening physical and emotional states suggest the disabling nature of dizziness. Dizziness is often described in various ways by patients. **Table 1** provides common feelings described by patients and what these may mean to a physician.[21,22]

Numerous diseases/disorders cause dizziness.[20–24] Central disorders can include, but are not limited to, cereberovascular disorders (eg, vertebrobasilar insufficiency [VBI]) (see article by Ishiyama and Ishiyama in this publication), anterior and posterior inferior cerebellar artery stroke, migraine, multiple sclerosis, neurodegenerative disorders (eg, Parkinson disease), central positional nystagmus, and central vestibular disorders.[21,24] In older adults, migraine is not common as the primary cause of dizziness. Bath and colleagues[23] determined that the most common central diagnoses linked to dizziness were vestibulocerebellar degeneration (3.3%), followed by cerebrovascular accident/VBI (3.1%), and multiple sclerosis (2.2%).

Peripheral vestibular disorders are common causes of dizziness among older adults.[10,23,25–27] Dizziness in older adults may also be related to cardiovascular disorders[28] and the use of medications[29] (see article by Shoair and colleagues in this publication). People who report a history of dizziness are likely to have evidence of vestibular dysfunction.[10] In addition, patients with a history of more than 1 fall within the past year were often found to have vestibular dysfunction.[10] Disorders of the vestibular system are responsible for 40% to 50% of dizziness in patients referred to otolaryngology and primary care clinics.[30–32] Bath and colleagues[23] reported that the most common vestibular disorder is benign paroxysmal positional vertigo (BPPV). However, in addition to disorders that affect central or peripheral vestibular function, vestibular dysfunction can be caused by age-related structural deterioration of the vestibular system.[33–35] Elderly patients with labyrinthine diseases secondary to metabolic or vascular issues also benefit from a vestibular rehabilitation program.[36]

Table 1
Typical words used to describe dizziness in older adults

Descriptor of Symptom	Definition	Most Likely Cause
Vertigo	Illusion of movement either of the person or of the visual surround	Peripheral or central vestibular disorder
Disequilibrium	Imbalance or unsteadiness but without vertigo	Somatosensory abnormality Visual illusions Cerebellar disorders
Presyncope	Lightheadedness that occurs just before fainting without vertigo	Vascular problem
Psychophysiologic	Refers to combination of symptoms like floating, rocking, swimming, or internal spinning or a feeling of being removed from one's body	Anxiety disorders Central disorders

Data from Karatas M. Central vertigo and dizziness: epidemiology, differential diagnosis, and common causes. Neurologist 2008;14(6):355–64; and Kerber KA. Dizziness in older people. In: Eggers SDZ, David SZ, editors. Vertigo and imbalance: clinical neurophysiology of the vestibular system. Handbook of clinical neurophysiology, vol. 9. Amsterdam: Elsevier; 2010. p. 491–501.

INDICATORS OF QUALITY OF LIFE AND RISK OF FALLING IN OLDER ADULTS

Age-appropriate gait speed requires body support, timing, and muscle power. Gait speed is a suitable measure to assess an older adult's general health status and quality of life. Assessing gait speed provides quick, inexpensive, and reliable information regarding quality of life and risk of falling.[37,38] Similar to measuring blood pressure and body temperature to screen patients' general health status, gait speed can also be used to assess general health status and disability in older adults.[39] Improvement in gait speed has been shown to be a good indicator of treatment effectiveness, and slowing of gait speed can indicate a worsening medical condition.[39]

The Timed Up and Go (TUG) test is often used to assess a persons' ability to ambulate, rise from a chair, and turn, which can be difficult for persons with vestibular disorders. The time (in seconds) that is taken to perform the test is strongly correlated with functional mobility.[40] People who are able to complete the TUG within 20 seconds are found to be independent in transfer tasks such as moving from the wheelchair to a bed, and have sufficient gait speed (0.5 m/s) for limited community mobility.[40] At 0.5 m/s, subjects in this study were walking very slowly and were not able to ambulate freely in the community. Older adults who took 13.5 seconds or longer to perform the TUG test were classified as frequent fallers with an overall correct prediction rate of 90%.[38] Generally, the slower people move on the TUG, the more impaired they are functionally. Whitney and colleagues[41] investigated the sensitivity of the TUG test in identifying the likelihood of falling in people with vestibular disease. Persons who took longer than 13.5 seconds to perform the TUG were 3.7 times more likely to have reported a fall in the previous 6 months. They concluded that the sensitivity of the TUG test for fall prediction was 80% and the specificity was 56% in patients who scored greater than 11.1 seconds on the test.[41]

As mentioned, older adults who fall more than twice a year are considered frequent fallers.[9] Falls cause restriction of activities and thus a lower quality of life.[5,8] However, falls are often not reported by patients. A thorough multifactorial fall-risk assessment should be initiated when a patient reports having fallen.[35,42] Patients should be asked about their history of falls during the initial interview. Factors such as the fallers' vital signs, visual acuity, cognitive status, need of an assistive device and most importantly gait speed and balance should be included in the history and examination.[42] Assessment of medication use and obtaining orthostatic vital signs should be included in the initial physical examination of the older adult (**Table 2**).[35]

| Table 2 |
Older adults should be referred to vestibular physical therapy if they demonstrate the following
A positive Dix-Hallpike test
A positive Romberg test
Dizziness with movement of the head
Dizziness associated with neck pain
Slow gait
A history of fall more than 1 time per 6 months
An in ability to rise from a chair without using arm support

THE ROLE OF REHABILITATION IN PATIENTS WITH VESTIBULAR DYSFUNCTION

Dysfunction in the vestibular system can result in multiple impairments that lead to dizziness, an increased risk of falling, and ultimately a lower quality of life. Vestibular physical therapy plays a key role in improving function. Exercises, samples of which are described in **Table 3**, are provided for patients who report dizziness to eliminate or markedly reduce their perceived dizziness and to prevent falls. The use of vestibular exercises dates back to the 1940s when exercises were first introduced by Cawthorne[43] and Cooksey to rehabilitate patients with vestibular disorders. Currently, these exercises are used by various practitioners but mainly physical therapists who specialize in vestibular physical therapy.

Improvements after vestibular rehabilitation have been well documented, regardless of the patient's age and gender.[44–46] Exercises were found to be effective in people with chronic vestibular disorders (even with a history of symptoms lasting more than 20 years), patients with conditions that affect the function of the balance system (eg, stroke, Parkinson disease), and in people with anxiety and depression.[47–49] Telian and colleagues[50] found that 59% of patients with vestibular dysfunction had dramatic improvements in their dizziness and resolution of symptoms that affect their lifestyle after vestibular rehabilitation. In the same report, 23% of patients, despite some residual symptoms, had considerable improvement after therapy. Jung and colleagues[46] compared outcomes of vestibular rehabilitation in patients with dizziness versus those who did not receive therapy. The group receiving vestibular rehabilitation had significant improvement in dizziness and balance compared with the control group. Moreover, dizziness and balance improvement was reported 3 weeks after

Table 3
Exercises commonly used in vestibular physical therapy management of older adults with balance and vestibular disorders

Type of Exercise	Reason for the Exercise	Description
VOR adaptation exercises	Assist the central nervous system to adapt to a change or loss in vestibular system input	VOR x 1: The patient moves the head to both sides (yaw or pitch) while keeping their eyes fixed on a stationary target (**Fig. 1**) and (**Fig. 2**) VOR x 2: The head and the hand holding the target are moving in opposite directions with the eyes fixated on the target
Habituation exercises	Involves repeated exposure to a provoking stimuli or movement so the pathologic response to the stimulus is reduced	The therapist selects movements that provoke the patient's symptoms and the patient repeats these motions until the patient no longer reacts adversely to the stimuli
Substitution exercises	Promotes the use of the remaining sensory systems to assist with postural control	The therapist attempts to have the patient optimize use of an intact sensory system to substitute for a sensory system that may be providing either no input or an error message to the CNS

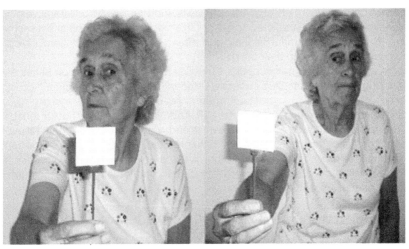

Fig. 1. Vestibulo-ocular reflex exercise (VOR x 1). An older woman performing VOR x 1 adaptation exercises in the yaw plane. The patient holds the target in her hand and moves the head to the right and left while fixating the eyes on the target.

vestibular rehabilitation compared with 3 months in the nonvestibular rehabilitation group, suggesting that vestibular physical therapy expedites improvement. Vertigo has been reported to be dramatically improved after vestibular rehabilitation and has been associated with significant increases in independence in ADL.[46,51] Significant improvements are evident in functional, physical, and emotional aspects of perceived dizziness and quality of life following vestibular rehabilitation.[47,49,51–54]

Exercises that focus on postural stability, gait, and gaze stabilization (see **Table 3**) contribute to the patient's ability to maintain balance and prevent falling.[55,56] Patients at 98% risk of falling, as measured by Berg balance test scores, responded to rehabilitation after one course of physical therapy, and the risk of falling dropped to 67%.[57] Macias and colleagues[57] determined that patients who had diagnoses such as stroke combined with vestibular dysfunction showed improvement without needing

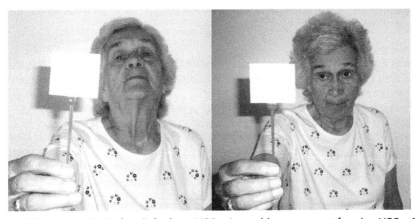

Fig. 2. VOR x 1 exercise in the pitch plane. VOR x 1: an older woman performing VOR x 1 in the pitch plane. The patient holds the target in her hand and moves the head up and down while fixating the eyes on the target.

to increase the number of physical therapy visits. Individuals with unilateral vestibular hypofunction who were predicted to be at high risk of falling on initial assessment, showed a 42% improvement in their gait after vestibular rehabilitation, indicating substantial improvement in their fall risk.[58]

Improving static and dynamic postural stability has positive effects on balance and risk of falling.[45] In a randomized controlled study, Yardley and colleagues[59] provided evidence of improvement in postural control, reports of dizziness symptoms, and emotional status in a primary care setting after administration of vestibular rehabilitation. The improvement was evident at 6 weeks and was retained at 6-month follow-up. Shepard and Telian[56] demonstrated that patients' static and dynamic postural control plus dizziness improved after vestibular physical therapy. Sense of disequilibrium and gait patterns improved after resection of acoustic neuromas after participation in vestibular exercise programs.[60]

THE EFFECT OF VESTIBULAR REHABILITATION ON VARIOUS CONDITIONS

Table 4 summarizes conditions that improve with vestibular rehabilitation and the positive outcomes that were found with each condition.

Peripheral Vestibular Disorders

Vestibular neuritis

Vestibular rehabilitation can assist a patient to recover functional abilities following vestibular neuritis (see article by Goddard and Fayad in this publication). The aim of vestibular rehabilitation is to promote neural plasticity in the central nervous system (CNS) and accelerate compensation (**Table 5**). Strupp and colleagues[61] reported improvements in postural stability in stance and vestibulospinal compensation after administration of vestibular rehabilitation exercises. Patients in the treatment group recovered faster in balance function and were able to resume normal daily activities (eg, playing tennis or returning to work) after rehabilitation.[61] Rehabilitation exercises, which are described in **Table 3**, are prescribed for a patient to accelerate central compensation via adaptation of the vestibulo-ocular (VOR) reflex, through habituation, and through use of the vestibulospinal reflex (see **Table 5**).[61,62] In a retrospective study, Komazec and Lemajic[62] concluded that early rehabilitation exercises are beneficial for patients with vestibular neuritis and satisfactory achievements were reported in an average treatment time of 2 months.

Ménière's disease

Patients with Ménière's disease should be referred to a vestibular rehabilitation therapist during an inactive phase of the disease to obtain support and education about the disease process. The rehabilitation therapist assesses the patient's balance abilities, strength, and provides advice regarding fall prevention during active attacks of the disease.[63] People with Ménière's disease with vertigo controlled by medical therapy or minimally invasive techniques can effectively benefit from vestibular rehabilitation to address disequilibrium symptoms associated with the disease. Exercises such as gaze stabilization, visual acuity, and static and dynamic postural exercises (see **Table 3**) were found to have some effect on the patient's balance function and gait.[64,65]

Chronic unilateral vestibular dysfunction (uncompensated lesion)

Patients with chronic unilateral vestibular dysfunction are good candidates for vestibular rehabilitation and have a good prognosis. Ninety percent of patients dramatically improve or completely recover postural control and disability status after rehabilitation

Table 4
Conditions that improve with vestibular rehabilitation

Patient Diagnosis	Noted Improvement with Vestibular Physical Therapy
Benign paroxysmal positional vertigo (BPPV)[a]	Subjective report of vertigo,[73,137–142] nystagmus,[73,138] quality of life[137]
Unilateral vestibular disorders	Fall risk,[45,143] vision[69,143,144] balance,[102,145] quality of life[53]
Chronic peripheral vestibular dysfunction	VOR gain and dizziness,[51,67] standing balance,[53,55,66] emotional status (ie, anxiety)[49]
Bilateral vestibular dysfunction	Postural control,[58,70,146] gait speed,[58,70] dizziness,[58,70,146] vision[147]
Vestibular neuritis	Ocular torsion (ie, nystagmus[61]), postural control,[60,61] ambulation skills, gait[148]
Postacoustic neuroma resection	Postural control,[60,149,150] dizziness,[77] motion sensitivity[60]
Ménière's disease	Self-report of symptoms,[64] balance,[64] dizziness, motion sensitivity[76]
Anxiety associated with vestibular disorder	Anxiety,[151] subjective report,[152] postural control,[151] presence of nystagmus, ability to cope with dizziness[59]
Cervical vertigo	Postural stability,[94] decreased neck pain,[153] intensity of dizziness,[94,153] postural sway[94]
Head injury	Gait improved,[82] postural stability,[82,154] less dizziness,[91] gaze stability[155]
Cerebellar disease and dysfunction	Self-perception of symptoms,[93,96] postural control,[93,96] gait,[96] decreased risk of falling[93,96]
Multiple sclerosis	Subjective report of dizziness and postural control[86,87]
Parkinson disease	Subjective complaint of vertigo[48]

[a] Medline search on July 27, 2010 revealed 512 papers on the search word "BPPV." Search was limited to randomized controlled trials in the past 10 years for the same search word and 17 papers were identified. Afterwards, only relevant papers were chosen.

provided they have no central disorders.[56] In a randomized controlled study, Giray and colleagues[55] provided evidence that patients with chronic vestibular dysfunction significantly improved with vestibular rehabilitation. Improvements were reported in dizziness symptoms, postural control, and physical and emotional status after physical therapy. Improvements after vestibular rehabilitation are correlated with plasticity and compensation mechanisms in the CNS.[66] Szturm and his colleagues[66] assessed changes in the VOR and found that vestibular rehabilitation exercises can induce compensation at the level of the CNS with resultant enhanced balance and less retinal slip. Moreover, a fast recovery in dizziness and visual analog scale scores has been reported in a patient with a history of more than 46 months of symptoms.[67]

Bilateral vestibular dysfunction
Although full recovery of symptoms does not occur in people with bilateral vestibular hypofunction, patients can benefit from vestibular exercise therapy.[58,68,69] Kerbs and

Table 5
Theories underlying vestibular rehabilitation

Theory	Brief Description	Function	Malfunction	Exercises
VOR adaptation	A reflex mediated by a 3-neuron arc including the vestibular afferent, the vestibular efferent, and the oculomotor motor neuron	Enables the stabilization of the image on the retina during head movement. Produces an eye movement of equal velocity to head movement but in the opposite direction. When the head moves to the right, the eyes instantaneously move to the left at the same speed of the head. This ratio of eye movement velocity opposite to head movement velocity is referred to as the VOR gain. In normal individuals, VOR gain should always equal 1	The eyes and head movement are not coordinated. The image stabilization on the retina during head movement is affected resulting in nystagmus and the sensation of oscillopsia	VOR x 1 and VOR x 2 (see **Figs. 1** and **2** demonstrating VOR x 1). It is thought that these exercises decrease symptoms of dizziness and improve function in elderly patients with vestibular hypofunction
Cervico-ocular reflex (COR)	Eye movement induced by neck stimulation during trunk rotation about a stationary head	The COR interacts with the VOR to drive eye movement based on input from the cervical proprioceptors	The COR may be adaptable in some people with vestibular hypofunction but not all patients. The COR is a response that is called for when needed and not all patients have the ability to use the COR	Body moving with the head stable

Vestibular spinal reflex	Input about body position is sent from the semicircular canals and vestibular nuclei to the medial and lateral vestibulospinal tracts to the spinal cord	Stabilize the body via increasing extensor muscle activities on the side to which the head is turned with flexion activity to the other side	Inability to maintain balance	Balance training and gait exercises
Sensory reweighting	Sensory reweighting consists of the 3 sensory systems: somatosensation, vision and vestibular	There are 3 sensory modalities through which the body maintains balance or controls posture	When somatosensation, vision, or vestibular function is lost or reduced, the central nervous system readjusts to become more reliant on the 2 remaining intact modalities	During vestibular rehabilitation the patient is repeatedly exposed to various sensory information so the brain can optimize postural responses to maintain balance

colleagues[70] performed a double-blind study in patients with bilateral vestibular loss and found improvements in ambulation speed, stair negotiation, and postural stability. Others have reported comparable results.[71]

BPPV

BPPV is common in older adults. Patient reports of vertigo or spinning sensations associated with changes in head position, which last up to 1 minute, are classic. Clinically, BPPV can be easily identified by provoking symptoms using the Dix-Hallpike maneuver. The Dix-Hallpike maneuver should be performed on all older adults complaining of dizziness. If BPPV is noted, patient referral to clinicians who are trained in canalith repositioning maneuvers is warranted (see article by Cho and White in this publication). Shepard and Telian[56] reported complete resolution of symptoms in 100% of their population after canalith repositioning maneuvers were performed. In a systematic review, Helminski and colleagues[72] established that there is strong evidence that canalith repositioning maneuvers are very effective in treating BPPV. In addition, Angeli and colleagues[73] have shown that 64% of older adults (age 70 years or older) improved with repositioning maneuvers. In patients who did not respond to repositioning maneuvers, 77% responded to another type of vestibular rehabilitation. Angeli and colleagues[73] concluded that a combination of the canalith repositioning maneuver and vestibular rehabilitation may improve outcomes in older adults.

Special consideration must be given when testing or treating older adults with BPPV. Because these maneuvers typically require approximately 30 degrees of neck extension and 45 degrees of neck rotation, patients with cervical issues must be repositioned cautiously. The treating clinician should consider having the older person's neck well supported during the Dix-Hallpike maneuver to prevent neck pain. Also, patients with low back pain or limited trunk/neck mobility should be cautiously treated with repositioning maneuvers because quick, unanticipated trunk movement might reproduce or increase their pain. Patients with osteoporosis or Paget disease are at risk for pathologic fractures. Thus, it is important to screen people with BPPV for these conditions before beginning testing or treatment. Most importantly, patients with severe rheumatoid arthritis must be treated with care because ligamentous laxity, especially within the upper cervical spine, is common and moving the neck beyond normal limits might cause serious injury to the spinal cord. Again, a tilting table should be used throughout the maneuvers to provide the desired outcome in persons with coexisting spine conditions.

In a study of persons not presenting to a clinic with a balance or vestibular disorder, 61% of older adults reported dizziness when asked.[74] Oghalai and colleagues[74] also reported that 9% of older adults had BPPV, plus those with BPPV had a higher percentage of falling in the last 3 months. These findings suggest that older adults should be screened for BPPV with Dix-Hallpike maneuvers. A Swedish study determined that BPPV is underestimated among older patients who present to primary care physicians with complaints of dizziness.[75]

Postsurgical conditions

The use of vestibular rehabilitation therapy aids in optimizing results after ablative vestibular surgery. Vestibular rehabilitation is recommended especially if reduction of symptoms (ie, vertigo or postural instability) after the ablative surgery does not match the surgeon's expectations, and the patient's condition does not improve. Dizziness after ablative surgery can be the result of incomplete or delayed postoperative compensation and thus, instead of proceeding to additional surgery, a trial of vestibular rehabilitation therapy (VRT) is advised when incomplete compensation is suspected.[56] Mruzek and colleagues[76] determined that less motion sensitivity and self-reported dizziness were seen in patients who received VRT after ablative surgery. Improved postural stability and decreased sense of disequilibrium were also reported in patients after acoustic neuroma resection.[60]

Patients with vestibular schwannoma resection noted significant improvements postsurgically after administration of a simple VRT exercise program and education.[77] The main improvements were reduced nystagmus at 2 to 3 weeks, less dizziness, and improved postural control.[77] Reduction of dizziness and improved postural control support the hypothesis that postsurgical VRT enhances central compensation mechanisms and suggest that simple VRT exercises such as VOR exercises should be prescribed after surgery.

El-Khashlan and colleagues[78] found that 89% of patients treated with VRT after surgery for acoustic neuroma reported improvements in their condition, and 86% of them walked independently one week after surgery. Functional improvements achieved through VRT after surgery occur relatively quickly (2–3 weeks) and can be accomplished with a simple exercise program.[60,77] Patients with Ménière's disease are excellent candidates for VRT after surgery and have a good prognosis.[78]

A few recent reports suggest that preoperative vestibular physical therapy may shorten the course of recovery after ablative schwannoma surgery.[79–81] Exercises that include movement of the head performed preoperatively helped patients avoid postoperative vertigo and symptoms of acute vestibular loss.[80] This pretreatment, also known as prehab, starts 14 days before the surgery and continues in the first weeks after surgery. Tjernstom and colleagues[81] reported that prehab treatment improved postural stability for up to 6 months after surgery in patients who underwent vestibular schwannoma surgical resection.

Central Vestibular Disorders

Patients who complain of dizziness caused by central disorders are harder to treat with VRT than those with only peripheral disorders.[82] Patients who have mixed peripheral and central disorders are challenging because of the complexity of their dysfunction[24] (see article by Cherchi in this publication).

Parkinson disease

Loss of postural reflexes and falling are cardinal manifestations of Parkinson disease (PD).[83] Koller and colleagues[84] reported that 38% of patients with PD fall, with 13% of them falling more than once a week. Thirteen percent of patients with PD who fall will sustain a fracture.

Vestibular rehabilitation exercises are believed to play a key role in plasticity and in central vestibular compensation.[66] Head and eye movement exercises were shown to be clinically beneficial in a patient diagnosed with PD with resting tremor and vertigo.[48] The patient's subjective complaints of vertigo were reported to be improved after VRT, and objective measures of gait and posture also demonstrated improvement. The use of VRT may promote the central compensatory mechanism by means of neural plasticity.[48]

Rossi-Izquierdo and colleagues[85] studied vestibular rehabilitation in a group of patients with PD who were at risk of falling using the TUG test. Patients who had scores greater than 15.9 seconds on the TUG were selected for the study. Investigators also assessed the patients' dizziness using the Dizziness Handicap Inventory (DHI) and the ability to control balance using computerized dynamic posturography (CDP). Vestibular rehabilitation exercises were effective in improving dizziness, ADL, gait velocity, and balance, plus reducing the risk of falling; changes persisted 1 year after treatment.[85]

Multiple sclerosis

Dizziness is a common complaint of patients with multiple sclerosis. Vertigo is the initial symptom in approximately 5% of patients with multiple sclerosis and 50% of people with multiple sclerosis experience dizziness at some time during the course of the disease.[21] Although it is still difficult to determine the effectiveness of vestibular rehabilitation for these patients because of the small sample sizes used in different studies, improvement after VRT has been reported.[86,87] Pavan and colleagues[87] reported a series of 4 patients in which vestibular rehabilitation was effectively used in patients with relapsing-remitting multiple sclerosis. Improvements were demonstrated after 2 months of vestibular rehabilitation with reports of less dizziness and improved postural control.[87] (Editor's note: anecdotal experience in our clinic suggests increased incidence of BPPV and BPPV recurrence in patients with multiple sclerosis, postulated to be the result of altered vitamin D and/or calcium metabolism in some patients with multiple sclerosis.)

Head injuries

Dizziness and vertigo are common with head injuries, especially in older adults after a fall. In cases where there are no severe consequences such as fracture or hemorrhage, 78% of people with head injury experience vertigo and approximately 20% continue to experience vertigo 6 months after the event.[63,88] Reports have demonstrated that the possibility of posttraumatic BPPV, Ménière's disease, and perilymphatic fistula occur after traumatic brain injury (TBI).[89] In addition, lesions of the CNS might impair the compensatory mechanisms in the central vestibular apparatus.[90]

In a patient with unilateral vestibular dysfunction after TBI, Herdman[91] illustrated that vestibular exercises improved the patient's symptoms. Although there was not complete balance recovery, the patient's postural stability improved considerably. Recent evidence suggests that persons can benefit from vestibular rehabilitation after mild TBI.[92] Age was not a significant factor related to recovery in persons with mild TBI[92] (see article by Akin and Murnane in this publication).

VRT is not limited to the conditions already discussed, although this review presents common examples of central disorders affecting vestibular system function that can be improved with vestibular rehabilitation. Patients with cerebellar disorders,[93] cervical vertigo,[94,95] vertebrobasilar artery insufficiency, and stroke can all develop dizziness that is amenable to improvement with vestibular rehabilitation.[24,95–97]

CONSIDERATIONS WITH VESTIBULAR REHABILITATION EXERCISES

Although improvements after vestibular exercise are established,[44–46] there are several other variables that affect the outcome of rehabilitation. As noted, people with bilateral vestibular dysfunction, despite reported benefit after therapy,[70] do not respond as quickly and as favorably to VRT as those with unilateral vestibular dysfunction.[98,99] Similarly, patients with central or mixed central and peripheral vestibular disorders show less successful rehabilitation outcomes compared with patients with peripheral vestibular lesion. Shepard and colleagues[100] reported that patients with pretherapy disability or a history of head injury are harder to treat. However, there has been improvement reported by persons with posttraumatic head injury.[92,100] Medications such as meclizine have been found to reduce or delay improvement.[101,102]

Customized or supervised exercises seem to be superior to generic or home-based exercises.[59,66,103,104] Customized exercises are believed to increase the patient's compliance. With customized exercise programs, the therapist regularly assesses patient progress and provides feedback to the patient regarding proper form while performing the exercises.[104] Szturm and colleagues[66] found significant improvement in patients with chronic unilateral vestibular dysfunction who were provided customized exercises versus those who received a general exercise program (Cawthorne-Cooksey exercises). Compensation mechanisms can be effectively induced by exercises that provide sensory feedback appropriate for behavioral changes to promote sensory-motor reorganization. Other variables that may delay compensation can be fear of falling, anxiety, multiple vestibular dysfunction, late physical therapy intervention,[105] impaired sensation including peripheral neuropathy,[106] and use of psychotropic and vestibular suppressant medications.

NOVEL INTERVENTIONS IN TREATING OLDER ADULTS WITH VESTIBULAR DISORDERS

In addition to the exercises prescribed to treat patients with vestibular disorders, there are new technologies that are promising for vestibular rehabilitation.

Virtual Reality

Virtual reality has long been used in the treatment of motor or psychological dysfunction.[107] This is a human-computer interaction-based technology (**Fig. 3**) allowing patients to participate actively in a real time three-dimensional virtual world, using images and graphics generated by the computer, creating the illusion of immersion in a real environment.

Patients who experience balance problems in a real environment can be trained to overcome these problems using virtual reality. Virtual reality provides an environment (eg, supermarket) similar to the real world environment, except that a patient is immersed in the environment in the safety of the clinic. Virtual reality technologies are decreasing in price and becoming easier to use in clinics.[108,109]

Use of virtual reality technology in vestibular rehabilitation may promote adaptation and compensation by creating retinal slip, which is an error signal occurring when eye

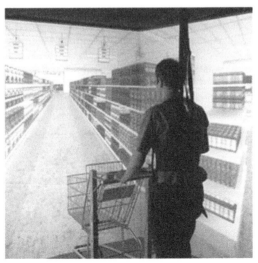

Fig. 3. A virtual reality grocery store. The patient is pushing the grocery cart at the self-selected gait speed and the scene moves at the same velocity.

velocity does not match visual target velocity, resulting in distortion or reduced distinction of objects of visual regard. Induction of retinal slip has been shown to improve balance in patients with uncompensated peripheral vestibular lesion.[66] Pavlou and colleagues[103] suggested that physical therapy involving conflicting visual environments may be more effective than traditional exercises. Virtual reality allows clinicians to control the treatment environment for patients in a safe manner.

Virtual reality may be used to provoke stimuli repetitively and quickly. Habituation exercises involve repeated exposure to provoking stimuli and are suggested to promote compensation and adaptation in patients with vestibular dysfunction.[110] Many patients complain of dizziness in places with complex visual sensory stimulation, such as supermarkets or shopping malls.[111] Postural sway in young and older persons with and without vestibular disorders has been shown to be affected by visual scenes in an immersive virtual environment.[109] However, it is impractical for vestibular physical therapists to monitor patient performance in real-life situations. Whitney and colleagues[112] reported that patients with unilateral vestibular lesions reported symptoms (ie, visual vertigo, space and motion discomfort) in a virtual reality grocery store that were similar to the symptoms they experienced in real-life grocery stores. With virtual reality, the therapist can dose the exercise in a safe environment and control the stimulation that provokes the patient's symptoms. Because maintenance of balance relies on sensory input from vision, proprioception, and vestibular function, virtual reality can work to reprioritize these senses when one or more are compromised. Patients who have compromised proprioceptive function and rely on vision to maintain balance can be immersed in a virtual reality environment to train the use of proprioception for balance control by frequently being presented with challenging proprioceptive cues. The exercises can increase the patients' ability to enhance postural control.[108] Suarez and colleagues[112,113] demonstrated that virtual reality can be used to treat older patients with balance problems and those at risk for falling. Patients showed less trunk sway and better postural responses after 6 weeks of treatment.[113]

Balance-enhancing Insoles

Reduction or loss of distal sensation in the lower extremities has been associated with aging.[114–116] Studies of patients with loss of distal sensation have shown a correlation of impairment of distal sensation with gait abnormalities, impaired balance, and increased risk of falling.[117–119] One promising technology that might enhance peripheral sensation is the stimulation of mechanoreceptors in the sole of the foot using a balance-enhancing insole (**Fig. 4**). The footwear insoles have a raised ridge around the perimeter to increase stimulation of the receptors in the vicinity of the outer ridge.

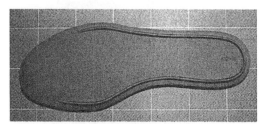

Fig. 4. Balance-enhancing insoles. The balance-enhancing insole is placed inside the shoe. The outer edge provides feedback to the patient about their postural stability. (*Courtesy of* Dr Stephen Perry.)

Perry and colleagues[120] investigated if these insoles improved medial-lateral balance control during gait, and whether benefits persisted after 12 weeks of wearing the insoles in daily life. The use of insoles influenced the ability to control body motion when walking over uneven surfaces. The stabilizing effect occurred during the most unstable phase of gait (ie, single support). The results were significant 12 weeks after use, which indicates that the brain did not habituate to cutaneous stimulation produced by the insole. Footwear insoles may play an essential role in maintaining dynamic balance and enhancing stability for older adults in the future.

Tai Chi

Tai chi is a traditional Chinese martial art that features slow movements, breathing exercises, and meditation. Breathing is coordinated with slow movement to achieve mind tranquility. It is practiced in a semi-squat position with adjustable intensities by increasing or decreasing the knee angle. Older adults tend to remain in the high-squat position.

Evidence in the literature supports the use of tai chi in people with a vestibular disorder.[121] McGibbon and colleagues[122] demonstrated that tai chi intervention resulted in improved gait speed and postural stability[123] in people with vestibulopathy; however, improvement in gaze stability was not evident after tai chi, and thus tai chi should be considered as an adjunct to vestibular rehabilitation.[122,123]

Tai chi has been shown to be effective at reducing the number of falls in older adults.[124] After tai chi training, both balance ability and plantar sensory function improved suggesting decreased risk of falling. Intensive tai chi training, performed for 1.5 hours in the morning 6 times a week, has been shown to be sufficient to improve balance in elderly individuals.[125] Balance improved with tai chi training, plus muscle strength, gait, lower extremity flexibility, and general mobility were enhanced.[126,127] One report advocates the use of tai chi to prevent decline in balance and gait in healthy older individuals.[127] Performing tai chi has also been shown to reduce the number of falls in healthy individuals.[128] Wu and colleagues[128] used telerehabilitation technology to exercise their patients using tai chi. Using telerehab increases compliance, and using tai chi resulted in a reduction in the risk of falling and improvements in balance. Tai chi once a week for 16 weeks significantly reduced the chances of falling in people older than 60 years.[129] Although further investigation is needed, these studies provide preliminary evidence of a promising intervention technique for older adults with vestibular disorders who are at risk of falling.

Vibrotactile Feedback Devices

Vibrotactile feedback devices (**Fig. 5**) are prosthetic devices currently being developed to help replace loss of self-motion information caused by disease, injuries, and aging. These prosthetic devices have been shown to influence postural control in standing and walking, and to reduce the risk of falling in older adults.[130] Wall and Kentala[131] demonstrated that vibrotactile feedback improved anteroposterior trunk tilt and trunk sway. Vestibulopathic patients were able to use information from the vibrotactile devices to reduce sway and imbalance deficits. Wall[130] also demonstrated improvement in tandem walking in vestibulopathic patients wearing the vibrotactile device. Trunk sway during tandem walking in vestibulopathic patients was significantly reduced, which suggests that risk of falling during ambulation may also be reduced. In older adults, gait was also significantly improved using the vibrotactile device.[130] Vibrotactile feedback devices might be used to enhance postural control under a variety of conditions and tasks. Patients with unilateral vestibular dysfunction who used a vibrotactile device demonstrated improved accuracy of stepping during

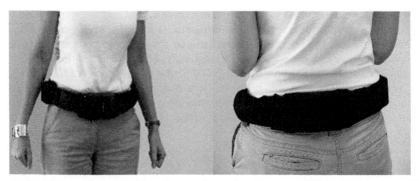

Fig. 5. A vibrotactile device. The vibrotactile device fits around the waist and provides augmented feedback about body tilt position. The anterior view (*left*) and the posterior view (*right*) of the vibrotactile device. (*Courtesy of* Conrad Wall III.)

walking and reduced trunk tilt.[132] In the future, vibrotactile biofeedback may be helpful with older adults to improve balance, although a recent report suggested that vibrotactile feedback might not be as effective in improving trunk sway and balance control when used in combination with a cognitive task (eg, counting backward).[133]

Optokinetic Stimulation

Visual vertigo is seen in some patients with vestibular dysfunction in which symptoms are provoked by strong visual-vestibular interactions (eg, supermarkets).[111] Habituation exercises aim to desensitize patients through continuous exposure to stimuli that provoke symptoms, and require patients to maintain balance when one or more sensory input is disturbed. Habituation exercises can improve patients' symptoms when they are combined with optokinetic stimulation. Pavlou and colleagues[103] concluded that customized vestibular rehabilitation using optokinetic stimuli is more beneficial than vestibular rehabilitation without optokinetic stimulation.

The Nintendo Wii

Several studies have investigated the use of the Nintendo Wii Fit to improve patient balance and standing posture.[134–136] Although no controlled trials have been published to support the use of Nintendo Wii Fit in patients with vestibular and/or balance disorders, some reports have shown significant improvements in patients with balance and standing posture.[134,135] The Wii Balance Board is a valid tool for assessing standing balance.[136] It is cost-convenient and easy to relocate compared with other laboratory equipment (ie, force platforms). The Wii is a promising technology that needs further statistically powered studies in patients with vestibular and balance dysfunction.

SUMMARY

Older adults with vestibular dysfunction can be helped with targeted exercise programs. Vestibular rehabilitation has demonstrated effectiveness in the treatment of older persons with peripheral and central vestibular disorders, but there is less evidence for the effectiveness of vestibular rehabilitation in older adults with central vestibular disorders and bilateral peripheral vestibular hypofunction. Dizziness and enhanced postural stability are typical outcomes of VRT. Improved quality of life and lower levels of anxiety have been shown after vestibular rehabilitation. Improvement in distal sensation and gait speed and marked reduction in the risk of falling have also been reported in older adults after VRT. There is strong evidence supporting the use of canalith repositioning maneuvers in older adults with BPPV. Innovative technologies in vestibular rehabilitation promise new interventions that may enhance treatment effectiveness for older adults with balance and vestibular disorders.

REFERENCES

1. Gordon M. Falls in the elderly: more common, more dangerous. Geriatrics 1982; 37(4):117–20.
2. Nevitt MC, Cummings SR. Type of fall and risk of hip and wrist fractures: the study of osteoporotic fractures. The study of osteoporotic fractures research group. J Am Geriatr Soc 1993;41(11):1226–34.
3. Nevitt MC, Cummings SR, Hudes ES. Risk factors for injurious falls: a prospective study. J Gerontol 1991;46(5):M164–70.
4. Sattin RW, Lambert Huber DA, DeVito CA, et al. The incidence of fall injury events among the elderly in a defined population. Am J Epidemiol 1990;131(6):1028–37.
5. Tinetti ME, Speechley M, Ginter SF. Risk factors for falls among elderly persons living in the community. N Engl J Med 1988;319(26):1701–7.
6. Watters CL, Moran WP. Hip fractures–a joint effort. Orthop Nurs 2006;25(3): 157–65 [quiz: 166–7].
7. Todd CJ, Freeman CJ, Camilleri-Ferrante C, et al. Differences in mortality after fracture of hip: the East Anglian audit. BMJ 1995;310(6984):904–8.
8. Gunter KB, White KN, Hayes WC, et al. Functional mobility discriminates nonfallers from one-time and frequent fallers. J Gerontol A Biol Sci Med Sci 2000; 55(11):M672–6.
9. Legters K, Whitney SL, Porter R, et al. The relationship between the activities-specific balance confidence scale and the dynamic gait index in peripheral vestibular dysfunction. Physiother Res Int 2005;10(1):10–22.
10. Agrawal Y, Carey JP, Della Santina CC, et al. Disorders of balance and vestibular function in US adults: data from the National Health and Nutrition Examination Survey, 2001–2004. Arch Intern Med 2009;169(10):938–44.
11. Sloane P, Blazer D, George LK. Dizziness in a community elderly population. J Am Geriatr Soc 1989;37(2):101–8.
12. Colledge NR, Wilson JA, Macintyre CC, et al. The prevalence and characteristics of dizziness in an elderly community. Age Ageing 1994;23(2):117–20.
13. Boult C, Murphy J, Sloane P, et al. The relation of dizziness to functional decline. J Am Geriatr Soc 1991;39(9):858–61.
14. Lasisi AO, Gureje O. Disability and quality of life among community elderly with dizziness: report from the Ibadan study of ageing. J Laryngol Otol 2010;124(9):957–62.
15. Hsu LC, Hu HH, Wong WJ, et al. Quality of life in elderly patients with dizziness: analysis of the Short-Form Health Survey in 197 patients. Acta Otolaryngol 2005; 125(1):55–9.
16. Olmos Zapata P, Abad Mateos MA, Perez-Jara J. [Fear of falling in the elderly with recurrent dizziness: a descriptive study]. Rev Esp Geriatr Gerontol 2010; 45(5):274–7 [in Spanish].
17. Perez-Jara J, Enguix A, Fernandez-Quintas JM, et al. Fear of falling among elderly patients with dizziness and syncope in a tilt setting. Can J Aging 2009;28(2):157–63.
18. Ekwall A, Lindberg A, Magnusson M. Dizzy - why not take a walk? Low level physical activity improves quality of life among elderly with dizziness. Gerontology 2009;55(6):652–9.

19. Burker EJ, Wong H, Sloane PD, et al. Predictors of fear of falling in dizzy and nondizzy elderly. Psychol Aging 1995;10(1):104–10.
20. Grimby A, Rosenhall U. Health-related quality of life and dizziness in old age. Gerontology 1995;41(5):286–98.
21. Karatas M. Central vertigo and dizziness: epidemiology, differential diagnosis, and common causes. Neurologist 2008;14(6):355–64.
22. Kerber KA. Dizziness in older people. In: Eggers SDZ, David SZ, editors. Vertigo and imbalance: clinical neurophysiology of the vestibular system, Handbook of clinical neurophysiology, vol. 9. Amsterdam: Elsevier; 2010. p. 491–501.
23. Bath AP, Walsh RM, Ranalli P, et al. Experience from a multidisciplinary "dizzy" clinic. Am J Otol 2000;21(1):92–7.
24. Furman JM, Whitney SL. Central causes of dizziness. Phys Ther 2000;80(2): 179–87.
25. Davis LE. Dizziness in elderly men. J Am Geriatr Soc 1994;42(11):1184–8.
26. Hoffman RM, Einstadter D, Kroenke K. Evaluating dizziness. Am J Med 1999; 107(5):468–78.
27. Chan Y. Differential diagnosis of dizziness. Curr Opin Otolaryngol Head Neck Surg 2009;17(3):200–3.
28. Maarsingh OR, Dros J, Schellevis FG, et al. Causes of persistent dizziness in elderly patients in primary care. Ann Fam Med 2010;8(3):196–205.
29. Tinetti ME, Williams CS, Gill TM. Dizziness among older adults: a possible geriatric syndrome. Ann Intern Med 2000;132(5):337–44.
30. Baloh RW. Vertigo. Lancet 1998;352(9143):1841–6.
31. Fuoco GG, Segal BN, Sweet R. Objective identification of dizzy patients by vestibulo-ocular and vestibulospinal testing. J Otolaryngol 1996;25(4):239–42.
32. McGee SR. Dizzy patients. Diagnosis and treatment. West J Med 1995;162(1): 37–42.
33. Matheson AJ, Darlington CL, Smith PF. Further evidence for age-related deficits in human postural function. J Vestib Res 1999;9(4):261–4.
34. Paige GD. Senescence of human visual-vestibular interactions. 1. Vestibulo-ocular reflex and adaptive plasticity with aging. J Vestib Res 1992;2(2): 133–51.
35. Furman JM, Raz Y, Whitney SL. Geriatric vestibulopathy assessment and management. Curr Opin Otolaryngol Head Neck Surg 2010;18(5):386–91.
36. Mantello EB, Moriguti JC, Rodrigues-Junior AL, et al. Vestibular rehabilitation's effect over the quality of life of geriatric patients with labyrinth disease. Braz J Otorhinolaryngol 2008;74(2):172–80.
37. Guralnik JM, Ferrucci L, Pieper CF, et al. Lower extremity function and subsequent disability: consistency across studies, predictive models, and value of gait speed alone compared with the short physical performance battery. J Gerontol A Biol Sci Med Sci 2000;55(4):M221–31.
38. Shumway-Cook A, Brauer S, Woollacott M. Predicting the probability for falls in community-dwelling older adults using the timed up & go test. Phys Ther 2000; 80(9):896–903.
39. Studenski S. Bradypedia: is gait speed ready for clinical use? J Nutr Health Aging 2009;13(10):878–80.
40. Podsiadlo D, Richardson S. The timed "Up & Go": a test of basic functional mobility for frail elderly persons. J Am Geriatr Soc 1991;39(2):142–8.
41. Whitney SL, Marchetti GF, Schade A, et al. The sensitivity and specificity of the Timed "Up & Go" and the dynamic gait index for self-reported falls in persons with vestibular disorders. J Vestib Res 2004;14(5):397–409.

42. Chang JT, Ganz DA. Quality indicators for falls and mobility problems in vulnerable elders. J Am Geriatr Soc 2007;55(Suppl 2):S327–34.
43. Cawthorne T. Vestibular injuries. Proc R Soc Med 1946;39(5):270–3.
44. Whitney SL, Wrisley DM, Marchetti GF, et al. The effect of age on vestibular rehabilitation outcomes. Laryngoscope 2002;112(10):1785–90.
45. Hall CD, Schubert MC, Herdman SJ. Prediction of fall risk reduction as measured by dynamic gait index in individuals with unilateral vestibular hypofunction. Otol Neurotol 2004;25(5):746–51.
46. Jung JY, Kim JS, Chung PS, et al. Effect of vestibular rehabilitation on dizziness in the elderly. Am J Otolaryngol 2009;30(5):295–9.
47. Cowand JL, Wrisley DM, Walker M, et al. Efficacy of vestibular rehabilitation. Otolaryngol Head Neck Surg 1998;118(1):49–54.
48. Zeigelboim BS, Klagenberg KF, Teive HA, et al. Vestibular rehabilitation: clinical benefits to patients with Parkinson disease. Arq Neuropsiquiatr 2009;67(2A):219–23.
49. Meli A, Zimatore G, Badaracco C, et al. Effects of vestibular rehabilitation therapy on emotional aspects in chronic vestibular patients. J Psychosom Res 2007;63(2):185–90.
50. Telian SA, Shepard NT, Smith-Wheelock M, et al. Habituation therapy for chronic vestibular dysfunction: preliminary results. Otolaryngol Head Neck Surg 1990;103(1):89–95.
51. Cohen HS, Kimball KT. Increased independence and decreased vertigo after vestibular rehabilitation. Otolaryngol Head Neck Surg 2003;128(1):60–70.
52. Zanardini FH, Zeigelboim BS, Jurkiewicz AL, et al. Vestibular rehabilitation in elderly patients with dizziness. Pro Fono 2007;19(2):177–84 [in Portuguese].
53. Meli A, Zimatore G, Badaracco C, et al. Vestibular rehabilitation and 6-month follow-up using objective and subjective measures. Acta Otolaryngol 2006;126(3):259–66.
54. Patatas OH, Gananca CF, Gananca FF. Quality of life of individuals submitted to vestibular rehabilitation. Braz J Otorhinolaryngol 2009;75(3):387–94.
55. Giray M, Kirazli Y, Karapolat H, et al. Short-term effects of vestibular rehabilitation in patients with chronic unilateral vestibular dysfunction: a randomized controlled study. Arch Phys Med Rehabil 2009;90(8):1325–31.
56. Shepard NT, Telian SA. Programmatic vestibular rehabilitation. Otolaryngol Head Neck Surg 1995;112(1):173–82.
57. Macias JD, Massingale S, Gerkin RD. Efficacy of vestibular rehabilitation therapy in reducing falls. Otolaryngol Head Neck Surg 2005;133(3):323–5.
58. Brown KE, Whitney SL, Wrisley DM, et al. Physical Therapy outcomes for persons with bilateral vestibular loss. Laryngoscope 2001;111(10):1812–7.
59. Yardley L, Beech S, Zander L, et al. A randomized controlled trial of exercise therapy for dizziness and vertigo in primary care. Br J Gen Pract 1998;48(429):1136–40.
60. Herdman SJ, Clendaniel RA, Mattox DE, et al. Vestibular adaptation exercises and recovery: acute stage after acoustic neuroma resection. Otolaryngol Head Neck Surg 1995;113(1):77–87.
61. Strupp M, Arbusow V, Maag KP, et al. Vestibular exercises improve central vestibulospinal compensation after vestibular neuritis. Neurology 1998;51(3):838–44.
62. Komazec Z, Lemajic S. [Specific vestibular exercises in the treatment of vestibular neuritis]. Med Pregl 2004;57(5–6):269–74 [in Serbian].
63. Whitney SL, Rossi MM. Efficacy of vestibular rehabilitation. Otolaryngol Clin North Am 2000;33(3):659–72.

64. Gottshall KR, Hoffer ME, Moore RJ, et al. The role of vestibular rehabilitation in the treatment of Meniere's disease. Otolaryngol Head Neck Surg 2005;133(3): 326–8.

65. Clendaniel RA, Tucci DL. Vestibular rehabilitation strategies in Meniere's disease. Otolaryngol Clin North Am 1997;30(6):1145–58.

66. Szturm T, Ireland DJ, Lessing-Turner M. Comparison of different exercise programs in the rehabilitation of patients with chronic peripheral vestibular dysfunction. J Vestib Res 1994;4(6):461–79.

67. Topuz O, Topuz B, Ardic FN, et al. Efficacy of vestibular rehabilitation on chronic unilateral vestibular dysfunction. Clin Rehabil 2004;18(1):76–83.

68. Minor LB. Gentamicin-induced bilateral vestibular hypofunction. JAMA 1998; 279(7):541–4.

69. Telian SA, Shepard NT, Smith-Wheelock M, et al. Bilateral vestibular paresis: diagnosis and treatment. Otolaryngol Head Neck Surg 1991;104(1):67–71.

70. Krebs DE, Gill-Body KM, Riley PO, et al. Double-blind, placebo-controlled trial of rehabilitation for bilateral vestibular hypofunction: preliminary report. Otolaryngol Head Neck Surg 1993;109(4):735–41.

71. Smith-Wheelock M, Shepard NT, Telian SA. Physical therapy program for vestibular rehabilitation. Am J Otol 1991;12(3):218–25.

72. Helminski JO, Zee DS, Janssen I, et al. Effectiveness of particle repositioning maneuvers in the treatment of benign paroxysmal positional vertigo: a systematic review. Phys Ther 2010;90(5):663–78.

73. Angeli SI, Hawley R, Gomez O. Systematic approach to benign paroxysmal positional vertigo in the elderly. Otolaryngol Head Neck Surg 2003;128(5):719–25.

74. Oghalai JS, Manolidis S, Barth JL, et al. Unrecognized benign paroxysmal positional vertigo in elderly patients. Otolaryngol Head Neck Surg 2000;122(5): 630–4.

75. Ekvall Hansson E, Mansson NO, Hakansson A. Benign paroxysmal positional vertigo among elderly patients in primary health care. Gerontology 2005; 51(6):386–9.

76. Mruzek M, Barin K, Nichols DS, et al. Effects of vestibular rehabilitation and social reinforcement on recovery following ablative vestibular surgery. Laryngoscope 1995;105(7 Pt 1):686–92.

77. Enticott JC, O'Leary SJ, Briggs RJ. Effects of vestibulo-ocular reflex exercises on vestibular compensation after vestibular schwannoma surgery. Otol Neurotol 2005;26(2):265–9.

78. El-Kashlan HK, Shepard NT, Arts HA, et al. Disability from vestibular symptoms after acoustic neuroma resection. Am J Otol 1998;19(1):104–11.

79. Magnusson M, Kahlon B, Karlberg M, et al. Preoperative vestibular ablation with gentamicin and vestibular 'prehab' enhance postoperative recovery after surgery for pontine angle tumours–first report. Acta Otolaryngol 2007;127(12): 1236–40.

80. Magnusson M, Kahlon B, Karlberg M, et al. Vestibular "PREHAB". Ann N Y Acad Sci 2009;1164:257–62.

81. Tjernstrom F, Fransson PA, Kahlon B, et al. Vestibular PREHAB and gentamicin before schwannoma surgery may improve long-term postural function. J Neurol Neurosurg Psychiatry 2009;80(11):1254–60.

82. Gizzi M. The efficacy of vestibular rehabilitation for patients with head trauma. J Head Trauma Rehabil 1995;10(6):60–77.

83. Bloem BR, van Vugt JP, Beckley DJ. Postural instability and falls in Parkinson disease. Adv Neurol 2001;87:209–23.

84. Koller WC, Glatt S, Vetere-Overfield B, et al. Falls and Parkinson's disease. Clin Neuropharmacol 1989;12(2):98–105.
85. Rossi-Izquierdo M, Soto-Varela A, Santos-Perez S, et al. Vestibular rehabilitation with computerised dynamic posturography in patients with Parkinson's disease: improving balance impairment. Disabil Rehabil 2009;31(23):1907–16.
86. Zeigelboim BS, Arruda WO, Mangabeira-Albernaz PL, et al. Vestibular findings in relapsing, remitting multiple sclerosis: a study of thirty patients. Int Tinnitus J 2008;14(2):139–45.
87. Pavan K, Marangoni BE, Schmidt KB, et al. [Vestibular rehabilitation in patients with relapsing-remitting multiple sclerosis]. Arq Neuropsiquiatr 2007;65(2A): 332–5 [in Portuguese].
88. Tuohimaa P. Vestibular disturbances after acute mild head injury. Acta Otolaryngol Suppl 1978;359:3–67.
89. Davies RA, Luxon LM. Dizziness following head injury: a neuro-otological study. J Neurol 1995;242(4):222–30.
90. Furman JM, Balaban CD, Pollack IF. Vestibular compensation in a patient with a cerebellar infarction. Neurology 1997;48(4):916–20.
91. Herdman SJ. Treatment of vestibular disorders in traumatically brain-injured patients. J Head Trauma Rehabil 1990;5(4):63–76.
92. Alsalaheen BA, Mucha A, Morris LO, et al. Vestibular rehabilitation for dizziness and balance disorders after concussion. J Neurol Phys Ther 2010;34(2): 87–93.
93. Gill-Body KM, Popat RA, Parker SW, et al. Rehabilitation of balance in two patients with cerebellar dysfunction. Phys Ther 1997;77(5):534–52.
94. Karlberg M, Magnusson M, Malmstrom EM, et al. Postural and symptomatic improvement after physiotherapy in patients with dizziness of suspected cervical origin. Arch Phys Med Rehabil 1996;77(9):874–82.
95. Revel M, Andre-Deshays C, Minguet M. Cervicocephalic kinesthetic sensibility in patients with cervical pain. Arch Phys Med Rehabil 1991;72(5):288–91.
96. Gill-Body KM, Krebs DE, Parker SW, et al. Physical therapy management of peripheral vestibular dysfunction: two clinical case reports. Phys Ther 1994; 74(2):129–42.
97. Cass SP, Borello-France D, Furman JM. Functional outcome of vestibular rehabilitation in patients with abnormal sensory-organization testing. Am J Otol 1996; 17(4):581–94.
98. Macias JD, Lambert KM, Massingale S, et al. Variables affecting treatment in benign paroxysmal positional vertigo. Laryngoscope 2000;110(11):1921–4.
99. Whitney SL, France DB. Bilateral vestibular disease: an overview. J Neurol Phys Ther 1996;20(3):41–5.
100. Shepard NT, Telian SA, Smith-Wheelock M, et al. Vestibular and balance rehabilitation therapy. Ann Otol Rhinol Laryngol 1993;102(3 Pt 1):198–205.
101. Konrad HR, Tomlinson D, Stockwell CW, et al. Rehabilitation therapy for patients with disequilibrium and balance disorders. Otolaryngol Head Neck Surg 1992; 107(1):105–8.
102. Horak FB, Jones-Rycewicz C, Black FO, et al. Effects of vestibular rehabilitation on dizziness and imbalance. Otolaryngol Head Neck Surg 1992;106(2): 175–80.
103. Pavlou M, Lingeswaran A, Davies RA, et al. Simulator based rehabilitation in refractory dizziness. J Neurol 2004;251(8):983–95.
104. Black FO, Angel CR, Pesznecker SC, et al. Outcome analysis of individualized vestibular rehabilitation protocols. Am J Otol 2000;21(4):543–51.

105. Bamiou DE, Davies RA, McKee M, et al. Symptoms, disability and handicap in unilateral peripheral vestibular disorders. Effects of early presentation and initiation of balance exercises. Scand Audiol 2000;29(4):238–44.

106. Vrancken AF, Franssen H, Wokke JH, et al. Chronic idiopathic axonal polyneuropathy and successful aging of the peripheral nervous system in elderly people. Arch Neurol 2002;59(4):533–40.

107. Rothbaum BO, Hodges LF. The use of virtual reality exposure in the treatment of anxiety disorders. Behav Modif 1999;23(4):507–25.

108. Virk S, McConville KM. Virtual reality applications in improving postural control and minimizing falls. Conf Proc IEEE Eng Med Biol Soc 2006;1:2694–7.

109. Whitney SL, Sparto PJ, Brown KE, et al. The potential use of virtual reality in vestibular rehabilitation: preliminary findings with the BNAVE. J Neurol Phys Ther 2002;26(2):72–8.

110. Norre ME, De Weerdt W. Treatment of vertigo based on habituation. 2. Technique and results of habituation training. J Laryngol Otol 1980;94(9):971–7.

111. Bronstein AM. Visual vertigo syndrome: clinical and posturography findings. J Neurol Neurosurg Psychiatry 1995;59(5):472–6.

112. Whitney SL, Sparto PJ, Hodges LF, et al. Responses to a virtual reality grocery store in persons with and without vestibular dysfunction. Cyberpsychol Behav 2006;9(2):152–6.

113. Suarez H, Suarez A, Lavinsky L. Postural adaptation in elderly patients with instability and risk of falling after balance training using a virtual-reality system. Int Tinnitus J 2006;12(1):41–4.

114. Gescheider GA, Edwards RR, Lackner EA, et al. The effects of aging on information-processing channels in the sense of touch: III. Differential sensitivity to changes in stimulus intensity. Somatosens Mot Res 1996;13(1):73–80.

115. Gescheider GA, Beiles EJ, Checkosky CM, et al. The effects of aging on information-processing channels in the sense of touch: II. Temporal summation in the P channel. Somatosens Mot Res 1994;11(4):359–65.

116. Verrillo RT, Gescheider GA, Bolanowski SJ, et al. Erratum; "When feeling is failing - the effects of aging on the sense of touch [J. Acoust. Soc. Am. 93, 2360 (1993)]. J Acoust Soc Am 1993;94(6):3518.

117. Richardson JK, Hurvitz EA. Peripheral neuropathy: a true risk factor for falls. J Gerontol A Biol Sci Med Sci 1995;50(4):M211–5.

118. Lord SR, Menz HB, Tiedemann A. A physiological profile approach to falls risk assessment and prevention. Phys Ther 2003;83(3):237–52.

119. Resnick HE, Vinik AI, Schwartz AV, et al. Independent effects of peripheral nerve dysfunction on lower-extremity physical function in old age: the women's health and aging study. Diabetes Care 2000;23(11):1642–7.

120. Perry SD, Radtke A, McIlroy WE, et al. Efficacy and effectiveness of a balance-enhancing insole. J Gerontol A Biol Sci Med Sci 2008;63(6):595–602.

121. Wayne PM, Krebs DE, Wolf SL, et al. Can Tai Chi improve vestibulopathic postural control? Arch Phys Med Rehabil 2004;85(1):142–52.

122. McGibbon CA, Krebs DE, Parker SW, et al. Tai Chi and vestibular rehabilitation improve vestibulopathic gait via different neuromuscular mechanisms: preliminary report. BMC Neurol 2005;5(1):3.

123. McGibbon CA, Krebs DE, Wolf SL, et al. Tai Chi and vestibular rehabilitation effects on gaze and whole-body stability. J Vestib Res 2004;14(6):467–78.

124. Richerson S, Rosendale K. Does Tai Chi improve plantar sensory ability? A pilot study. Diabetes Technol Ther 2007;9(3):276–86.

125. Tsang WW, Hui-Chan CW. Effect of 4- and 8-wk intensive Tai Chi training on balance control in the elderly. Med Sci Sports Exerc 2004;36(4):648–57.

126. Choi JH, Moon JS, Song R. Effects of Sun-style Tai Chi exercise on physical fitness and fall prevention in fall-prone older adults. J Adv Nurs 2005;51(2): 150–7.

127. Lin MR, Hwang HF, Wang YW, et al. Community-based Tai Chi and its effect on injurious falls, balance, gait, and fear of falling in older people. Phys Ther 2006; 86(9):1189–201.

128. Wu G, Keyes L, Callas P, et al. Comparison of telecommunication, community, and home-based Tai Chi exercise programs on compliance and effectiveness in elders at risk for falls. Arch Phys Med Rehabil 2010;91(6):849–56.

129. Voukelatos A, Cumming RG, Lord SR, et al. A randomized, controlled trial of tai chi for the prevention of falls: the Central Sydney tai chi trial. J Am Geriatr Soc 2007;55(8):1185–91.

130. Wall CI. Application of vibrotactile feedback of body motion to improve rehabilitation in individuals with imbalance. J Neurol Phys Ther 2010;34(2):98–104.

131. Wall C, 3rd, Kentala E. Control of sway using vibrotactile feedback of body tilt in patients with moderate and severe postural control deficits. J Vestib Res 2005; 15(5–6):313–25.

132. Dozza M, Wall C, 3rd, Peterka RJ, et al. Effects of practicing tandem gait with and without vibrotactile biofeedback in subjects with unilateral vestibular loss. J Vestib Res 2007;17(4):195–204.

133. Verhoeff LL, Horlings CG, Janssen LJ, et al. Effects of biofeedback on trunk sway during dual tasking in the healthy young and elderly. Gait Posture 2009; 30(1):76–81.

134. Shih CH, Shih CT, Chiang MS. A new standing posture detector to enable people with multiple disabilities to control environmental stimulation by changing their standing posture through a commercial Wii Balance Board. Res Dev Disabil 2010;31(1):281–6.

135. Shih CH, Shih CT, Chu CL. Assisting people with multiple disabilities actively correct abnormal standing posture with a Nintendo Wii balance board through controlling environmental stimulation. Res Dev Disabil 2010;31(4):936–42.

136. Clark RA, Bryant AL, Pua Y, et al. Validity and reliability of the Nintendo Wii Balance Board for assessment of standing balance. Gait Posture 2010;31(3):307–10.

137. Salvinelli F, Casale M, Trivelli M, et al. Benign paroxysmal positional vertigo: a comparative prospective study on the efficacy of Semont's maneuver and no treatment strategy. Clin Ter 2003;154(1):7–11.

138. Cohen HS, Kimball KT. Effectiveness of treatments for benign paroxysmal positional vertigo of the posterior canal. Otol Neurotol 2005;26(5):1034–40.

139. Munoz JE, Miklea JT, Howard M, et al. Canalith repositioning maneuver for benign paroxysmal positional vertigo: randomized controlled trial in family practice. Can Fam Physician 2007;53(6):1049–53, 1048.

140. Richard W, Bruintjes TD, Oostenbrink P, et al. Efficacy of the Epley maneuver for posterior canal BPPV: a long-term, controlled study of 81 patients. Ear Nose Throat J 2005;84(1):22–5.

141. von Brevern M, Seelig T, Radtke A, et al. Short-term efficacy of Epley's manoeuvre: a double-blind randomised trial. J Neurol Neurosurg Psychiatry 2006;77(8):980–2.

142. Simhadri S, Panda N, Raghunathan M. Efficacy of particle repositioning maneuver in BPPV: a prospective study. Am J Otolaryngol 2003;24(6):355–60.

143. Hall CD, Heusel-Gillig L, Tusa RJ, et al. Efficacy of gaze stability exercises in older adults with dizziness. J Neurol Phys Ther 2010;34(2):64–9.

144. Herdman SJ, Schubert MC, Das VE, et al. Recovery of dynamic visual acuity in unilateral vestibular hypofunction. Arch Otolaryngol Head Neck Surg 2003; 129(8):819–24.

145. Corna S, Nardone A, Prestinari A, et al. Comparison of Cawthorne-Cooksey exercises and sinusoidal support surface translations to improve balance in patients with unilateral vestibular deficit. Arch Phys Med Rehabil 2003;84(8): 1173–84.

146. Asai M, Watanabe Y, Shimizu K. Effects of vestibular rehabilitation on postural control. Acta Otolaryngol Suppl 1997;528:116–20.

147. Herdman SJ, Hall CD, Schubert MC, et al. Recovery of dynamic visual acuity in bilateral vestibular hypofunction. Arch Otolaryngol Head Neck Surg 2007; 133(4):383–9.

148. Cohen HS, Kimball KT. Decreased ataxia and improved balance after vestibular rehabilitation. Otolaryngol Head Neck Surg 2004;130(4):418–25.

149. Cakrt O, Chovanec M, Funda T, et al. Exercise with visual feedback improves postural stability after vestibular schwannoma surgery. Eur Arch Otorhinolaryngol 2010;267(9):1355–60.

150. Levo H, Blomstedt G, Pyykko I. Postural stability after vestibular schwannoma surgery. Ann Otol Rhinol Laryngol 2004;113(12):994–9.

151. Gurr B, Moffat N. Psychological consequences of vertigo and the effectiveness of vestibular rehabilitation for brain injury patients. Brain Inj 2001;15(5):387–400.

152. Jacob RG, Whitney SL, Detweiler-Shostak G, et al. Vestibular rehabilitation for patients with agoraphobia and vestibular dysfunction: a pilot study. J Anxiety Disord 2001;15(1–2):131–46.

153. Wrisley DM, Sparto PJ, Whitney SL, et al. Cervicogenic dizziness: a review of diagnosis and treatment. J Orthop Sports Phys Ther 2000;30(12):755–66.

154. Telian SA, Shepard NT. Update on vestibular rehabilitation therapy. Otolaryngol Clin North Am 1996;29(2):359–71.

155. Gottshall KR, Hoffer ME. Tracking recovery of vestibular function in individuals with blast-induced head trauma using vestibular-visual-cognitive interaction tests. J Neurol Phys Ther 2010;34(2):94–7.

Appendix:
PATIENT QUESTIONNAIRES
Dizziness/Vertigo

Because patients presenting with dizziness can harbor serious, if not life-threatening, conditions, several experts from this publication have provided sample patient questionnaires to guide the physician to better examine, diagnose, and treat the patient with vertigo.

Questionnaires provided by the **House Ear Clinic** and **University of Virginia** focus on important questions for the adult patient. The questionnaire provided by **Gianoli and Soileau of The Ear and Balance Institute,** in addition to providing essential questions, is useful for physicians evaluating the litigating patient presenting with dizziness. The questionnaire provided by **McCaslin and colleagues of Vanderbilt University** is suitable for children and adults. **O'Reilly and colleagues of Alfred I. duPont Children's Hospital** provide useful questions appropriate for pediatric patients.

Each questionnaire may also be downloaded from this publication online at www.oto.theclinics.com.

Otolaryngol Clin N Am 44 (2011) 497–507
doi:10.1016/j.otc.2011.02.002
0030-6665/11/$ – see front matter © 2011 Elsevier Inc. All rights reserved.

oto.theclinics.com

Questionnaire: Dizziness in Children

Structured Questionnaire for Differential Diagnosis of Dizziness in Chilldren

Nature of Symptoms					
Vertigo	☐ Yes	☐ No	Dizziness	☐ Yes	☐ No
Acute	☐ Yes	☐ No	Chronic	☐ Yes	☐ No
Paroxysmal	☐ Yes	☐ No	Continuous	☐ Yes	☐ No
Hearing loss	☐ Yes	☐ No			
Age, years	☐ >5	☐ ≤5			
Change of symptoms with head position	☐ Yes	☐ No			
Associated symptoms					
Headache	☐ Yes	☐ No			
Fever	☐ Yes	☐ No			
Vomiting	☐ Yes	☐ No			
Anxiety	☐ Yes	☐ No			
Depression	☐ Yes	☐ No			
Change in consciousness	☐ Yes	☐ No			
Head trauma	☐ Yes	☐ No			
Drugs	☐ Yes	☐ No			
Family medical history					
Hearing loss	☐ Yes	☐ No			
Migraine	☐ Yes	☐ No			
Seizures	☐ Yes	☐ No			
Neurologic examination	☐ Normal	☐ Abnormal			
Physical examination	☐ Normal	☐ Abnormal			

Provided by Devin L. McCaslin PhD, Gary P. Jacobson PhD, Jill Gruenwald AuD

Dizziness Questionnaire

A series of focused questions will differentiate the nature of the pathology in most patients.

Based on the work of G. Michael Halmagyi GH. History II. Patient with Vertigo. In: Disorders of the Vestibular System. Baloh RW, Halmagyi GH, Editors. Oxford University Press 1996. p. 171-177.

QUESTION	CLINICAL INFORMATION
What does it feel like?	• Is this vestibular / labyrinthine (vertigo) or something else (presyncope, syncope, seizure)
What other symptoms are associated with it?	• Declining hearing after head trauma (EVA) • Tinnitus, hearing loss (hydrops) • Dysarthria, diplopia, paresthesias(vertibrobasilar disease) • Cranial nerve weakness (skull base, intracranial lesions) • Headache, paroxysmal torticollis (migraine, BRVC) • Sweating, palpitations, dyspnea (orthostasis, panic, attacks)
How long do the symptoms last and how many have occurred?	• Seconds – minutes (BPPV) • Hours (TIA, migrant, hydrops) • Days – weeks (labyrinthitis, vestibular neuritis)
What makes it better or worse?	• Vestibular generated vertigo always worse with movement • Rolling, bending (BPPV) • Valsalva (PLF)
What is the background history?	• Otologic disease (PLF, labyrinthitis, BPPV) • SNHL (syndromic/ non-syndromic / congenital vs. acquired /), ototoxic medications, congenital or acquired vestibular hypofunction • Neuropathies (peripheral neuropathy) • Vascular disease (congenital cardiopulmonary disease, von Hippel-Lindau with, intracranial vascular lesions) • Family history neoplasms (NF-2, Gorlin's syndrome, Costello Syndrome) (acoustic neuroma, medulloblastoma) • Anxiety/depression (panic attacks) • Motion intolerance (migraine) • Family history of balance disorders (periodic ataxias, migraine, hereditary vestibulopathy) • Autoimmune disease (autoimmune inner ear disease) • Seizure history (temporal lobe seizures) • Ophthalmologic disease (Oculomotor anomaly, amblyopia, disorders of acuity,depth perception

HOUSE EAR CLINIC, INC.
2100 West Third Street, 1st Floor
Los Angeles, California 90057

DIZZINESS QUESTIONNAIRE

Name_____ Date_____

I   When you are "dizzy" do you experience any of the following sensations? Please read the entire list first.

Then check **yes** or **no** to describe your feelings most accurately.

Yes ☐ No ☐   1. Lightheadedness or swimming sensation in the head.

Yes ☐ No ☐   2. Blacking out or loss of consciousness.

Yes ☐ No ☐   3. Tendency to fall: To the right?

Yes ☐ No ☐   To the left?

Yes ☐ No ☐   Forward?

Yes ☐ No ☐   Backward?

Yes ☐ No ☐   4. Objects spinning or turning around you.

Yes ☐ No ☐   5. Sensation that you are turning or spinning inside, with outside objects remaining stationary.

Yes ☐ No ☐   6. Sensation of the environment moving up and down while you walk.

Yes ☐ No ☐   7. Loss of balance when walking: Veering to the right?

Yes ☐ No ☐   Veering to the left?

Yes ☐ No ☐   8. Headache.

Yes ☐ No ☐   9. Nausea or vomiting.

Yes ☐ No ☐   10. Pressure in the head.

Yes ☐ No ☐   11. Palpitations, perspiration, shortness of breath, or a feeling of panic.

II   Please check **yes** or **no** and fill in the blank spaces. **Answer all questions.**

                1. My dizziness is:

Yes ☐ No ☐   Constant?

Yes ☐ No ☐   In attacks?

                2. When did dizziness first occur?_____

                3. If in attacks: How often?_____

                    How long do they last?_____

                    When was the last attack?_____

Yes ☐ No ☐   Do you have any warning that the attack is about to start?

Yes ☐ No ☐   Do they occur at any particular time of day or night?

Yes ☐ No ☐   Are you completely free of dizziness between attacks?

Yes ☐ No ☐   4. Does change of position make you dizzy?

Yes ☐ No ☐   5. Do you have trouble walking in the dark?

Yes ☐ No ☐   6. When you are dizzy, must you support yourself when standing?

(Please turn page and finish questionnaire.)

Yes ☐ No ☐ 7. Do you know of any possible cause of your dizziness? What?_____

8. Do you know of anything that will:

Yes ☐ No ☐   Stop your dizziness or make it better?_____

Yes ☐ No ☐   Make your dizziness worse?_____

Yes ☐ No ☐   Precipitate an attack?_____

(Fatigue? Exertion? Hunger? Menstrual Period? Stress? Emotional? Upset?)

Yes ☐ No ☐ 9. Were you exposed to any irritating fumes, paints, etc., at the onset of dizziness?

Yes ☐ No ☐ 10. **If you are allergic** to any medications, please list: _____

_____

Yes ☐ No ☐ 11. If you ever injured your head, were you unconscious?

Yes ☐ No ☐ 12. **If you take any medications** regularly, for any reason, please list: _____

_____

Yes ☐ No ☐ 13. Do you use tobacco in any form?_____ How much?_____

III Do you have any of the following symptoms? Please check **yes** or **no** and check **ear** involved.

Yes ☐ No ☐ 1. Difficult in hearing?   Both ears ☐ Right ☐ Left ☐

Yes ☐ No ☐ 2. Noise in your ears?   Both ears ☐ Right ☐ Left ☐

2a. How loud is your tinnitus or head noise most of the time?

☐ None   No head noise.

☐ Very Soft   Heard only in a quiet situation.

☐ Moderate   Heard only in an ordinary situation.

☐ Loud   Heard and noticed in all situations, even
                when concentrating on something else.

2b. Describe the noise_____

2c. Does noise change with dizziness? If so, how?_____

_____

Yes ☐ No ☐ 3. Fullness of stuffiness in your ears?   Both ears ☐ Right ☐ Left ☐

Yes ☐ No ☐ 4. Pain in your ears?   Both ears ☐ Right ☐ Left ☐

Yes ☐ No ☐ 5. Discharge from your ears?   Both ears ☐ Right ☐ Left ☐

IV Have you ever experienced any of the following symptoms? Please check **yes** or **no** and check **constant** or in **episodes.**

Yes ☐ No ☐ 1. Double Vision, blurred vision or blindness. Constant ☐ In Episodes ☐

Yes ☐ No ☐ 2. Numbness of face.   Constant ☐ In Episodes ☐

Yes ☐ No ☐ 3. Numbness of arms or legs.   Constant ☐ In Episodes ☐

Yes ☐ No ☐ 4. Weakness in arms or legs.   Constant ☐ In Episodes ☐

Yes ☐ No ☐ 5. Clumsiness of arms or legs. Constant ☐ In Episodes ☐

Yes ☐ No ☐ 6. Confusion of loss of consciousness. Constant ☐ In Episodes ☐

Yes ☐ No ☐ 7. Difficulty with speech.   Constant ☐ In Episodes ☐

Yes ☐ No ☐ 8. Difficulty with swallowing. Constant ☐ In Episodes ☐

Yes ☐ No ☐ 9. Pain in the neck or shoulder. Constant ☐ In Episodes ☐

Yes ☐ No ☐ 10. Seasickness or car sickness Constant ☐ In Episodes ☐

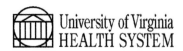 **University of Virginia HEALTH SYSTEM**

Vestibular & Balance Center
415 Ray C. Hunt Drive
University of Virginia Medical Center,
PO Box 800871, Charlottesville, Virginia 22908
(434) 924-2050   FAX (434) 982-0700

Dizziness Questionnaire

Name:_____ Age: _____ Date: _____

Please answer these questions as completely as possible **and bring with you to your scheduled appointment**. If you are unsure of any questions, please discuss them at the time of your evaluation.

When did your symptoms begin? _____
Did they begin gradually _____ or suddenly _____?
Is your dizziness constant _____ or in spells _____?
  If spells, how often do the spells occur? _____
  How long does each spell last? _____
  In between spells, are you free of your dizziness? Yes ____ No____
Are your symptoms getting better ____, worse ____, or are they the same ___?
Does motion cause your symptoms? Yes _____ No ____
Does motion make your symptoms worse? Yes ____ No ____
  If yes, which direction, right, left or both? _____

Describe your dizziness (check all that apply):

__Spinning of yourself   __Lightheadedness
__Objects spinning around you   __Swimming sensations in your head
__Imbalance or unsteadiness   __Weakness
__Blackout or faint   __Other

Do you experience any other symptoms before, during or after your dizziness?

__Headaches   __Nausea
__Pressure in the head   __Vomiting
__Ear pain or pressure   __Weakness in arms or legs
__Numbness in your face, arms, or legs __Difficulty speaking or swallowing
__Blurred or double vision

Do you experience loss of balance while walking? Yes _____No ____
  If yes, do you veer more often to the right ____or left ____?
Do you have difficulty walking in the dark? Yes ____ No ____
Have you fallen? No__ Yes__ How many times? _____ Which direction? _____

over

Medical History

Do you have any difficulty hearing? Yes _____ No_____
  If yes, which ear? Right _____ Left _____ Both_____
  If yes, does your hearing fluctuate (go up and down)? Yes ____ No ____
Do you have any noises in your ears? Yes _____ No _____
  If yes, is it constant _____ or intermittent _____?
   Right ear _____ Left ear _____ Both ears _____
Do you ever feel fullness or stuffiness in your ears? Yes ____ No ____
Have you ever had any ear surgery? Yes ____ No ____
  If yes, please describe (which ear, type of surgery, and when)

_____

_____

Do you have, or have you ever had, any of the following?

    __Diabetes   __High blood pressure
    __Asthma   __Heart attack
    __Sinus problems   __Stroke
    __Head injury   __Cataract
    __Neck or back injury   __Glaucoma
    __Seizures   __ Arthritis
    __Osteoporosis

What medications do you take on a regular basis? (prescription and over–the-counter)

_____

_____

_____

On a scale of 0 to 10, indicate the influence your dizziness has on your life.
(Circle your answer)

It doesn't   *I cannot*
bother me   *function*

0   **1**   **2**   **3**   **4**   **5**   **6**   **7**   **8**   **9**   **10**

UNIVERSITY OF VIRGINIA VESTIBULAR & BALANCE CENTER

The Ear and Balance Institute, Inc.

James S. Soileau, M.D.   Gerard J. Gianoli, M.D.
17050 Medical Center Drive, Suite 315
Baton Rouge, LA 70816
Phone (225) 293-6973 Fax (225) 293-0788

Name: Age: _____ ⬜Male ⬜Female

Occupation: _____ **Date:** _____

Name of Referring Dr.: _____ **Account#:** _____

Please circle either a Yes or No and reply to the following questions. Where indicated, fill in the blanks with your own words as completely as possible, or circle the appropriate word or words.

Audiology

1.   Y   N   Do you have any trouble hearing?
              Right   Left   Both Ears

2.   When did you first notice you had a loss of hearing?

              _____
              Describe onset: Sudden   Gradual

3.   Which is your "better" ear
              Right   Left   Same

4.   Y   N   Does your hearing seem better on some days than others?
              Right   Left   Both Ears

5.   Y   N   Do you seem to hear any noises such as buzzing, ringing, roaring, popping?

              _____
              Right   Left   Both Ears
              Describe the noise: _____
              Describe the onset: _____
              Is this noise continuous or intermittent? _____

6.   Y   N   Have you noticed a fullness or stiffness in your ears?
              Right   Left   Both Ears

7.   Y   N   Do you ever have pain in your ears?
              Right   Left   Both Ears

8.   Y   N   Have you ever had drainage or discharge from your ears?
              Right   Left   Both Ears

9.   Y   N   Have you ever had ear surgery?
              Right   Left   Both Ears
              Type of Surgery: _____
              Surgeon: _____ When: _____ Where: _____
              Type of Surgery: _____
              Surgeon: _____ When: _____ Where: _____

10.	Y	N	Have you ever been exposed to loud noise(s)?
			Please describe: _____
11.	Y	N	Does any member of your family have a hearing problem?
			Which family members? _____
12.	Y	N	Have you ever worn a hearing aid?

Vestibular

13.	Y	N	Have you ever suffered with dizziness or unsteadiness?
			Please describe: _____
14.	Y	N	Does any change in head or body position make the dizziness worse?
			Please describe: _____
15.	Y	N	Does your dizziness or unsteadiness come in attacks? If so, please describe:
			When was the <u>very first</u> attack? _____
			How long do they usually last? _____
			How long was your last attack? _____
			What makes it worse? _____
	Y	N	Do you have any warning before an attack?
	Y	N	Are you completely free of dizziness between attacks?
16.	Y	N	When you are dizzy, do you have to support yourself when standing or walking?
17.	Y	N	Do you know of anything that will stop your dizziness?
			What? _____
18.			When you are dizzy, do you experience any of the following sensations?
	Y	N	Light-headedness or swimming sensation?
	Y	N	Blacking out or loss of consciousness?
	Y	N	Tendency to fall? If so, which way? _____
	Y	N	Objects spinning or turning around you?
	Y	N	Sensation that you are turning or spinning inside?
	Y	N	Nausea or vomiting?
	Y	N	Headache?
	Y	N	Pressure in your head?
	Y	N	Change in hearing?
19.	Y	N	Has your dizziness ever caused you to fall?
			When? _____
			How often? _____
			Any injuries? _____

20.   Have you ever experienced any of the following symptoms? Please circle
       if constant or in episodes.

   Y   N   Double vision, blurred vision, or blindness?   Constant   Episodes

   Y   N   Numbness of face or extremities?   Constant   Episodes

   Y   N   Weakness in arms or legs?   Constant   Episodes

   Y   N   Clumsiness in arms or legs?   Constant   Episodes

   Y   N   Confusion or loss of consciousness?   Constant   Episodes

   Y   N   Difficulty with speech?   Constant   Episodes

   Y   N   Difficulty in swallowing?   Constant   Episodes

21. Y   N   Does fatigue, emotional stress, hunger, anxiety or menstrual periods have any
       affect on your dizziness? Please describe: _____

       _____

22. Y   N   Just before the menstrual period, do you have: dizziness, change in your
       hearing, fullness in the ears or increased ringing in the ear? Please describe:

       _____

       _____

23. Y   N   Does heat or being warm make your symptoms worse?

24. Y   N   Have you ever injured your head? Please list every incident and explain in detail?

       When? _____ Unconscious? Y   N   Fracture? Y   N

       When? _____ Unconscious? Y   N   Fracture? Y   N

       When? _____ Unconscious? Y   N   Fracture? Y   N

       _____

       _____

       _____

       _____

25. Y   N   Have you been in an auto accident within the last 5 years? If yes, list date(s):

       1) _____ 2) _____ 3) _____ 4) _____ 5) _____

26. Y   N   Have you ever fallen and/or hit your head? If yes, list date(s) and explain:

       1) Date _____ Explain: _____

       2) Date _____ Explain: _____

       3) Date _____ Explain: _____

       4) Date _____ Explain: _____

       5) Date _____ Explain: _____

27. Y   N   Have you ever been involved in any type of accident while at work? If yes, list
       date(s) and explain:

       1) Date _____ Explain: _____

       2) Date _____ Explain: _____

28. Y   N   Have you had any other type of head injury? If yes, list date(s) and explain:

1) Date _____ Explain: _____

2) Date _____ Explain: _____

Allergies

29. Y   N   Do you have any allergies? _____

30. Y   N   Do you ever have itching of the skin, palate or roof of the mouth?

31. Y   N   Do you have marked fatigue two or three hours after meals?

32. Y   N   Do you eat snacks frequently between meals?

33. Y   N   Do you have frequent migraine headaches or pain in the back of the neck?

General

34. Y   N   Do you ever experience a tremor, feeling of faintness or blacking out a few hours after meals?

35. Y   N   Do you perspire easily or have night sweats?

36. Y   N   Do you experience any of the following? Dry skin, irregular menstrual periods, sudden change in mood or muscle pain? Please explain:

_____

_____

_____

37. Y   N   Have you ever received radioactive iodine for treatment of the thyroid gland or had thyroid surgery? _____

38. Y   N   Have you ever experienced pain or swelling in the neck or voice box?

39. Y   N   Have you ever received a prolonged course of antibiotics? Please list below:

Medication   Date

_____   _____

_____   _____

_____   _____

_____   _____

_____ _____

Patient Signature   Date

_____ _____

Witness Signature   Date

Index

Note: Page numbers of article titles are in **boldface** type.

A

Adolescent(s), brain of, 310–311
    chronic daily headaches in, 314–315
    dizziness and vertigo in, case illustrating, 309–310
        etiologies of, 311–313, 316
        head imaging in, 316–318
        incidence of, 311
    migraine in, 313–314
    postural orthostatic tachycardia syndrome in, 315–316
    vertigo in, diagnosis and treatment of, 313–314
Adult(s), infrequent causes of disequilibrium in, **405–413**
    older, dizziness in, diseases/disorders causing, 474
        vestibular rehabilitation in, **473–496**
      falls by, 473–474, 475
      medication-related dizziness in, **455–471**
      vestibular disorders in, novel interventions in, 485–488
Antiepileptic drugs, and dizziness in older adult, 463–465
    side effects of, 463–464
Antihypertensive drugs, and dizziness in older adult, 459–462
Anxiolytic drugs, and dizziness in older adult, 463
Artery(ies), vertebral, 416
      or basilar, stenosis of, recurrent stroke and, 425–426

B

Balance, static, assessment of, in vestibular disorders, 260–261
Balance and motor development, 257
Balance function, and development of vestibular system, differential
    diagnosis in pediatric population, **251–271**
Balance function testing, findings on, in vertigo in children, **291–307**
Basilar migraine, 266, 430–431
Benign paroxysmal positional vertigo, in children, 264, 266, 297–298
    in elderly, 439, 444
    vertebrobasilar insufficiency and, 425
    vestibular rehabilitation in, 482
Benzodiazepines, and dizziness in older adult, 462
Beta-blockers, and dizziness in older adult, 461
Blast exposure, and head injury, vestibular consequences of, **323–334**
    otologic injuries caused by, 324
    vestibular test findings following, 328–331
    victims of, special testing considerations for, 331

Otolaryngol Clin N Am 44 (2011) 509–517
doi:10.1016/S0030-6665(11)00027-2
0030-6665/11/$ – see front matter © 2011 Elsevier Inc. All rights reserved.
oto.theclinics.com

Moving?

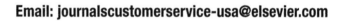

Make sure your subscription moves with you!

To notify us of your new address, find your **Clinics Account Number** (located on your mailing label above your name), and contact customer service at:

Email: journalscustomerservice-usa@elsevier.com

800-654-2452 (subscribers in the U.S. & Canada)
314-447-8871 (subscribers outside of the U.S. & Canada)

Fax number: 314-447-8029

Elsevier Health Sciences Division
Subscription Customer Service
3251 Riverport Lane
Maryland Heights, MO 63043

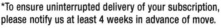

*To ensure uninterrupted delivery of your subscription, please notify us at least 4 weeks in advance of move.

Printed and bound by CPI Group (UK) Ltd, Croydon, CR0 4YY

03/10/2024

01040458-0007

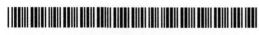